MEN'S HEALTH 1999 TODAY

Exciting New Strategies to Build a Stronger Body, Enjoy Great Sex, Eat Healthier, Look Younger, and Dress with Style

Edited by Michael Lafavore, Men'sHealth® Magazine

 Rodale Press, Inc.
Emmaus, Pennsylvania

─── OUR PURPOSE ───

*"We inspire and enable people to improve
their lives and the world around them."*

Contents

STYLE

Introduction

Knowledge Is Power

Power. To a senator, it represents steering money to his pet project back home. To a baseball player, it means driving a pitch into the upper deck. To a general, it translates into maximum ordnance on target.

Here at *Men's Health*, we have a different slant on what power means. We believe a man is powerful when he is armed with knowledge. Specifically, health knowledge. With this information at hand, you can make intelligent decisions about your life. Decisions that translate into getting the most out of every minute you spend exercising. Eating the right foods at precisely the right times to fuel muscle growth and boost energy and stamina. Finding creative new ways to keep sex satisfying for you and your partner. Staying healthy while others around you get sick. Keeping mentally sharp. Even dressing in style for every occasion.

In today's hectic world, we realize that men don't exactly perk up at the thought of diving through murky studies to recover the pearls of wisdom. That's where we come in. We tracked down the latest health studies and findings. We read the dense books. We talked to the top health professionals. We checked into exciting developments on the horizon for men.

The result? A powerful collection of the most up-to-date, actionable health information that you'll find anywhere. And we've packaged it so that you can tap into this amazing power source quickly. No windbags allowed in this book.

In an effort to provide a well-rounded package of useful knowledge, we've included a style section in this year's edition. After all, how you groom and dress yourself is part of the total health picture. But style is more than snappy dressing. It's also how you carry yourself and interact with others. Ordering wine, for example. It's covered in the "Style" chapter's "Vital Reading" section.

Here's some more of what you can expect to find inside.

"Benchmarks" is a feature that appeals to men's innate curiosity with seeing how they measure up to other men. Each one is a list of averages and oddball facts that provides an intriguing look into what men do. Want to know how long sexual sessions last for single and married men? Or what sport causes more injuries than karate, bowling, and horseback riding combined? Or how many people are seriously considering quitting their jobs? Then you need to check these out.

In "Vital Reading," we present the very best advice from a variety of publications. Many of these pieces are from *Sex and Health: The Newsletter of the Men's Health Institute*, which comes from the publisher of *Men's Health* magazine. There also is a growing field of books that address the health concerns of men. We culled the best parts of the best books, and you can read them in "Best Reads." Find out how to dress right on casual days at the office, quickly cure the most common headache, or get her to overcome her sexual inhibitions.

We went right to the experts in "Interviews." These engaging talks with top researchers, doctors, and authors tackle such topics as evaluating good and bad multivitamins, managing in-laws, and the best routines to build a strong body.

One of the biggest services that we can do for readers is provide up-to-date, breaking news about what's going on in men's health research. Check out "News Flashes" to discover the latest findings on Viagra, how to fend off Alzheimer's disease, a possible cure for baldness, and the dangers of a low-fat diet.

Even more exciting than the latest findings are what researchers and doctors are cooking in their laboratories. "Soon to Be News" reveals fascinating studies and research in the works. In the near future, you can expect to see such amazing discoveries as a pill to boost immunity, a clearer link between eating potatoes and preventing Parkinson's disease, a nasal spray that will end impotence, drugs that boost memory, and an acne med-

icine that can combat rheumatoid arthritis.

For a look at the latest trends, how they got started, and whether they are legitimate, check out "Fad Alerts." You'll get the real scoop on creatine; find out if the latest gimmick on infomercials, air gliders, are worth the money; and get the lowdown on whether energy bars really give you a boost.

"New Tools" is one of our favorite features. Why? Because we love gadgets and gizmos. And that's exactly what these sections showcase. Some of the cool stuff that we found is: a radio-wave treatment to cure snoring, 100-percent cotton-twill khaki pants like we used to wear in our younger days, antibacterial paint that can kill 99 percent of bacteria and viruses, and training aids to lower your golf score.

Between periodic surveys and letters to the editor, a large number of questions roll into our office. We love to read them because they give us great insights into what's on our readers' minds. We collected the best of the bunch and present them in "The Answer Man" section of each part.

Topping off each part is a very useful section called "Actions." Here you'll find great tips to change your lifestyle for the better—right now. From how to fit a great workout into a busy day to dealing with stress from work and home to eating common foods that will ward off disease, you really get your money's worth with this feature.

So there you have a taste of what's inside. The book is arranged so that you can access the information quickly and easily. Whether you read it for a few minutes before you hit the sack or crack it open on a lazy Sunday afternoon, there will always be entertaining reading ahead. And interesting pieces to start you on the road to power.

In *Men's Health Today 1999*, we arm you with the knowledge to make it a short trip.

Michael Lafavore
Editor-in-Chief, *Men's Health* Magazine

1

FITNESS

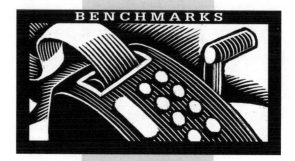

- Percentage increase in sales of ab machines from 1995 to 1996: 200

- Chance that someone who frequently works out with exercise equipment will be seriously injured: 1 in 400

- Percentage of the 47.3 million frequent exercisers in America who are men: 44

- Number of 12-ounce beers a man would have to drink to fuel up on carbs for a marathon: 52

- Times greater than the force of gravity when astronauts can black out: 6

- Times greater than the force of gravity that football players may routinely take hits: 13

- Number of recreational baseball players injured each year from sliding into bases: 1.7 million

- Sport that causes more injuries than karate, bowling, and horseback riding combined: golf

- Percentage of nudists who rank cycling as one of their favorite sports: 32

- Estimated percentage of runners who are injured every year: 50

- Percentage of Americans who own running shoes but don't run: 87

- Estimated amount of body fluid in cups perspired during one hour of exercise in hot weather: 6¾

- Percentage of Americans who are completely sedentary: 40

- Percentage of people whose biggest obstacle to exercise is lack of time: 47

- Number of Americans who are overweight or obese: 58 million

- Percentage of older gardeners who do it for fitness: 44

- Percentage of Americans who believe that mowing the lawn is risky: 54

Quick Way to a Flat Stomach

These exercises will have your gut packing its bags in no time.

No part of your body says more about what you do behind closed doors than your gut does. Lead a balanced life and your belly will tell no tales, but if you spend too many evenings at home with a spray can of cheese and several yards of beef jerky, the truth becomes impossible to hide.

A low-fat diet, a top-flight abdominal routine, and regular aerobic exercise are the only long-term solutions to a burgeoning belly. But don't fret: While you wait for your new lifestyle to take effect, there are some other slightly devious ways to take the Buddha out of your belly.

Work both sides. "Weak lower-back muscles allow the spinal column to sway, and that can make the stomach protrude," says John Abdo, certified fitness trainer and the author of *Body Engineering*. Whenever you work the front of your torso, work the back as well.

Build up to look slimmer. The appearance of your waist is relative to the condition of your back and shoulders. "If you increase the width of your shoulders and upper back, your waistline will look narrower," says Abdo.

Smoke your hams. Weak, tight hamstrings can also lead you to arch your back, forcing your stomach forward (and putting you at serious risk of back trouble). They should be stretched and strengthened regularly.

With the help of Abdo and Alex Signorello, a personal fitness trainer at Strong Heart Strong Body in San Francisco, we've put together a workout designed to quickly bulk up your back and shoulders while strengthening the muscles that keep your gut in its proper place. For the weight exercises, you should lift enough to bring your muscles to exhaustion within the recommended number of repetitions. (This may mean using a different weight for different sets of the same exercise.) And remember that this is only a temporary fix. If you don't accompany these exercises with an honest-to-gut anti-fat program, your belly will catch up in no time.

INCLINE SHOULDER PRESS
(works the fronts and sides of your shoulders)

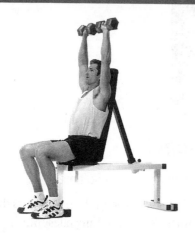

Adjust an incline bench to about a 60-degree angle. Grab a dumbbell in each hand and sit with your back against the angled part of the bench and your feet flat on the floor. With your elbows bent and your palms facing forward, hold the dumbbells next to your shoulders. Extend your arms straight up, touch the dumbbells together above your head, then bring them down to your shoulders with a slow, controlled movement. Do three or four sets of 10 to 12 repetitions.

DUMBBELL REVERSE FLY
(works the backs of your shoulders)

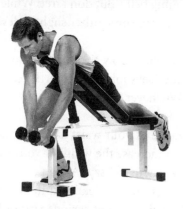 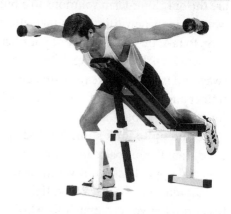

Adjust an incline bench to a 30- to 45-degree angle and grab a dumbbell in each hand. Facing the slanted part of the bench, place your left knee on the horizontal part, keeping your right foot on the floor. Press your left thigh and chest against the slanted part of the bench and allow your arms to hang on both sides.

With your elbows slightly bent, bring the dumbbells up and extend your arms out to the sides until they are just about parallel to the floor. Slowly bring them back down so that they're hanging at your sides again. Do three sets of 8 to 10 repetitions, switching legs after each set.

SIDE LATERAL RAISE
(works the tops and sides of your shoulders)

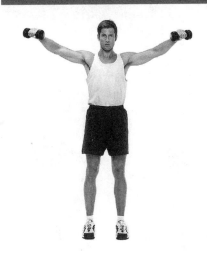

Stand with your feet about shoulder-width apart. Grab a dumbbell in each hand, with your palms facing your thighs. Keeping your elbows bent slightly but rigid, extend both arms to the sides and raise the dumbbells. Rotate your arms slightly as you lift, so that by the time they're just higher than your ears, your palms are facing the floor. Bring the dumbbells back down to your thighs with a slow, controlled motion. Be sure to hold yourself as rigid as possible throughout the exercise to keep your body from swaying. Do three sets of 10 to 12 repetitions.

LAT CABLE CROSSOVER
(works the sides of your upper back)

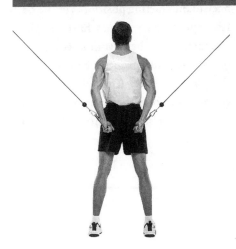

Use a cable-crossover machine with two high pulleys. Attach a handle to each pulley. Grab a handle in each hand, with your palms down, and stand midway between the towers and just in front of the weight stacks, with your feet slightly more than shoulder-width apart. Extend your arms up and slightly behind your body. With your elbows slightly bent but rigid, pull both handles down and behind your buttocks. Let the resistance pull your arms back up slowly. Do three sets of 10 to 12 repetitions.

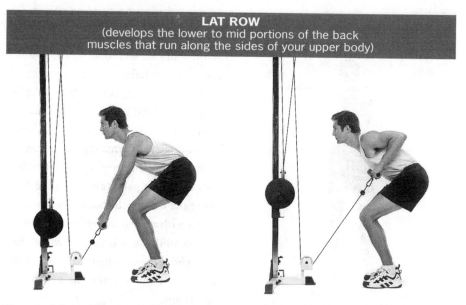

LAT ROW
(develops the lower to mid portions of the back muscles that run along the sides of your upper body)

Use a weight-pulley machine with a low cable. Attach a straight bar to the machine, then grab the bar palms-down with a grip slightly narrower than shoulder width. Bend forward until your upper body is almost parallel to the floor. Extend your arms and step back from the machine until the weight is a few inches off the stack. Keep your legs about shoulder-width apart, your knees slightly bent and your head looking straight ahead or slightly up.

Pull the bar toward your knees, slide it up close to your thighs, and bring it in to your belly. Reverse the movement and go back to the starting position. For the first few repetitions, you may have to adjust your stance and bend your knees slightly in order to find a properly balanced position for your body. If you don't have access to a weight-pulley machine, you can also use dumbbells. Do three sets of 10 to 12 repetitions.

UPRIGHT ROW
(develops the fronts and sides of the shoulders and the trapezius, the muscle that runs from the base of your skull to the center of your back)

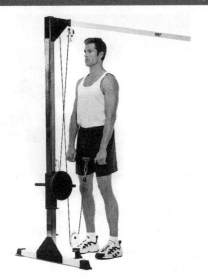 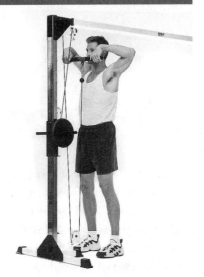

Use a weight-pulley machine with a low cable. Stand facing the pulley and grab the bar with your hands about six inches apart, palms down. Stand straight and hold the bar at thigh level.

Now raise it, lifting your elbows to the sides and curling your wrists slightly inward so the bar stays close to your body. Continue to raise your elbows and lift the bar until it's in front of your face, between your nose and chin. Be sure to look straight ahead throughout this movement. If you feel discomfort in your wrists or shoulders, try adjusting the spacing of your grip. You can also do this exercise with dumbbells if you don't have access to a weight-pulley machine. Do three sets of 10 to 12 repetitions.

CABLE DEADLIFT
(works your lower back)

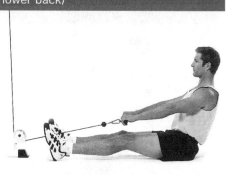

Sit facing the low cable at a weight-pulley machine, your legs extended in front of you and your knees slightly bent. Grab a straight bar, palms down. Adjust the pulley cable so that you're far enough away from the machine to feel the weight pulling your upper body forward. (If the weight is touching the stack, you're too close.)

Without bending your arms, lean back with a slow, controlled motion until your back is at a 90-degree angle to the floor. Now lean back slightly farther to break this perpendicular position. Do three sets of 10 to 15 repetitions.

SIDE KNEE CROSSOVER
(stretches your lower back and buttocks)

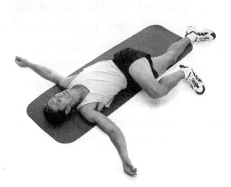

Lie faceup on the floor with your arms extended to the sides so that your body forms a cross. Bend your left knee and bring it as close to your chest as possible without lifting your lower back off the floor. Keeping your knee bent and both shoulders on the floor, slowly cross your knee over to the right side of your body. Hold the stretch for 7 to 12 seconds before releasing the position very slowly. Repeat with the right knee.

HYPEREXTENSION
(works your lower back)

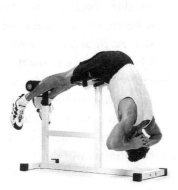
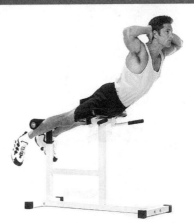

Caution: If you have back problems, this exercise can make them worse. If not, proceed to the back-extension machine. Position your ankles under the padded bars and rest your upper thighs on the padded platform. Cross your arms over your chest or place them behind your head and allow your hips and upper body to hang down over the platform so that they form a 90-degree angle with your lower body.

Slowly raise your torso until it's aligned with the rest of your body, and then go slightly higher. Slowly lower yourself back to a 90-degree angle.

If you don't have access to a back-extension machine, you can also use a bench. (The back-injury warning applies here, too.) Lie facedown on the bench and wrap your legs around the middle—or, if you have a training partner, have him hold your legs. Position yourself with your hips and upper body hanging off one end of the bench. Lower your upper body slowly toward the floor, then return to the starting position. Do two to four sets of as many repetitions as you can handle. Once you can do 15 per set, try holding a weight plate against your chest.

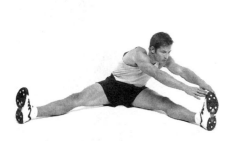

SPREAD SIT-AND-REACH
(stretches your hamstrings and lower back)

Sit on the floor and spread your legs as far apart as possible. Make sure your knees are locked before you begin the movement. Slowly reach along your left leg with both hands and try to touch your toes. Hold the stretch for 7 to 10 seconds. Slowly return to the starting position and repeat the stretch to your right foot. Alternate the stretch to each side until you've done a minimum of three per side.

The Perfect Body

Pay attention to these overlooked muscle groups and build a body that looks great.

When most men exercise, they target the vanity muscles: pecs, abs, quads, calves, biceps, and triceps. Soon, however, they find that their bodies are as one-dimensional as their workouts.

Consider your chest: If you neglect to balance your bench presses with upper-back exercises, you could end up pec-less. Here's how: Weak back muscles will allow your pectorals to pull your shoulders forward, according to Alan Mikesky, Ph.D., director of the human performance and biomechanics laboratory at Indiana University–Purdue University at Indianapolis. "This actually de-emphasizes the size of your chest."

The same goes for other body parts. If you spend hours on your biceps and triceps but neglect your forearms, your arms will look like drumsticks instead of meat hooks. And if all you do is squats, you'll neglect your lower legs, too. Worse, all this muscular imbalance makes you a prime candidate for injuries.

Dr. Mikesky and Timothy N. Ziegenfuss, Ph.D., an exercise physiologist at Eastern Michigan University in Ypsilanti, have designed one great exercise for each neglected area. Start with a weight you can lift for one set of 8 to 12 repetitions to fatigue for the first few weeks, then add a few more sets.

BEHIND-THE-BACK WRIST CURL
(If you're doing biceps curls and triceps extensions,
you need to build size and strength in your forearms.)

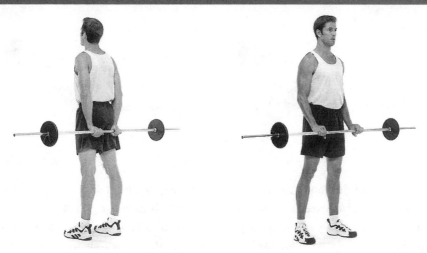

Place a light barbell on the floor and stand with your back to it, a few inches from the center of the bar. Position your feet slightly more than shoulder-width apart. Squat and grab the barbell with an underhand grip, a little less than shoulder-width apart, and slowly stand. Keeping your arms straight and your forearms and wrists pressed against your lower back and buttocks, slowly curl the barbell up as high as possible.

Hold this position for a moment, and then slowly lower the weight. After you finish your repetitions, place the barbell on the floor and stand so that it's in front of you. Squat again, grab the barbell with a narrow overhand grip and stand. With your forearms and wrists pressed against your hips, curl the bar as far as possible. Make sure that you hold the weight for a second before lowering it.

REAR SHOULDER EXTENSION
(If you're doing military presses, you need to work the backs and fronts of your shoulders.)

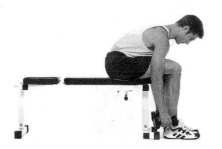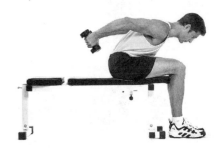

Holding a light dumbbell in each hand, sit on the end of an exercise bench with your feet flat on the floor. With your arms hanging down, bend forward at the waist until your chest is touching your thighs.

Keeping your head down and your elbows slightly bent but rigid, slowly lift your arms straight back along the sides of the bench. Raise them as high as possible, hold for a moment, then slowly return to the starting position.

ALTERNATING ARM/LEG LIFT
(If you're doing bunches of crunches, you need to strengthen your lower back.)

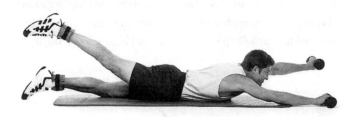

Attach a light ankle weight to each ankle and lie facedown on the floor within easy reach of two light dumbbells. Grab a dumbbell in each hand and extend your arms straight out in front of you. You should be looking down at the floor, with your arms locked and your feet about shoulder-width apart. With a slow, controlled motion, simultaneously lift your right arm and left leg as high as possible without bending either. Pause for a second, and then lower them. Repeat with your left arm and right leg to complete one repetition.

ONE-ARM PULLDOWN
(If you're doing bench presses, you need to build
a back that's as strong as your chest.)

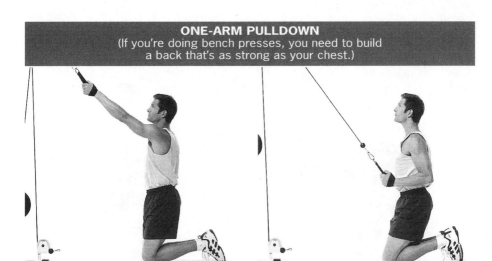

Attach a strap to the high cable of a weight-pulley machine and loop it around your left wrist. Face the weights and kneel about two feet in front of them. Your right arm should be at your side, and your left arm should be pointing toward the pulley.

Keep your back straight and slowly pull the cable toward your body. Maintain a slow, controlled movement as you allow the weight to pull your arm to the starting position. Repeat, then switch arms.

SHOULDER BENCH PRESS
(If you're doing twisting crunches, you need to develop the muscles that wrap
around from your shoulder blades to your pectorals.)

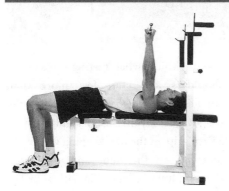
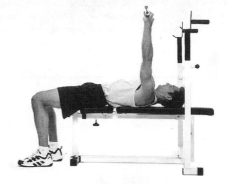

Lie faceup on a bench-press bench with your feet flat on the floor. Lift the barbell off the rack and, with your arms straight, hold the bar directly above your shoulders.

Keep your head, neck, and back flat against the bench, and try to lift your shoulders slightly off the bench. Hold the weight for a moment, then lower it.

STIFF-LEGGED DEADLIFT
(If you're doing leg extensions, you need to strengthen your hamstrings, which oppose the quadriceps muscles.)

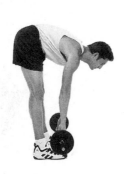
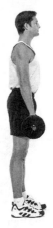

Caution: If you have lower-back problems, avoid this exercise. Place a light barbell on the floor and stand facing it with your feet hip-width apart. Bend at the waist and grab the barbell with your hands slightly more than shoulder-width apart. Keep your back flat, your knees unlocked but rigid, and your arms extended.

Slowly rise until the bar is resting in front of your thighs. Slowly lower it to the floor. If you have trouble keeping your back flat, use a lighter weight.

LATERAL LUNGE
(If you're doing squats, you need to build your inner and outer thighs for a more powerful-looking leg.)

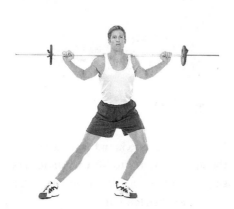

Stand with a barbell resting across your shoulders and your feet more than shoulder-width apart. Make sure that the weight is evenly distributed and you have a firm grip on the bar. Keeping your right foot flat on the floor and your back straight, lunge to the side with your left leg. Your right foot should be pointing to the side at about a 45-degree angle, with your left leg bent at a 90-degree angle. Use your right leg to draw you back to the starting position, then lunge to the other side.

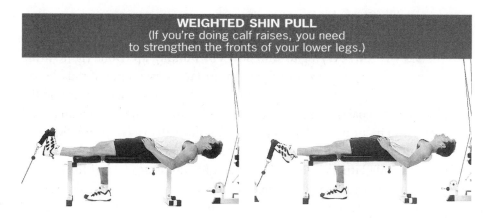

WEIGHTED SHIN PULL
(If you're doing calf raises, you need
to strengthen the fronts of your lower legs.)

Place a flat bench in front of a weight-pulley machine and attach an ankle strap to the low cable. Sit on the end of the bench, facing the weight stack, and loop the strap around your left foot close to your toes. Slide back and lie down. Keeping your right foot flat on the floor and your left leg flat against the bench (only your foot and ankle should extend beyond the bench), slowly pull your left toes as far toward your shin as possible.

Hold for a moment, then let the weight slowly pull your foot back down. Switch to the other foot.

Seven Costly Workout Sins

Avoid these mistakes and get the best results for your time.

For some guys, finding time to exercise isn't much of an issue. In between hanging out in the yard and working on their appeals, they can always fit in a leisurely workout.

For the rest of us, though, getting 30 minutes in the gym is a superhuman achievement, and we're determined to spend every second burning flab, sculpting muscle, and drawing wistful glances from lithe yoga instructors. Yet on a tour of our company gym, we saw men wasting precious time by misusing equipment, doing pointless exercises, and leering at a woman whom we later saw in the parking lot writing down their license numbers.

Don't be like one of those guys. Ask yourself: Do any of the following moves sound familiar?

Mistake #1: You're trying to slim down by bulking up. Done right, lifting weights is a great weapon in your fight against fat. Every pound of muscle you put on increases your resting metabolism, so you burn more calories around the clock. But if your goal is a leaner, tighter body, the worst thing you can do is load the bar with so many plates that you can't lift it more than a few times. "Men lift too much weight, thinking it will firm them up," says Edward Jackowski Jr., founder of Exude Fitness in New York City and author of *Hold It! You're Exercising Wrong.* "But excess bulk can make some men grow thicker and look fatter."

To build lean muscle, use moderate weight—light enough to do at least 15 repetitions of an exercise with good form, but heavy enough so that the 15th one really burns. Do three sets of each exercise, two if you're pressed for time.

Mistake #2: You're fixated on the gym. It's easy to become so intrigued by all the robo trainers in a gym that you forget there's any other way to exercise. "It's all those great displays and flashing lights," says Jan Griscom, a personal trainer in Las Vegas. "Guys are hypnotized."

But when a hard-core gym rat finally breaks a sweat outside the gym, he often experiences an agonizing condition known as gym-shock. It's that moment when you face the great outdoors and discover that you're not in nearly as good shape as you thought you were—that riding a mountain bike through a stream is a lot tougher than pedaling that stationary bicycle, even at a high tension. That climbing 200 floors on a stairclimber doesn't mean you'll last 20 minutes hiking uphill.

"Machines are designed to isolate and work specific areas," says Lisa Jamison, a personal trainer in Tampa, Florida. But if you play sports, you're involving several different muscle groups as well as the skeletal system, tendons, ligaments, and joints—and you attain a whole different level of fitness than the guy who works out on just a stairclimber.

No matter how hard you work in the gym, set aside a little time for climbing rocks, running hills, or chewing up the trails on a mountain bike. Not only will you boost your fitness but you'll feel better, too. "The gym is an artificial environment, and you can be your own worst enemy," says Rick O'Bryan, a personal trainer in Hollywood, California. "Guys who work out only in the gym can end up obsessing about how they look, instead of focusing on how they perform. Fortunately, though, there are no mirrors outdoors."

Mistake #3: You take a nice long rest between sets. You've just finished a heavy set of biceps curls, and your muscles are pumped and quivering. Time to towel off, grab some water, and spend a minute or two chatting about Vivaldi with the vixen on the VersaClimber. You'll get around to that next set soon enough, right?

Wrong. "All that time between sets compromises the exercise," says Jamison. Within a minute, your body recovers 72 percent of its strength. Within three, you've recovered all the strength you're going to recover without an extended rest. To build strength, you need to stimulate and fatigue the maximum number of muscle fibers. With each set, your muscles become more fatigued, so your body uses additional fibers to pick up the slack. Keep the breaks to a minute or less. You will push your muscles and make real progress.

Mistake #4: You're coasting along on the treadmill. When you're on that treadmill, you're not really running. You're just picking up your feet while the ground moves underneath you.

And if you think you're going to train for the New York Marathon on your treadmill, forget it. Running outdoors is a lot tougher than raising your feet and waiting for the ground to roll on underneath. "The treadmill is a useful tool," says Jamison, "but it's nowhere near as strenuous as running on the pavement."

If you're training for a race, whether it's the Olympic Trials or the annual Turkey Trot, Jamison suggests doing at least 50 percent of your training outdoors, particularly your longer runs. Spend your treadmill time on speed or hill work, she advises. "If you're not confident about your times, a treadmill is a lot less threatening than doing intervals with a group at the track."

Mistake #5: You're stuck in a routine. "Men are creatures of habit," says Jamison. "I often have men come to me and say, 'This program worked great when I started it.' I ask when that was, and they say, 'Nine years ago.'"

The problem with sticking to the same routine is that after a few months, your muscles become used to it. "Your body is on autopilot and probably has been since about three months into the program," says Jamison. "It may be a great maintenance routine, but you're not gaining."

She recommends changing your program every three months or so.

Mistake #6: You're too tense. Yes, you can up the level on a stationary bike and make those pedals very, very hard to turn. Does that mean you're getting a better workout than those other "wimps" with lighter tension?

"Nope," says Chris Kostman, a spinning instructor and veteran bicycle racer in Los Angeles. "You're putting a huge amount of pressure on your knees and not getting a better workout." Usually, he says, guys who ride a stationary bike on level nine or set a spinning bike to very high tension end up compromising their riding position to push the pedals, increasing knee pressure. Maybe your best bet is to find a cadence you can maintain, then gradually increase the resistance.

Mistake #7: You've fallen in love with your stairclimber. Most guys think that one aerobic machine is every bit as good as another, and that's partially true: Any one of them can give you a good cardiovascular workout. But by sticking with the same machine, you're not benefiting as much as you could from your gym time.

"Each cardiovascular machine in a gym trains us in a different way, uses the same muscle group at a slightly different angle," says O'Bryan. "It makes more sense, muscle-wise, to use each of the machines for 15 minutes than to spend your entire workout on one machine."

If you have a half-hour to spend on aerobic exercises, he suggests spending 10 minutes each on the treadmill, stairclimber, and stationary bike. Tomorrow, you might opt for the rower, skier, and VersaClimber. "Not only do you get a much better workout," he says, "but it's a lot less boring. You always have that next machine to look forward to."

Diversify Your Interests

Recharge your workouts with some cross-training.

Maybe you're a runner. Maybe you're the best damn runner since Secretariat. But if running is the extent of your exercise program, then you're probably not in great physical condition. Oh, sure, your cardiovascular fitness may be second to none, and you have hamstrings to rival Baryshnikov's. But are your shoulders strong enough to carry life's heavy loads? Are your abdominals tough enough to protect your lower back from injury? And, come on, aren't you becoming a little bored with running?

What you need is a little cross-training. By identifying what your current workout program lacks—and adopting some new exercises to round it out properly—you can bring your whole body into line and reach fitness levels you've never seen before. Plus, you'll be less likely to fall prey to tedium or, worse, overuse injuries. All you need to do is find your current activity, then try these suggestions for enhancing it. Mixing it up at least twice a week ought to do the trick.

Walking

Keep the pace to at least 3.5 miles per hour, or your pulse at 55 to 75 percent of its maximum (to find your max, subtract your age from 220), and you'll tone your lower body—especially your calves, quadriceps, and hamstrings—while receiving a decent cardiovascular workout.

Like most aerobically oriented activities, walking firms your muscles but won't give you brawn. (Your upper body, especially, tends to be left out of the picture.) And although it does get your heart pumping, it's not the most challenging of exercises, so there's little opportunity to measure your improvement.

How to cross-train: Once a week, strap on a 5- to 10-pound day pack and head for a hill with at least a 5 to 7 percent grade. The extra weight, plus the added intensity of walking on an incline, will raise your heart rate and draw more muscle involvement from your back, abdominals, and quadriceps.

Weather allowing, you can add intensity by snowshoeing for a half-hour a few days a month. Snowshoeing mimics the motions of walking but adds more of an emphasis to the hip and thigh muscle involvement.

Running

Running improves your cardiovascular fitness, helps lower blood pressure, and shapes your calves, hamstrings, and buttocks. Plus, it's one of the fastest ways to burn off extra pounds.

Michael Johnson aside, most runners don't have the upper body or abdominals of an Adonis. Many running enthusiasts also have tight hamstrings and underdeveloped quadriceps.

How to cross-train: Running in deep water (get some tips on proper form from that aquarobics instructor in the clingy swimsuit) once a week for 30 to 40 minutes will provide the same muscle involvement and aerobic benefits as exercising on land, with none of the impact. It will also call the quads into play and help beat the muscle imbalances that runners develop. To work your upper body, hit the weight room twice a week for the basics—12 to 15 repetitions each of biceps curls, triceps extensions, chest presses, lat pulldowns, and dumbbell rows. Finish with 20 crunches.

Swimming

Swimming not only helps shape your shoulders, calves, and nearly every major muscle group in between but also gets your heart pumping. And your chances of injury are somewhere between "very low" and "only if you dive in shallow water."

Swimming burns a lot of calories, but it doesn't burn fat like other sports do. And because so much movement comes from the upper body, swimmers often have beautifully developed shoulders, chests, and torsos but disappear from the waist down.

How to cross-train: Two or three times a week, split your workout by swimming 5 minutes freestyle, 5 minutes with a kickboard and fins; another 5 minutes freestyle, and 5 minutes with a pull-buoy to concentrate on your upper body. Work up to 10-minute segments.

To help yourself burn fat faster, come up for air once a week and spend 30 to 45 minutes on the rowing machine or cross-country ski machine, keeping your heart rate at 70 to 80 percent of maximum.

Rowing

Whether you're stroking on the open water or sweating it out on a rowing machine, you get a great aerobic workout and tone your arms, legs, abdomen, torso, and buttocks. All the better if there's a fetching coxswain ordering you, "Stroke!"

If you have perfect form, this is a pretty complete exercise. But most of us use our backs too much, risking strain while minimizing the exercise's effect on the rest of our bodies. And, let's face it—if you're not cruising the Charles, it can get a little dull.

How to cross-train: Twice a week, try interval training. After a 10- to 15-minute warmup, maintain a moderate rate of 20 strokes for one minute. Increase your pace to 35 to 40 strokes for one minute, then go back to 20 strokes for a minute. Alternate these paces for 15 minutes, then cool down.

For a change, try cross-country skiing in the great outdoors or in the gym. Like rowing, it works a wide variety of muscle groups and offers similar aerobic benefits.

Cross-Country Skiing

Believe it or not, cross-country skiing is the gold standard of fitness activities. Many exercise physiologists rank it as the most effective cardiovascular workout. Sliding along (on snow or a ski machine), you condition your calves, quadriceps, triceps, shoulders, abdomen, chest, and back, and at the same time put your heart and lungs through a powerful workout as well.

Cross-country skiing bothers beginners, who haven't quite gotten the hang of the arm-swing and foot glide, and frequent skiers, who plead boredom with the somewhat monotonous movements of the indoor machine.

How to cross-train: Once a week, step off the machine and onto a slide board. Sliding works the abductor and adductor muscles of the hips (less emphasized by skiing), along with calves, quadriceps, hamstrings, and lower back. After a 5-minute warmup, spend 20 minutes at 60 to 70 percent of your maximum heart rate. (Talk to a trainer about the variety of moves you can use on this piece of equipment.) You may also want to do abdominal crunches and grab some dumbbells and do upper-body work.

If there's enough snow, take your skiing skills outside a few times this winter. Using a skating style (which emphasizes a sideways push for forward motion, much like ice or inline skating) will also put more emphasis on the buttocks and inner/outer thigh muscles.

Cycling

Pedaling a road bike or upright stationary bike will work most of your lower body, especially your quadriceps and buttocks. It will also burn fat quickly and keep your cardiovascular system in good order. And if you take to the road, boredom is usually not a problem.

Although your quadriceps will be mighty, your hamstrings will never receive much of a workout, leading to muscle imbalance. And if you limit your ride to stationary bikes, your upper body will take it a little too easy.

How to cross-train: Recumbent bikes, those strange recline-and-pedal contraptions at most gyms, will give you the same pedaling pleasure but put more emphasis on your hamstrings and less on your quadriceps. You can also shock the neighbors by buying a recumbent for outdoor use; just make sure that tractor trailer sees you before you pull into the intersection. A couple times a week, intensify your indoor workout with interval training.

For a more complete workout, try mountain biking. Jumping out of the saddle improves your range of motion, dancing on the pedals helps you maintain your balance, and you'll even work your upper body as you chug up the slopes.

Stairclimbing

A stairclimber can give your buttocks, hamstrings, quadriceps, and calves a killer workout. It'll also burn calories quickly and strengthen your heart. But don't cheat by draping your arms over the frame and using the machine as a crutch. Your lower body should be supporting most of your weight, or you won't get the workout you need.

While stairclimbing is a pretty complete lower-body workout, your upper body is being neglected.

How to cross-train: Once a week, spend 45 minutes on a full-body climbing machine such as the VersaClimber. You'll do the step movements, but your arms, shoulders, and chest will see some action, too.

In addition, spend one day a week in the weight room. No need to get fancy with your lifts. One set of exercises each for your shoulders, biceps, triceps, chest, back, and abdominals ought to be enough to keep you from becoming bottom-heavy.

Weight Training

Working against a resistance load expands muscle cells. If you do a variety of exercises, you'll pump up the major muscle groups.

The body's most important muscle—the heart—is pretty much left out of the equation.

How to cross-train: To add aerobic intensity, cut the rest periods between sets to less than 30 seconds. And keep the blood pumping through all the muscle groups by switching off between lower- and upper-body exercises. For example, switch from a leg press to a seated row, then go for lunges, chest presses, leg curls, and shoulder presses. Do one set of 10 to 15 repetitions, then repeat the cycle.

Or you can alternate lifts with brief aerobic activity. Jump rope or hit the heavy bag for two minutes, do 50 pushups or situps, run in place, or hop on a stationary bike. Mixing up the aerobic activities keeps your whole workout fresh.

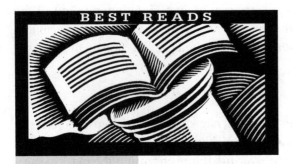

BEST READS

The Real Power Lunch

As men try to cram more activities into their days, workouts sometimes make the expendable list. But Brian Paul Kaufman and Sid Kirchheimer point out in Stronger Faster: Workday Workouts That Build Maximum Muscle in Minimum Time *(Rodale Press, 1997) that lunchtime is enough time not only to eat but also to fit in meaningful exercise.*

Okay, so maybe working out at lunchtime isn't your first choice, but it just may be the best time for you to squeeze in a little exercise.

"Think about it. How long does it take you to eat your lunch—not wolf it down, but casually eat it? Probably 15 minutes, tops," figures Adele Pace, M.D., a fitness consultant in Ashland, Kentucky, and author of *The Busy Executive's Guide to Total Fitness.*

If you get an hour for lunch, that leaves you 45 minutes of exercise time. That's time enough for a good workout, even if you never leave the confines of your office building.

Although it's right in the middle of the day, lunchtime actually tends to be a popular time for busy guys to exercise, says John Amberge, a certified strength and conditioning specialist and director of corporate programs for the Sports Training Institute in New York City. "It's a great way to recharge your batteries after a hard morning, and that pick-me-up can carry through the rest of the day."

Making It Work

Cramming a lunchtime workout into your schedule is eminently doable, says Amberge.

"If your exercise facilities are within 10 minutes of your office, you have plenty of time to work out and eat lunch," he says. "We get a lot of executives in here at around 11:30 A.M. They work out for a half-hour to 45 minutes, then they grab lunch on the way back to the office."

Maybe that's not an option for you; maybe your office is miles from a club; or maybe your job demands that you be close by, just in case. Well, you can always work out in the office. If you do, that's almost better, in a way. Since you don't have to go anywhere, you'll have even more time for more exercise.

"Of course, if you exercise around the office, you'll probably want to modify your workout a little bit. You'll want to do enough so that you feel like you're getting some benefit from the activity, but not so much that you end up all sweaty going into your afternoon meetings," says Amberge.

Whatever type of exercise you have time for, heed the following advice. These tips should help you make the most of your midday muscle building.

Drink before noon. Even before the lunch whistle blows, you can start preparing for exercise by making sure that you have plenty of fluids in your system.

"If you're not well-hydrated, it may adversely affect your performance," says Barry Franklin, Ph.D., director of cardiac rehabilitation and exercise laboratories at William Beaumont Hospital Rehabilitation and Health Center in Birmingham,

Michigan. "You won't be able to make the most of your workout time. I definitely recommend getting some fluids into you." And he means water, not coffee.

The caffeine in coffee will actually cause your body to get rid of more fluids, not to mention the fact that caffeine can increase stress on your heart, Dr. Franklin says. "A couple cups in the morning is fine. But after that, switch to water."

Munch at midmorning. Roughly an hour before you exercise, start fueling for your workout. "If you're doing any kind of serious weight training or heavy exercise, do not eat lunch before you do it. You'll be too loaded down with food—you'll feel awful," Amberge says. But you have to have some fuel in you, so he recommends eating something easy to digest but high in carbohydrates, such as a bagel or a piece of fruit.

Eat afterward. After your workout, your body will practically be starving for more fuel. And chances are that you'll be feeling hungrier, so go ahead and eat your lunch afterward. Just be sure that your heart rate is out of its aerobic zone, says Joanne Curran-Celentano, R.D., Ph.D., associate professor of nutrition and food science at the University of New Hampshire in Durham. She suggests that you cool down enough so that your heart rate is close to normal before you eat a full meal.

Take a stroll. If you did make it to the gym, odds are that you didn't have time to do much of a cooldown. So before you get back to the office to eat or resume work, walk an easy lap or two around the parking lot.

"It'll be a lot easier on your body—especially your heart and the muscles you just worked out—if you go for a walk or do some light stretching in your office than if you go back upstairs and sit still for the next four to five hours," says Dr. Pace.

Consolidate your efforts. Even if the gym is across the street, you may find yourself crunched for time, between changing, exercising, changing back, showering, *and* eating lunch. So cut some corners. When you work out, stick to a five-minute warmup and do lifts that only work compound muscle groups—squats, for example, work several muscles at once, says Amberge.

Bring your own. If you're really serious about working out where you work, bring in a pair of dumbbells and keep them in your office—10- to 15-pounders ought to do nicely. "Then there's any number of arm, shoulder, and chest exercises that you can do right in your own office chair," Amberge says. These range from basic curls to overhead presses. Whatever exercise you choose, you're bound to give new meaning to the term *power lunch.*

The Office Circuit

Unfortunately, all too many guys find themselves with some time to exercise at lunch but not enough to get to a gym and do a serious workout. That's okay. It doesn't mean that you can't get in some exercise at lunch anyway.

"There are a number of exercises that you can do at lunch right around your office, if you want to be creative about it," Amberge says. It doesn't take a lot of extra planning, just a willingness to do it. Most important, you won't break such a sweat that you'll be offending everyone when you walk into an afternoon meeting. Amberge, who helps corporations set up their own in-house exercise programs, suggests the following office circuit. See if you can complete it.

Note: On days that you plan to do an office workout—or any workout where you're on your feet—it pays to pack along a pair of walking shoes or cross-trainers. Your feet will thank you.

Warmup

This may be a fairly low-intensity exercise program, but it still pays to warm up your muscles before you use them. Here's how.

Visit your vehicle. You remembered to park your car at the furthest reaches of the lot and walk in, didn't you? Now, walk out to it, briskly, with a little bit of swing in your arms. From your desk chair to the driver's seat and back is one lap. Do at least two laps.

Walk the halls. Now do one circuit around the perimeter of the floor your office is located on.

"You can even mix it up with some interval training; sprint for a couple seconds, then slow back down to a brisk walk," suggests Amberge. Time those sprints so that you'll be dashing past the boss's office—you'll look like you're rushing to an important meeting, at lunch no less!—and you might even boost your career health, too.

Workout

Now that you're warmed up, you're ready to get down to business. Try these exercises.

Climb the corporate ladder. You don't want to look like you're roaming the floor lost and with nothing to do, so don't do multiple laps around your floor.

Instead, expand to other floors of your building. For this part of the workout, do a lap around your floor, then take the stairs up to the next floor, walk the circumference of that floor, then hit the stairs again for the floor above that. Do three to five floors, then come back down, taking the steps as fast as you can.

Step it up. Find an isolated stairwell and try this calf burner. Step up on a stair with your right foot, slowly raise your heel off the ground, then step up with your left foot, raising your left heel. Since you'll be walking on the balls of your feet, be sure to hold on to the railing for balance. Walk up one flight in this manner.

Make a conference call. If your work life revolves around a cubicle, seek out some privacy and exercise in an empty conference room. "Conference rooms make excellent exercise rooms," says Amberge. "There's plenty of room to maneuver, and they're usually empty at lunch."

For starters, do pushups and crunches, as many as you can. You can also do lunges and squats. Or grab two chairs (the nonrolling variety, please), position them on either side of you, put your hands on the seats, legs straight out on the floor in front of you, and do dips.

Cooldown

Don't head straight back to work after your workout. Take a few minutes to recover and prepare yourself for the rest of the workday. Here are two steps that will help ease you back to your desk, refreshed and ready to go.

Hit the water. If you've been doing these exercises at a brisk pace, you should actually feel a little winded. Don't park yourself at your desk just yet. Walk slowly to the water cooler. Fill your glass, drink it down. Have another. "It's always a good idea to rehydrate after any exercise," says Amberge.

Refuel. Now, to eat. Pick a spot a good 5- or 10-minute walk away and stroll over. Or if you brown-bagged it and weather permits, take your lunch and walk out to a nearby park. "The point is to do some slow, easy exercise that allows your heart rate to come down gradually, rather than abruptly stopping," Amberge says.

Pumped Up with a Goal in Mind

Men are bombarded with a dizzying array of fitness programs and routines almost on a daily basis. But according to Kenton Robinson in Banish Your Belly: The Ultimate Guide for Achieving a Lean, Strong Body—Now *(Rodale Press, 1997), before you can evaluate which ones are right for you, you have to get a handle on two critical items: motivation and realistic expectations. Without the first one, you don't stand a chance of lifting a single weight or running a single mile. Without the second, you'll soon lose heart and head back to the couch.*

You should know up front that the hardest part of belly banishing is just getting started. Once you've begun, it gets easier and easier.

Part of the reason is inertia: A body at rest tends to stay at rest. Even more powerful than inertia is the force of habit.

Every one of us is a collection of habits. Who we are and how we look are in many ways a product of that collection. If, for example, your particular collection of habits includes frequent trips to the icebox between innings on the idiot box, it's a pretty safe bet you have yourself a gut in progress.

The only way to redefine yourself—to start achieving leanness rather than merely worrying about being overweight—is to acquire a new set of habits. How do you do that? By doing things over and over again until they become habits.

Put succinctly, who you are is what you do. In other words, you can become some*one* else by doing some*thing* else.

Get Ready

How do you get yourself to take that first step? For starters, you need to decide whether you are really ready to do what it takes to banish that belly. According to Kelly Brownell, Ph.D., co-director of the Yale University Eating and Weight Disorders Clinic, a good way to do this is to make a list of the pros and cons of changing your ways.

A pro, for example, may be "I will look skinnier in my Skivvies." A con may be "the pains of Big Mac withdrawal." After you make your lists, look at which is longer. Are you ready? If the cons outnumber the pros, you're probably not.

If, however, the pros win, your next step is to figure out what's going to be the best motivator for you. Is it that you'll look better? Feel better? Be healthier? Live longer? Be a babe magnet? Be able to shoot hoops with the kid without losing your wind?

"Motivation is probably the most important factor," says Dragomir Cioroslan, head coach of the U.S. Weightlifting Federation and the 1996 U.S. Olympic weightlifting team. "And understanding the benefits is a strong motivating factor."

This is because regardless of what your biggest motivator is—and we'll talk later about what's realistic—it's something you're going to want to keep in the forefront of your mind for all those times when you just can't seem to shake off your inertia.

Believe in Yourself

Perhaps the hardest thing you have to do—harder than changing your eating habits, harder than working exercise into your life—is to change the way you talk to yourself.

Don't act innocent with us. Maybe you don't talk aloud, but if you're a human being, you do talk to yourself. Like cartoon characters who have an angel perched on one shoulder and a devil on the other, all of us carry on internal dialogues with ourselves.

Unfortunately for many of us, the devil often gives the angel the boot. And the devil is clever. Not only does he tempt us into sin ("Hey, you're fat already! What's another slice of cheesecake?"), he has an even more subtle tool for undercutting our self-confidence: the "if . . . then" way of thinking. "If you can just lose 20 pounds," he tells you, "then you'll feel great about yourself."

This kind of thinking will get you nowhere, says Daniel Kosich, Ph.D., senior consultant for the International Association of Fitness Professionals and author of *Get Real: A Personal Guide to Real-Life Weight Management.*

"What happens when people go into a weight-loss program with the 'I'll-feel-better-about-myself-when-I-get-there' sort of attitude is that it makes the program a punishment," Dr. Kosich says. "It's like they're a bad person now, but if they can get to a certain place, then they can be a good person. I think that really makes it difficult to achieve the long-term goal."

If you're going to stay motivated, Dr. Kosich says, you have to learn to like yourself first. Don't undertake this program because you can't stand the way you look right now. Do it because you like yourself for who you are and because you want to improve the quality of your life.

Dr. Kosich argues that this self-acceptance is key to any successful weight-maintenance program.

Accentuate the Positive

One of the most important things that you can do—indeed, you must do—is to keep reminding yourself of your accomplishments. Nothing will short-circuit your efforts more quickly than focusing on all the weight you haven't lost. Focus instead on the weight you've shed, and you'll find encouragement in each small victory.

People often overlook the benefits of even a small amount of weight loss, says Ronette Kolotkin, Ph.D., a clinical psychologist and director of behavioral programs at the Duke University Diet and Fitness Center in Durham, North Carolina.

So if, to invert the cliché, you can look at your gut as half empty instead of half full (and remember when it was all full), you'll keep yourself psyched to keep going.

Moving toward Realistic Expectations

Let's be brutally frank. Unless you're willing to devote enormous time and effort to working out, and unless you have just the right genetic makeup, you are probably never going to have abs like the washboards you see on male fashion models.

We'll say it again another way: You'll never have the "shredded" look of a bodybuilder unless you subject yourself to the regimen of a bodybuilder. And even then, you won't succeed unless you were born with the right type of muscular structure.

Why? The length of your muscle fibers is the single most important factor in determining potential muscle size. And muscle-fiber length is genetically predetermined. Sure, intense exercise can grow muscle significantly—but there is a limit. In other words, if you were born with average-length muscle fibers, you will never look like Stallone, who was blessed with unusually long muscle fibers.

In addition, you have two types of muscle fibers: fast-twitch and slow-twitch. Fast-twitch fibers provide tremendous force, the kind you need for sprints or lifting weights. Slow-twitch fibers provide endurance. Like muscle-fiber length, the ratio of fast-twitch to slow-twitch muscle in your body is genetically predetermined. Men with a greater proportion of fast-twitch fibers make better bodybuilders; guys with more slow-twitchers make better marathoners. So if you are a slow-twitcher, you are pretty much destined to a life of slow-twitching (of course, that means a fast-twitcher will rarely beat you in a mile run).

We don't mean to give you an excuse to stop working on your physique. Our point merely is that it is awfully tough to achieve the look of a bodybuilder. It is perfectly within your capacity, however, to add significant strength and definition to your body, and specifically, your belly, no matter what your genetics are.

"A flat stomach is very achievable for everyone," says Cioroslan.

How Much, How Soon?

Another question to ask yourself is how quickly can you realistically expect to lose all that flab that you have spent so many years collecting?

If you're thinking that you can drop 20 pounds in a month, we have bad news for you. While it may be possible to lose that kind of weight that fast, it is certainly not healthy to do so. Moreover, when you lose it that quickly, you're not likely to keep it off.

"Don't try to change everything overnight," says Michele Trankina, Ph.D., professor of biological sciences at St. Mary's University and adjunct associate professor of physiology at the University of Texas Health Science Center, both in San Antonio. "Gaining the weight didn't happen overnight, so you need to lose it in a systematic way that takes a lot of patience."

What, then, is a reasonable amount of weight to aim to lose each week?

"I would say 2 pounds at the most," says Dr. Trankina. "It depends on the person and it depends on how much water weight he is carrying. A person may lose weight, and it may be mostly water at first. If you lose 5 to 8 pounds a month, I think that's good. I think that's a healthy weight loss. For larger people, maybe 10 pounds."

And you're going to be healthier than if you followed a crash plan. Any program that promises you can lose 10 or more pounds a week, says Dr. Trankina, is going to require you to shun the nutrients that you need, which will "wreak havoc on the metabolic systems of the human body. Anytime you simulate starvation, that's an abnormal metabolic situation, and it should be avoided."

When you are losing weight at that rate, she says, you are most likely doing so at the expense of muscle mass (your body will burn it to give the brain the glucose it needs to keep running). Needless to say, if your goal is a lean, mean, muscular body, this is clearly the last thing you want to do.

Redefining "Comfort"

One fact you must face at the outset is that in order to lose weight, you're going to have to get comfortable with being uncomfortable.

More precisely, you're going to be redefining what feels comfortable to you.

"A lot of people don't have the heart to take some of the hard work that comes with it," says Cioroslan. "That's why you have procrastination. They don't want to get out of their comfort zones. But you must put yourself through some uncomfortable positions, spend time, work hard, sweat a little bit, control your diet. It takes a change in lifestyle. And that is the most difficult barrier to reaching consistent fitness: lifestyle."

So you must expect some initial difficulty in getting used to doing things that you didn't used to do. This is in part because you are redefining yourself and, in the process, redefining what feels good to you.

Stick with it, and you will discover that what seemed uncomfortable to you at the outset will become comfortable to you later on. In fact, it will be more than comfortable; after 6 to 12 weeks or so, says Cioroslan, you are likely to wonder how you got through a day without exercising.

Indeed, when you hit a day where you just can't make it to the gym, you may be surprised to discover that you feel frustrated, says Cioroslan. "You'll feel that something was taken away from you."

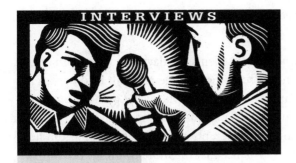

Weight-Training Experts on
Strengthening Every Part of Your Body

Men are a gender of do-it-yourselfers. Say what you will about men's refusal to ask for directions—the fact is, if it weren't for guys figuring out stuff for ourselves, we'd still be traveling to Europe by boat. Even so, if you want fast results, it pays to consult with the experts. Here some eminent fitness experts weigh in with answers to the toughest weight-lifting questions.

We've heard that it's good to vary weight routines, but how often? And what exactly should be varying?

"Varying your weight routine is crucial if you want to continue to build muscle," says Avery Faigenbaum, Ed.D., assistant professor of exercise physiology in the department of human performance at the University of Massachusetts in Boston. "Otherwise, your muscles become accustomed to your exercise program and may stop responding to it."

Changing your program—what experts call periodization—is pretty simple. There are five variables that determine the results you'll see with your weight-training program:

1. The exercises you do
2. The order in which you do them
3. The number of sets you perform
4. The number of repetitions/amount of weight you lift (higher weights mean fewer repetitions)
5. The amount of time you rest between sets

"If you take a look at these five variables and change them throughout the year, you'll probably have the best results and avoid overtraining," Dr. Faigenbaum says.

There's no cut-and-dried rule for how often you should change your program, but Trey Teichelman, fitness director of the Larry North Fitness Factory in Dallas, recommends changing one of these five factors every four to six weeks.

How much time can you take off from weight training before you start to lose the strength you've built?

"The longest break I'd prescribe to my clients is 7 days," says Teichelman. He estimates that after 10 days of not lifting, the average guy will find he can lift about 10 percent less weight than he used to. Stay out of the gym for a month, and you could end up losing as much as 25 percent of the strength you've gained.

The rate at which your strength declines, however, depends in part on how long you've been training. "There's evidence that the more training you have behind you, the slower you're going to lose your strength," says Michael H. Stone, Ph.D., professor of exercise science at Appalachian State University in Boone, North Carolina.

What is a "drop set"?

A drop set is an additional set that's performed right after you've completed your regular sets of a particular exercise. It's done to squeeze a little extra work out of a muscle—to "top it off," in musclehead lingo—after it has been put through its regular paces. This technique is a great way to shake up your routine when you've hit a plateau. "Drop sets are ideal when your program becomes stagnant and you're looking to put in a little more variety," says Teichelman.

Here's a typical drop-set routine: Do your usual number of sets at your usual weight, then, without resting, reduce the weight by about 25 percent. Go for 12 to 15 repetitions at this weight, then reduce the weight by another 10 percent. Perform another 12 to 15 repetitions at this lighter weight and then, if your muscles can take it, reduce the weight again and do another 12 to 15 repetitions.

Drop sets are tough, so Teichelman doesn't recommend trying them with free weights. Use machines instead: They make it easier to control the weight when your muscles are spent.

And don't overdo the drop-set strategy. It may be something you want to incorporate from time to time, but our experts advise against using it as part of your everyday routine.

What exactly is circuit training? Is it as good for building muscle as regular weight training?

Circuit training is a full-body workout in which you perform a single set of several different strength exercises, one right after the other. Generally, you do one set of an exercise, then move on to the next exercise with little or no rest in between. One time around all of the exercises is one circuit.

Circuit training won't build as much size or strength as straightforward weight lifting will, and it won't give you all the cardiovascular benefits of a regular aerobic workout. But it is an effective way to derive some of the benefits of both, especially if you're pressed for time. It's also an excellent starting point if you're new to exercise. "Circuit training is appropriate for a health-related approach to fitness," says Terry J. Housh, Ph.D., director of the exercise physiology laboratory at the University of Nebraska at Lincoln. "Research shows that in people who haven't weight trained before, circuit training can improve strength, muscle endurance, and maybe even body composition."

If it seems like you're lifting more weight than you were three months ago, but your muscle size is exactly the same, what gives?

The answer depends on where you are in your training. "During the first couple months of a strength training program, the gains made involve what we call neuromuscular factors," Dr. Faigenbaum says. "The exercise becomes easier, but it's mostly because you've become more efficient at recruiting the muscle fibers that are involved in a certain lift. Sure, you may have gotten a little stronger, but mostly you've become more skillful."

This is the point when beginners start to wonder why their muscles haven't grown any bigger. Usually, the gains are still a few months away. "After you've recruited more and more muscle fibers while performing a given activity, then muscle growth kicks in," says Dr. Faigenbaum. Be patient, and eventually your muscles will start to grow.

If you've been lifting for awhile and your muscles just stop increasing in size, the problem may be your diet. "If you aren't taking in enough carbohydrates and protein, it can hinder muscle growth," says Teichelman. You may also need to introduce some variety into your workout.

Finally, it's possible that you've reached your genetic potential. "If your parents aren't very big, then it's possible your muscles have reached their maximum size."

We've read that different exercises work a muscle "from different angles." What does that mean, and why is it good?

A man's muscles are more complex than you might think, and they need to be challenged from a variety of angles in order to grow.

"Take the pectoralis major, for example—the chest muscle," says Gary Dudley, Ph.D., professor of exercise science at the University of Georgia in Athens. "It has fibers that run horizontally and others that run vertically. No one exercise can hit both sets of muscle fibers. By doing an incline bench exercise, you hit a greater number of horizontal fibers; with a flat bench, you hit more vertical fibers. So if you have an interest in developing the entire muscle, you'll work it from different angles."

But you don't necessarily have to master every piece of equipment in the gym. "In some cases, you can activate a different part of the muscle simply by putting your hands in different positions," says Dr. Stone. For instance, a biceps curl performed with an underhand grip emphasizes the short head of the biceps; but a hammer curl, done with your palms facing in toward each other, works the long head of the biceps.

If you run, should you still do weight training on your calves? Will making your calves too strong put you at risk of getting shinsplints?

Having strong calves does not mean you'll be more susceptible to shinsplints. In fact, Teichelman encourages runners to work their calves diligently.

If you're prone to shinsplints, it probably has more to do with the kind of ground you're running on, according to Teichelman. Hard surfaces, such as concrete sidewalks, are the worst, he says, and your shins and tibial muscles absorb most of the impact. Running on grass or dirt tracks, alternating your running days with bicycling or water workouts, and taking at least one day off each week all seem to help with shinsplints, he adds.

Is it better to do a full-body workout three times a week, or just work certain parts (say, chest and biceps) on certain days? Does it matter which parts are grouped together?

The answer depends on what sort of body you're trying to create. "If you're looking simply to tone your muscles, you should work your entire body three times a week, using different exercises in all three workouts," says Teichelman. "If you are looking to gain strength and size, I would recommend training four to six times per week, and targeting different muscle groups on different days."

As for which muscle groups you train together on any given day, there's no right or wrong answer. Some experts train the chest and triceps together on one day, back and biceps the next. The reason? Chest exercises like the bench presses also work the triceps, while back exercises like seated rows stress the biceps. Other lifters, including Teichelman, train the chest and back on the same day since these two muscle groups oppose each other, and training them together helps keep them equally strong.

We've read that you need to perform only one set of an exercise to build muscles. So why do all the serious lifters do four or five sets?

The answer depends on two factors: what kind of shape you're in, and what you hope to accomplish with your lifting program. For a guy who's out of shape or who hasn't lifted weights before, doing one set of each exercise will certainly produce strength gains, especially at the beginning, says Dr. Faigenbaum. It's also a useful, time-efficient strategy for maintaining the strength you've already built.

However, if you're trying to build a lot of muscle or enhance sports performance, doing just one set probably isn't enough. "Generally, when you're performing an exercise, some of the muscle fibers of a muscle group don't fire until a significant load has been placed on them," says Teichelman. "This usually happens on the third set." So it's a question of investment and return: If you want serious muscle, you have to take weight lifting seriously. But if you just want to stay in shape, just do one set.

Is it true that during a bench press, you should lower the weight very slowly because that is the most important part of the exercise? This doesn't seem to make sense since lowering the weight feels easy compared with the actual lifting part.

This is a true statement. Lowering the weight feels easy partly because of gravity. But even if it feels like your muscle isn't working very hard, the lowering phase actually puts about as much strain on the muscle as raising it does.

So make sure you give each half of your repetition equal time. "If you're letting the weight down quickly, you're shortchanging that negative phase where major strength and size gains occur," says Dr. Faigenbaum.

Is there a formula for a leg curl stating that you're supposed to lift a certain amount that corresponds with how much you can lift on a leg extension?

The "formula" is known as the 3–2 rule, says Budd Coates, a champion marathoner and corporate fitness director in Emmaus, Pennsylvania. "It means that you should be able to do a leg curl with about two-thirds the amount of weight you use for a leg extension," he says. Training the legs this way helps prevent a strength imbalance between the hamstring (the muscle that runs down the back of the thigh) and the quadriceps (the large muscle on the front of the thigh). An imbalance in the leg muscles can lead to lower-back and knee problems.

If you don't have the money or the time to buy a gym membership, what else besides crunches and pushups can you do around the house to help build muscle?

Some home gym machines are affordable, and free weights are even less expensive. Core moves—shoulder presses, lateral raises, front raises, biceps curls, and single arm rows—can be done with a cheap set of dumbbells.

Teichelman is a big fan of exercises that use your body weight for resistance. "For your chest, besides pushups, do decline pushups with your feet on the couch and your hands on the floor," he says. "For your triceps, do chair dips. For your legs, squats, lunges, and step-ups work well with or without weights." And of course, a pullup bar in the basement is the best 20 bucks you'll ever spend.

Dr. Faigenbaum also recommends inexpensive props like rubber tubing and medicine balls for at-home workouts.

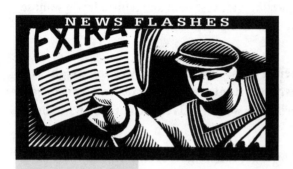

Running Can Prevent Heart Disease

BERKELEY, Calif.—A dash of medicine: How fast you run, and how far, can make all the difference in preventing heart disease. Research from the National Runners' Health Study may lead to new ways of "prescribing" exercise to help with specific problems. "We're finding that faster runners have lower blood pressure, while longer-distance runners have higher levels of high-density lipoprotein (HDL), or 'good' cholesterol," says Paul Williams, Ph.D., a biostatistician at the Lawrence Berkeley National Laboratory in California. During a study of 8,300 male runners in the trial, Dr. Williams found that running faster had 13.3 times greater impact on lowering blood pressure than running at a leisurely pace. Conversely, running farther at a slower pace didn't greatly affect blood pressure, but it had six times more effect on raising HDL cholesterol than short, quick runs.

"These principles should apply to any sustained and vigorous exercise, such as cycling and swimming," adds Dr. Williams. So if you want lower blood pressure, increase your intensity. If you want to raise your HDL cholesterol, add duration.

Replacing Salt after Exercise
Is as Important as Replacing Water

ABERDEEN, Scotland—Chugging water after exercise doesn't mean your body is ready to pound the pavement again. Replacing the salt you lost is also critical, according to researchers at the University of Aberdeen Medical School. "Salt acts as a sponge, holding the water in the tissues," says Ronald J. Maughan, Ph.D., professor of physiology and coauthor of the study. "If you don't consume enough salt along with water, you'll lose most of the water in urine in three hours and slip back into dehydration."

The amount of sodium you need depends on how much time you have to recover before exercising again, says Dr. Maughan. If you exercise more than once a day and always feel parched by day's end, try having at least one or two sports drinks that contain sodium, such as Gatorade. But if you work out only once a day, don't load up on salt. You probably already get enough from the food you eat.

Weight Lifting Belts May Do More Harm Than Good

COLUMBUS, Ohio—Don't count on that hefty lifting belt to protect you against injury. In fact, back-support belts may do more harm than good, according to William Marras, Ph.D., director of the Biodynamics Laboratory at Ohio State University. "Weight lifters need to be especially careful because leather support belts let you lift about 20 percent more weight, but don't offer any protection to the spine," he says. "You're lured into a false sense of security." The only people who should use them, Dr. Marras says, are those under the guidance of an occupational physician.

Exercise May Help Combat Chronic Fatigue Syndrome

DUBLIN, Ireland—It might sound counterintuitive, but it appears that exercise helps patients manage chronic fatigue syndrome. In a study of 66 patients, a 12-week aerobic-exercise program was twice as effective at fighting fatigue as 12 weeks of instruction in flexibility and relaxation. "The aerobics group reported feeling less tired," says Kathy Y. Fulcher, Ph.D., lead study author and general manager of Westpoint Health Club, also in Dublin. A follow-up showed sustained benefit after a year, she adds.

Aerobic Exercise Boosts Hearing

OXFORD, Ohio—And you thought that a daily run was just good for your heart. Regular aerobic exercise can improve hearing, according to Helaine M. Alessio, Ph.D., associate professor in the department of physical education, health, and sports studies at Miami University. Exercise increased patients' sensitivity to soft noises by as much as 75 percent, Dr. Alessio says. Exercise sends enriching blood to all the body's organs, researchers theorize, including the ears. "Sessions lasting 30 minutes will do it," says Dr. Alessio, who notes that weight training doesn't appear to confer the same benefits.

Shorter, More Frequent Workouts Are Better for You

BOSTON—Even a quick sweat can help keep your heart healthy. That news is from researchers at Brigham and Women's Hospital, who found in their 12-year survey of 22,000 men that exercising vigorously for 11 to 24 minutes twice a week reduced heart attack risk by 36 percent. Men who exercised for more than 24 minutes reaped no greater rewards, but those who did quick workouts five or more times per week cut their risk of heart attack by 46 percent. "This suggests that shorter, more frequent workouts may be better for your heart than longer, less frequent sessions," says study research fellow Claudia Chae, M.D.

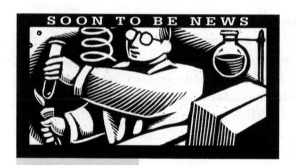

SOON TO BE NEWS

Stronger Calves Mean Better Balance?

You may have heard that your sense of balance comes from your inner ear. That's only part of it. It's largely your calf muscles—not your inner ear—that maintain your balance when you're standing still. Researchers who created an environment that deactivated the inner ear equilibrium of volunteers were surprised when the subjects didn't topple. They finally determined that muscular sensors in the volunteers' calves were keeping them upright.

Continuing experiments are focusing on whether calf exercises will improve balance, according to Richard Fitzpatrick, M.D., Ph.D., of the Prince of Wales Medical Research Institute in Sydney, Australia.

Check Your Heart at the Door?

Soon you may have to get your pump checked before pumping iron at a health club. The American Heart Association (AHA) and the American College of Sports Medicine (ACSM) have recommended in a joint statement that all facilities offering exercise equipment or services screen the heart health of new members.

About one in four adult Americans have some form of cardiovascular disease. And the fastest-growing segment of health club members is those over 34, an age when the risk of heart disease begins to rise. Some have even survived heart attacks and are following their doctors' orders to exercise more. During exercise, people with heart disease are at a 10-times-higher risk of having a heart problem, such as a heart attack, than people without heart disease. "But you can't tell who has heart disease just by looking at a person," says Gary J. Balady, M.D., chairman of the AHA's Committee on Exercise and Cardiac Rehabilitation, which helped develop the statement. "That's why screening new members of a facility is so important. If you can identify those who have been diagnosed with heart disease or are experiencing symptoms of heart disease, then you can find out from their doctors if they have any exercise limitations and monitor them more closely," he says.

The screening recommended in the joint statement includes a short questionnaire that asks about a person's medical history, symptoms, and cardiovascular risks. People with heart disease or anyone who answers "true" to a specified number of statements on the questionnaire are required to get a medical evaluation before starting an exercise program.

Because the health club industry is not regulated, clubs are not forced by law to follow the new screening recommendations. But the AHA and the ACSM hope most health clubs will keep their clients' interests at heart and implement the screening as soon as possible.

Pop a Pill to Boost Your Immunity?

Hard-core athletes may soon be able to give their immune systems a boost with a substance that's found naturally in the body. L-glutamine, an amino acid essential for immune function, may be the key to help athletes fight off infections. Intense training by professional and other serious athletes weakens their immune systems, leaving them more susceptible to infection and illness. Researchers theorize that as your overworked muscles use more of your body's L-glutamine, your immune system becomes weakened. Supplementing with the amino acid, they say, may prevent your natural supply from being tapped and your immune system from being sapped.

"There is some indication that supplementing with L-glutamine may help strengthen the immune system. It's not proven, but maybe in a few years we'll make that connection," says Peter W. R. Lemon, Ph.D., professor and chairman of exercise nutrition at the University of Western Ontario in London. "But until more research is done, it is premature to recommend taking L-glutamine supplements," he adds.

Jet Skis Running into Rough Waters?

The National Park Service (NPS) may soon put the brakes on a popular form of water recreation. The agency announced that it will place a ban on the use of personal watercraft such as Jet Skis as early as later this year.

The NPS cites safety, noise, and environmental concerns as the main reasons for the ban. Indeed, the safety record of personal watercraft is far from glowing. They account for 11 percent of all vessels registered in the country, yet they're involved in more than 35 percent of watercraft accidents.

Personal watercraft are currently used in 32 of the 87 NPS areas that allow motorized boating, including Big Bend, Mount Rainier, and Olympic National Parks. Even after the ban is in place, 13 parks could continue to allow the use of the craft in designated areas, while a dozen others will be given a two-year grace period. During that time, they can either develop special regulations to continue the vehicles' use or do nothing at all—in which case the ban would go into effect after the two-year period.

Although the official ruling that will ban personal watercraft from national parks may not be made until later this year, some areas such as Yellowstone, Glacier, and Canyonlands National Parks have already put bans in place. Other parks where little or no use of the craft has been observed have also issued the ban.

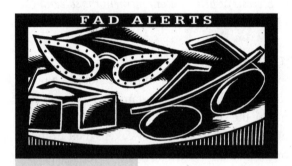

FAD ALERTS

Creatine

When creatine monohydrate first showed promise as a muscle enhancer, we read the studies, interviewed the doctors and athletes, and came to this conclusion: Creatine seemed to be safe for exercise junkies, though taking any supplement could have unforeseen side effects. Soon after we came to our conclusion, three wrestlers died and creatine was implicated. When several pro baseball players using creatine suffered muscle pulls, athletes began flushing their supplies.

"We've discouraged our players from using it," says A. Eugene Coleman, Ed.D., director of conditioning for the Houston Astros. Like others, he believes creatine forces muscles to retain too much water, inviting muscle strains and dehydration.

But according to Richard B. Kreider, Ph.D., a noted creatine researcher at the University of Memphis in Tennessee, that fear is unfounded. "There's no link between the wrestlers' deaths and creatine," he maintains. "Two weren't even taking creatine, and one had stopped months beforehand." He notes that the victims were trying to lose weight quickly through measures like fasting, not drinking, and exercising in rubber suits in heated rooms, which led to dehydration and dangerous increases in body temperature.

As for the ballplayers, Dr. Kreider points out that these isolated incidents of muscle cramping don't outweigh studies involving hundreds of men who showed no such problems. "If creatine caused cramping," he reasons, "two-thirds of the Nebraska football team would be hurt."

Still, no long-term studies on creatine supplementation have been concluded, so it's possible that negative side effects could pop up.

HMB

Flip through any muscle mag, and you'll see loads of ads for beta-hydroxy beta-methylbutyrate. Muscleheads, who tend to avoid multisyllabic words, just call it HMB. Supplement companies claim that this amino acid by-product stops muscle breakdown during exercise, which spurs faster muscle growth. As evidence, they point to a single preliminary study in the *Journal of Applied Physiology* that reported that 28 men who took HMB during a seven-week weight lifting program showed 20 percent less muscle breakdown than lifters taking a placebo, and gained an average of two kilograms (4.4 pounds) more lean muscle.

But these results are hard to interpret, says Peter Lemon, Ph.D., professor of applied physiology at Kent State University in Ohio. Some of the study subjects didn't consume enough calories or protein, so it's impossible to tell if HMB was solely responsible for the differences in muscle mass. "It's also possible that some subjects in the HMB group gained muscle mass due to a placebo effect," explains Dr. Lemon.

Finally, you don't need to drop $90 on a one-month supply of HMB for one simple reason: You already have it. "Our bodies produce all the HMB we need," says Kristine Clark, R.D., Ph.D., director of sports nutrition at the Pennsylvania State University Center for Sports Medicine in University Park. "Adding more won't enhance muscle growth; the excess will just be eliminated."

Air Gliders

Now that ab machines are filling Dumpsters, the infomercials have a new shtick: "air gliders." These contraptions look like cross-country ski machines with suspended foot pads. Some manufacturers claim that they deliver a full-body workout, burning 600 to 1,000 calories an hour, without harming your joints.

Don't dial up the home shopping channel yet. "You can probably expend about the same number of calories walking or jogging that you would by using one of these machines," says Steven F. Loy, Ph.D., an exercise physiologist at California State University at Northridge.

Further, while air glider workouts might help you break a sweat if you're out of shape, they may not give physically fit people much of a challenge, says Alan Mikesky, Ph.D., director of the human performance and biomechanics laboratory at Indiana University–Purdue University at Indianapolis, who tested one of the gliders on the market. "Even when using resistance, I had trouble elevating my heart rate," he said. If you're a well-trained runner, an air glider may provide only a weak aerobic workout.

Can air gliders really save your joints from stress? "Unless you're severely overweight or have specific problems with your joints, you're just as safe running or using a treadmill," says Dr. Mikesky.

Low-Oxygen Training

 To replicate the pulse-pounding, lung-searing effects of high-altitude exercise, New York's Crunch fitness club is offering the world's first hypoxic (low-oxygen) training room. The oxygen content within this vinyl cell has been cut to about 15 percent (normal sea level is around 21 percent). The result is an artificial atmosphere that makes your lungs feel as if they're on top of a 9,000-foot mountain. And you don't even have to pay the air fare to Denver.

We sent *Men's Health* magazine senior writer Joe Kita to pedal a stationary bike inside this room for 15 minutes, and he definitely felt the shortage of oxygen. Even at a moderate pedaling cadence, his well-trained heart was pounding and he couldn't maintain a conversation. Although the low-air chamber shelled him, it's doubtful that working out in such an environment will improve his fitness.

"I can't imagine that low oxygen could help anyone become more fit," says Jack Daniels, Ph.D., one of the world's foremost altitude-research experts. "In fact, some of the more recent research suggests that those who live at high altitude full-time should train at low altitude, where they'll be able to exercise more intensely." Sure, high-altitude training has been practiced by Olympic athletes for decades. The difference? They move to the mountaintop, training in the clouds for months before the event, which gives their bodies adequate time to adjust. Pedaling a bike in a room with thin air won't.

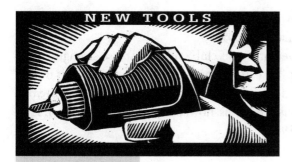

Lower Golf Scores

Golf Training Aids

Admit it. The boy in you sees a golf-training gadget and says, "I gotta try it." This, despite the fact that most resemble some type of bondage device. You're a reasonable man, so you don't mind looking like an idiot as long as the thing helps your game, right? And some of them can help.

"Teaching aids can be beneficial, but be careful not to wear the devices for an extended period during your practice sessions," says T. J. Tomasi, Ph.D., director of the Player's School at PGA National in Palm Beach Gardens, Florida. "Hit six or eight balls with the training aid on, then hit six or eight without it. If you come to rely too much on the device, you won't be able to hit a ball very well without it."

Here are Dr. Tomasi's opinions of 10 popular training gadgets.

1. The ProWedge Angel is a medieval-looking shackle intended to lock your forearms in the proper position throughout your swing. "I'm usually wary of devices that teach by restricting the golfer, but there's no question that the forearms need to stay together," says Dr. Tomasi. Price: $100

2. The Golf Foot is a giant plastic foot that straps onto any golf shoe to help you maintain better balance. Most beginners tend to rock up on the toe of their lead foot and lose balance. The Golf Foot prohibits such movement. "While this is one of the goofiest-looking products out there—I call it the agony of 'da-feet'—it is effective," says Dr. Tomasi. Price: $40

3. The John Daly Power Groove sounds more like a Friday night at the disco than a day on the green. You're tethered to a giant pole by something called the "Ingenious Gyro Coupler." Wow. With enough swings, the manufacturer guarantees you'll cut your handicap by one-third as you train your muscles to memorize the rhythm, balance, tempo, and feel of a great golf swing. That's a lofty claim, even for a product endorsed by Daly, a beefy pro who has won two major championships. "You have to

set the device in the correct position for your body type if it's going to work," cautions Dr. Tomasi. Price: $200

4. The Heavy Hitter is a weighted golf club said to increase strength, flexibility, and conditioning. "Be careful not to hurt yourself with this thing," says Dr. Tomasi. "It's fine for warming up, but you should build your strength in the gym." This product is, however, useful for fending off late-night intruders. Price: $90

5. The Impact Bag is a plastic sack that you fill with towels or other soft, heavy material; then you whack it. The idea is to get your hands and arms conditioned to the position and feeling of hitting a proper golf shot. (Of course, if a golf ball were the size of the Impact Bag, it would be a helluva lot easier to hit.) "Be careful not to hit this bag too hard," warns Dr. Tomasi, "and be sure it's correctly positioned in your stance—not too far back—or you'll learn a swing that leaves the club face wide open, and you'll acquire an awful slice." Price: $35

6. The Wonder Stick is just that—a stick. The maker designed it to promote proper body alignment and a correct swing plane. "Good product, bad name," says Dr. Tomasi. "It needs to be used exactly as instructed, or it could be more damaging than helpful. It's a good idea to use it with a teaching pro watching." Whatever you do, don't get it caught between your knees or in the steering wheel of your cart. Ouch. Price: $50

7. The Power Leg Coil is supposed to provide you with a solid base and convey the feeling of the proper weight shift essential to a good golf swing. It's a strap that attaches your right knee to your left foot. A right-knee brace is designed to teach the correct flex. "It's good for some; not good for others," says Dr. Tomasi. "Some body types require a straighter back leg. Tall players, for example, will often swing with a back leg that's nearly straight at the top of their backswing. A player who thinks 'coil' in his backswing will find this device helpful." Tip: Don't try walking anywhere while it's still attached. Price: $50

8. The Whippy TempoMaster looks like a gag club. The shaft is superflexible, so the clubhead sort of wobbles. But when swung slowly and smoothly, the TempoMaster will function as a normal club, while improving your tempo and timing. "This may seem like the silliest aid in the bunch, but it's not. It definitely helps with the average golfer's main problem of poor tempo," Dr. Tomasi says. "Yanking the club from the top of the backswing will ruin every good thing you might do during the rest of the swing. This device is very effective in helping golfers with this problem." Price: $109

9. The Master Putt, reminiscent of the handlebar on an old Schwinn Stingray, is designed to force you to use the large muscles of your back and shoulders while putting. "This device allows you to focus on the feel of using the big muscles," Dr. Tomasi says. "Don't worry about making putts with it; concentrate on the feeling of the correct stroke." Price: $30

10. Merlin's Laser Putter incorporates an infrared laser into the face of the putter head to improve your aim. "Good putting has always been mystical," Dr. Tomasi says. "Even though it's the closest you get to your target all day, most golfers find it hard to aim the putter face on the correct line. Merlin shows you exactly where you're aiming." It makes an impressive pointer for corporate presentations, too. Price: $200

Stronger Eyeglasses

Polycarbonate Lenses

Ask for polycarbonate lenses the next time you're shopping for eyeglasses. They're much stronger than any other type of lens, says ophthalmologist Paul F. Vinger, M.D., of Tufts University School of Medicine in Boston. In testing, regular glass and plastic lenses shattered during common types of abuse, but a polycarbonate lens was barely dented when struck by a baseball speeding at 94 miles per hour. "These fibrous lenses bend without breaking, like a piece of green wood," says Dr. Vinger. "They might cost a few dollars more, but if you're active, they're worth it."

Greater Speed and Agility

Cybex Reactor

You sweat. You lift. You have a body like the NBA's Grant Hill, but you move like you're carrying his yearly salary in your back pocket—all in loose change. Maybe the Cybex Reactor can help.

The Reactor, a new speed- and agility-training machine, consists of a floor platform dotted with up to four rows of circular pads that are wired to a computer. Each time a circle on the monitor lights up, you jump to the corresponding target on the floor. Depending on the program you choose, you can practice sequences of jumps to build agility, or hit as many targets as you can in a specified time.

In addition to basic fitness drills, there are sports-specific programs that mimic the movements you need for baseball, volleyball, tennis, soccer, basketball, skiing, football, and hockey. "If you choose the basketball program, the Reactor will measure your hang time between jumps so you can work on perfecting your vertical leap," says Jeff Glennon, fitness operations manager at the Sports Center at Chelsea Piers, New York City.

More Effective Exercise

Pulse Monitor

In the past few years, the price of pulse monitors has gone the way of those of VCRs and desktop calculators. It has almost gotten to the point where you expect to get one as a prize in your next box of Wheaties. Given that some of the more expensive monitors can retail for close to $400, we started wondering about the quality of the budget models that are selling for as little as $49.95.

We gathered eight units from a variety of manufacturers and distributors. We wore them while running, cycling, swimming, weight lifting, and, ahem, having sex. One staffer even wore his through an entire workday to gauge if it could help him control stress. (It did.)

Surprisingly, our favorite monitor was the least expensive one of the bunch: the $49.95 Nashbar NA-HRM. It has a nice big simultaneous display of pulse rate and elapsed time, programmable high- and low-limit settings so you'll know when you're in your target zone, a light for night viewing, and a memory that records and displays how long you've spent above, below, and inside your target zone. It's extremely easy to use, and it's all the average guy needs in a heart rate monitor, plus Nashbar throws in a handlebar mount so you can use it while you bicycle.

Although we did not test the Nashbar unit for accuracy, studies of heart rate monitors in general have found they're off by no more than six beats per minute, an insignificant amount for recreational purposes. This one seemed to perform no better or worse than the others in our review. We also didn't test its durability, but even if this Hong Kong–made unit goes "boing!" after its one-year warranty is up, you can buy another and still have spent significantly less than if you'd ordered an expensive model.

Training by heart rate has long been recognized as the most effective way to exercise since you always know your level of exertion. As always, if you're over 40 or have a family history of heart problems, you should consult your doctor before starting any exercise program, but overall, pulse monitors provide a useful and fascinating window into your heart that, at this price, shouldn't be ignored.

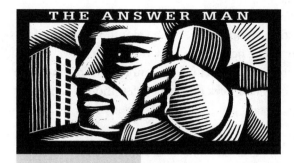

Nauseated while Lifting

Halfway through a weight training session, I become nauseated. I warm up, I drink plenty of water, and I don't eat too soon beforehand. So what gives?
—D. P., Portland, Ore.

Nausea during lifting may mean you're pushing too hard, says Carl Maresh, Ph.D., professor of exercise physiology at the University of Connecticut in Storrs. It's a fairly common response to lifting too much weight and not giving your body enough time to recover between sets. Also, pay attention to your breathing pattern during workouts. Holding your breath or hyperventilating can cause you to become nauseated and dizzy.

It's also important to make sure your diet is well-balanced. "Nausea can be a sign of low blood-glucose levels," says Dr. Maresh. Your body needs an adequate intake of carbohydrates throughout the day, not just before your workout. But eating a complex carbohydrate snack such as a bagel roughly an hour before your workout might alleviate the problem.

If none of this helps, see a doctor. "If you're doing everything right and you still find yourself becoming nauseated, it could signal something more serious," says Dr. Maresh.

Ace on the Court

The guy I play tennis with consistently beats me. I know I can take him if I just put a little more power in my serve. Is there an exercise that will help?
—J. L., Dallas

A serve is basically a throwing movement, so you'll need to strengthen your shoulders to produce more speed, says Pat Etcheberry, who has worked with tennis players Jim Courier and Monica Seles at L.G.E. Sports Science in Orlando, Florida.

Many pros use a medicine ball, says Etcheberry. "With both hands, hold a three- or four-pound medicine ball above and a little behind your head," he says.

"Then, bring it directly over your head and throw it forward with both hands." Do two or three sets of 15 repetitions, throwing with a smooth motion and increasing your distance gradually over a period of weeks. If you don't have a medicine ball, a gym pullover machine or a pullover using dumbbells works the same muscles. Do these exercises three times a week for the next few months, and your serve should be faster than ever, he says.

A Big Chest

I have rotator cuff problems and can't do any incline bench work. Is there any other way to build the upper chest besides incline bench routines?
—C. W., South Bend, Ind.

Actually, there are two ways, says John Abdo, certified fitness trainer and the author of *Body Engineering*. One is to use the chest fly machine but with the seat dropped lower than normal: Instead of bringing your hands together at chest height, Abdo advises you to find the seat position that lets your hands come together at a height between your clavicle and chin. This isolates the upper pectorals and takes a lot of the pressure off your rotator cuffs and shoulders. Do 10 to 12 repetitions at a light weight to make sure you're not stressing your shoulders.

Another option is a modified cable fly. Place an incline bench between the two weight stacks. Then lie on the bench, grab the two low cables, and do the fly move from this position. Complete 10 to 12 reps with a light weight. In both exercises, keep the motion slow and controlled to avoid straining your rotator cuff.

Early Riser

You recommend eating three to four hours before exercise, but I work out at 6:00 A.M. I'm not going to wake up at 3:00 in the morning for breakfast, so what should I eat, and when?
—M. H., Cleveland

Assuming you're not about to run in a marathon, it's okay to exercise on an empty stomach in the morning, says Richard Bullough, Ph.D., adjunct professor of nutrition at the University of Utah in Salt Lake City. "You just want to make sure you eat soon afterward." Here's why: Your muscles burn very little stored carbohydrate during the night. When you wake up, he says, you typically have enough stored carbohydrate to exercise for roughly an hour without collapsing in a soggy heap. Since running or lifting weights immediately after eating makes some people nauseated, you might as well wait until you've finished, and then have breakfast.

To make sure you wake up with energy to burn, eat a high-carbohydrate dinner the night before. Dr. Bullough recommends low-fat lasagna with salad, some whole-wheat bread, and fruit for dessert as a way to prime your muscles for an early-morning workout. Right after your workout, replenish your carbohydrate stores with a high-fiber, low-fat breakfast, like a whole-grain bagel with low-fat yogurt, and juice.

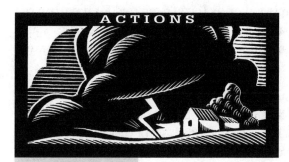

ACTIONS

Some days, finding time to work out is as tough as finding a New York cabbie with a name you can pronounce. So when you do make it to the gym or your basement to pump iron, you want to get the most out of it. Here are some tips to help you exercise smarter.

1. **Strengthen a key muscle.** We're talking about the serratus muscles, which extend from the bottoms of your shoulder blades through your armpits and attach to the sides of your rib cage. "Without them, you couldn't even lift your arms above your head," says Don Chu, Ph.D., registered physical therapist and president of the National Strength and Conditioning Association, based in Colorado Springs, Colorado. And because they visually link your chest and abs, developed serratus muscles can make your torso look tighter than ever.

You can build these oft-forgotten muscles with uneven pushups. Place something that's wide, stable and about four-inches high—a briefcase will do—on the floor. Assume the pushup position, but put your right hand on top of the object. Your hands should be slightly more than shoulder-width apart. Lower yourself to perform a regular pushup, but lower the left side of your body as close to the floor as possible. Push yourself up and repeat the movement. This motion helps isolate your left serratus. Do 12 repetitions, then slide the object over and place your left hand on it to work your right serratus. Hit each side for three sets.

2. **Press your tongue against the roof of your mouth while you do crunches.** "That'll prevent you from using your neck muscles to jerk yourself up," says Susan M. Kaschalk, an exercise physiologist in Pontiac, Michigan. Keep your eyes focused on the ceiling to further isolate your stomach.

3. **Focus on muscle groups.** Big areas of your body, such as the arms, legs, and back, aren't single muscles but groups of muscles. Attack as many of these as possible during a workout. Called compound exercises, these big-muscle exercises can get you in and out of the gym fast. A squat, for example, simultaneously works the quadriceps, hamstrings, and buttocks—more than a dozen muscles in all. It's equal to doing three exercises at once. If you're pressed for time, you can achieve a workout that hits all major muscle groups with only six exercises: squat, bench press, upright row, military press, pulldown, and crunch. Total workout time: 45 minutes.

4. **Employ the push-pull method.** Shorten a 45-minute full-body workout by alternating upper-body exercises with lower-body ones, and pushing movements with pulling movements. For example, after a set of chest-building bench presses (a compound exercise that calls for you to push, not pull, the weight), you can go directly to a squat (a lower-body blaster) or to a pulling movement such as the pulldown or upright row. By being smart about the way you work out, you'll need no more than a mere minute of rest between exercises. Total workout time: 30 minutes.

5. **Do one set.** Turn up your workout and get out of the gym in less time than it takes to watch the Super Bowl halftime show. A study conducted by the Colleges of Medicine and Health and Human Performance at the University of Florida in Gainesville found that doing one set of weight lifting exercises to fatigue builds as much muscle as doing the typical three-set regimen. That means you can complete an effective strength training program in a third of the time. Total workout time: approximately 15 minutes.

6. **Lose weight.** If you're lifting heavy weights that allow you to do just a few repetitions, cut your weight by a quarter and aim for three sets of 15 to 20 repetitions per set. When that becomes easy, add more repetitions, not more weight.

7. **Set yourself free.** It sounds obvious, but most men forget that machines and free weights are interchangeable. If you usually use a machine to work a particular body part, switch to barbells or dumbbells. If you normally use free weights, try a machine.

8. **Pull your own weight.** Set aside one or two workout days each month to do only body-weight exercises. A full routine can include overhand-grip pullups, underhand pullups, plyometric pushups (an explosive movement where the hands leave the floor), jump squats, dips, and crunches.

9. **Find your Achilles' heel.** To focus on a muscle group that needs work, try a technique called sandwich sets. Say you want to strengthen your hamstrings. Before you do your normal full-body routine, sneak in a set of hamstring curls, then move on. Once you've worked every muscle group, finish with three more good sets of hamstring curls. Because you've prefatigued that muscle, your final sets will be more challenging than ever.

10. **Record your reps.** Once you know how much you can lift, take a notebook to the gym and check off the exercises as you go through your routine. Make notes about whether the set was easy or brutal. The closer attention you pay, the better you'll know when it's time to increase the weight or change your routine.

11. **Broaden your horizons.** Go to the gym, do your new routine, and then check out that one machine you've always wanted to try but couldn't quite figure out. Ask someone to show you how to use it. Try to find one new thing to try at least every couple of weeks. It doesn't matter if you hate it—you don't have to do it again. "By doing something different, you'll keep from going stale," says Ed Burke, author of *The Complete Home Fitness Handbook.*

12. **First run, then iron.** According to researchers at California State University in Los Angeles, men perceived their workouts as harder when they did 50 minutes of weight training followed by 20 minutes of stationary cycling than when they did aerobics before weight training. This error could cause men to ditch an aerobic workout they really need, says Nazareth Khodiguian, Ph.D., a study author. So do your aerobics before weight training, or do the workouts on alternating days, to ensure that you get the maximum heart-training benefits from your aerobic exercise.

13. **Reestablish your aerobic routine.** If it has been awhile since you've done anything in this department, start out slow. "Do too much and you'll be sore and blow off the next workout," says Burke. Instead, take a walk. As you go, pick a landmark (a fire hydrant, a movie marquee, a lost wallet) and jog easily toward it—no sprinting. Once you reach your goal, return to a walking stride. Do this for about 30 minutes. Over the next month, gradually increase the proportion of time you spend running and eliminate the walking.

14. **Go easy on the ice.** We've been slapping ice bags on bumps and bruises for years. But a Swedish study suggests that you shouldn't ice an injury before exercise, or for more than 30 minutes in any case. Icing a sore muscle before exercise reduces its flexibility and makes it more prone to injury. Worse, icing too long can cause frostbite or nerve damage. And watch those synthetic cold packs. "They become much colder than ice and can cause frostbite faster," says Mike Ferrara, Ph.D., director of sports medicine at Ball State University in Muncie, Indiana. Use crushed ice in a plastic bag for 15 minutes, he advises.

15. **Rest.** But make it an active rest. "To maintain fitness without burning out, a guy needs active recovery," says Burke. That means doing something other than the typical workout—maybe just a long walk. Do something recreational, but not so intense that it feels like exercise. We're partial to croquet.

16. **Hydrate with carbos.** Don't just guzzle that fluorescent carbo drink after your workout. According to Australian researchers, ingesting carbohydrates throughout your exercise session will boost your power and endurance. Male cyclists who sipped carbo beverages every 15 minutes while pedaling had more sustained energy than cyclists who drank them only during the latter phases of exercise or who drank liquids without carbohydrates. "The regular intake helps keep your blood sugar levels steady," says Debra Wein, R.D., a sports nutritionist and exercise physiologist at the University of Massachusetts in Boston. During a long run, take in 30 to 60 grams of carbohydrates each hour (roughly two to four 12-ounce sports drinks).

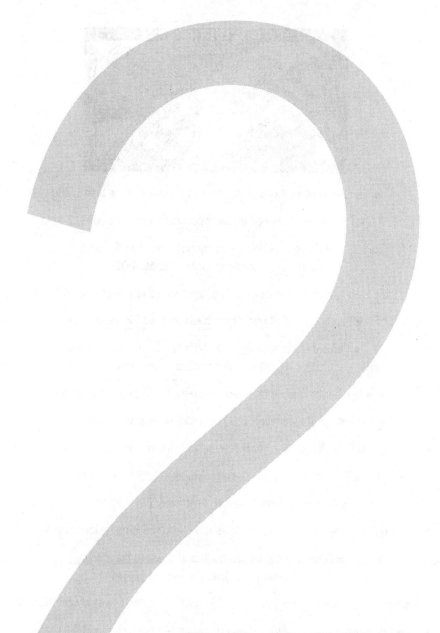

EATING

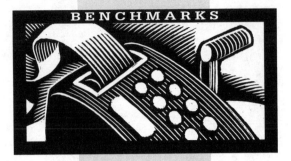

■ Number of natural chemicals in a cup of coffee: more than 1,000

■ Percentage of all edible plant species that humans eat: 0.2

■ Number of glasses of tap water you can drink
for the price of one six-pack of soda: 4,000

■ Estimated tons of food wasted in the United States in a given year: 48 million

■ Percentage of all restaurant meals ordered for takeout: 51

■ Percentage of men who admit they've eaten take-out food
that's been left out for more than two hours: 37

■ Number of lunches the average American skipped last year: 56

■ Percentage of Americans who eat at McDonald's on any given day: 7

■ Ratio of men who slurp their pasta to women who do: 3 to 1

■ Pounds of pasta the average American eats each year: 20

■ Amount of pizza Americans eat every day: 100 acres

■ Percentage of food budget Generation Xers spend on restaurants: 42

■ Estimated number of foodborne illnesses that occur
each year in the United States: 81 million

■ Percentage of medical schools that don't require students to study nutrition: 78

■ Number of states in which publicly disparaging a particular food is illegal: 13

■ Percentage by which the number of kosher delis
in New York City has fallen since 1965: 88

■ Average number of frogs eaten by the French each year: 200 million

■ Percentage of Americans who have eaten ground beef in the past 24 hours: 34

VITAL READING

Coffee's Bum Rap

Here's some compelling evidence to justify drinking java.

Call it the physics of vice: For every pleasurable action, there's an equal and opposite reaction. You smoke, and your lungs get tarred. Drink too many vodka tonics, and your liver turns to jelly.

But one vice no one ever explained the consequences of was coffee. It is a vice, right? Isn't this why your in-laws switched to decaffeinated when they hit 50, and why they cluck their tongues when you insist on stopping at Dunkin' Donuts for a hit of the hard stuff? Well, we decided to do a little research and get the scoop on coffee. It's about the best news you're going to read all month.

See, it turns out that coffee has gotten a bum rap. For example, there were reports a few years ago of a Danish study that found that coffee raises blood cholesterol. Papers all over America reported that Juan Valdez could do for your arteries what the *Exxon Valdez* did for Prince William Sound. But there's a catch: While coffee does indeed contain compounds that can raise your cholesterol levels, when you filter the coffee, these compounds are removed. But the Danes, like the Turks and Greeks, made their coffee by boiling it, and never ran it through a filter. So, yes, coffee can raise your cholesterol, but only if you forgo the filter or use a French press. In fact, coffee made in a French press (again, sans filter) can raise cholesterol as much as 20 points.

Assuming that you're filtering your brew, "It's very hard to come up with anything damning about coffee," says Harvey Wolinsky, M.D., Ph.D., a cardiologist, internist, and professor of medicine at Mount Sinai Medical Center in New York City. Coffee does cause heart palpitations in a small percentage of the population, which is why it's not recommended for heart arrhythmia patients. In the rest of us, coffee raises the pulse temporarily, as anyone who downs two cups on an empty stomach knows. "But after decades of heart-health studies, not one single heart condition could be linked to coffee consumption," says Dr. Wolinsky.

And although coffee can raise your blood pressure, the temporary rise brought on by a cup or two of coffee is less than the change in pressure when you stand up. Or sit down. So relax, because stress can push up your pressure a lot quicker than coffee.

If coffee has one great drawback, it's the fact that caffeine creates a physical dependence, according to Roland Griffiths, Ph.D., professor in the departments of psychiatry and neuroscience at Johns Hopkins University School of Medicine in Baltimore. "People who consume caffeine on a daily basis may experience headaches, muscle aches, and fatigue if they quit it abruptly," he says. Just going overnight without coffee can be long enough to induce mild caffeine-withdrawal symptoms, though most people start to feel crummy after about 18 caffeine-free hours. It doesn't matter how much coffee you consume per day—one, three, five cups—you can still become physically dependent on the stuff.

But why quit, when you consider what that morning cup can do for you?

Increase your endurance. Caffeine boosts endurance by delaying fatigue. Research shows that when consumed an hour before an endurance event, three or four cups of coffee (about 400 milligrams of caffeine) can help athletes run or cycle up to 20 minutes longer than their caffeine-free competitors. To achieve this boost, recommends Kristine Clark, R.D., Ph.D., director of sports nutrition at the Pennsylvania State University Center for Sports Medicine in University Park, daily caffeine users should abstain from caffeine for four days prior to the athletic event. "This way," says Clark, "your body is resensitized to the caffeine and you will receive a true benefit from it." But even if you don't swear off the sauce, a cup of coffee before heading out for your daily run may enhance your alertness. It won't help, however, in power sports or strength training.

Move things along. We don't want to dwell on something you've probably already discovered, but coffee is great for stimulating your bowels. Dr. Clark says this is the other reason that endurance athletes drink coffee before competition. They want to lighten their load before they start running or cycling for hours. And coffee does the trick. As for its diuretic effects, Dr. Clark advises all athletes to drink water regularly to replenish fluids lost during workouts, regardless of coffee intake.

Keep things in your head. Coffee was a staple in college when you were cramming for tests, and it may have done more than just keep you awake all night. Studies show that coffee also improves long-term memory. W. Scott Terry, Ph.D., professor of psychology at the University of North Carolina at Charlotte, suggests that coffee facilitates the storage of information in your long-term memory bank because it keeps the brain alert and attentive. The exact mechanism of coffee's effect on memory is still unknown, but it does seem to help people hold on to what they've learned.

Breathe easier. If you suffer occasional bouts of asthma, hit the coffee shop for some relief. "Caffeine acts as a mild bronchodilator, relaxing the spasm in the lungs' bronchi," says Marshall Plaut, M.D., chief of the allergic-mechanisms section at the National Institute of Allergy and Infectious Disease.

If you have moderate or severe asthma, don't forgo your medication for a cup of coffee. It's no miracle cure.

Flush your kidneys. You know that coffee is a diuretic. Pulling off the highway for a cup on a long trip means pulling off the highway an hour later for other reasons. But this stimulating effect may keep your kidneys stone-free. Researchers at the Harvard School of Public Health found that drinking coffee daily can reduce your risk of kidney stones by 10 percent. By the way, beer works, too.

Food as Medicine

Eats that are good for what makes you feel bad.

Like any good June Cleaver wannabe, most moms had a proven recipe for comforting you whenever you were down. Be it a cold or the flu, a runny nose or a sour stomach, or perhaps a full-contact introduction to pro wrestling courtesy of the Ahern boys next door, Mom's routine always involved the same foods.

Casting aside for a moment the magical powers of the slippers, the real question is this: Can certain foods actually make you feel better when your body is feeling beat up? Or is it a bunch of sentimental hooey to think that a glass of ginger ale and a few crackers can perk you up? Experts may debate forever the merits of cream of mushroom soup, but they agree on one thing: The right foods can indeed help speed recovery from a wide range of illness and misfortune, from a bruised head to a bruising headache. "Nutrition is extremely important during recovery from an illness," says Jane Lanzillotti, R.D., nutrition education manager at South Shore Hospital in the Boston area. "It may not work miracles, but it can certainly help."

It's worth noting that the primary nutrient our experts mentioned—no matter the ailment—was plain old water. Guzzling plenty of H_2O just may be the most important thing you can do to keep your body in good repair—and to mend it.

That said, here's what's good to eat when you're . . .

. . . fending off a cold. When you feel like the Eighth Army used your body as a proving ground, start looking around for a grapefruit. "The first thing you should do is eat a lot of foods rich in vitamin C," says Laima Wesson, R.D., health educator–dietitian at the University of California, Los Angeles's student health

service. "It's an antioxidant that helps strengthen your immune system." Citrus fruits and juices fit the bill here, as do sweet red peppers, broccoli, and strawberries.

If your appetite has been lousy thanks to the cold, you can recharge your batteries with an easy-to-digest meal. Like maybe a baked potato and a steaming bowl of soup. "Soups, especially tomato and vegetable soups, tend to be very rich in vitamin C, and they are a very palatable way of delivering nutrients," says Kristine Clark, R.D., Ph.D., director of sports nutrition at the Pennsylvania State University Center for Sports Medicine in University Park.

And if you're a big milk-drinker, there's probably no reason to stop now. "While some people, especially those with chronic asthma or other lung problems, report that drinking milk worsens their conditions, there's little in the scientific literature to indicate that milk promotes mucus," says Lanzillotti.

. . . doubled over with diarrhea. Maybe you drank the water. Maybe you've been munching Olestra-based snack chips. Maybe both. Whatever the reason, you're spending more time around johns than a lady of the night. Just remember these two simple rules:

- **Rule number one:** Your body is starved for calories, so feed it (and again, don't forget to drink lots of water since you'll likely be dehydrated, too).
- **Rule number two:** Avoid foods high in fiber and in fat. They're both hard to digest, and the last thing you want to do now is make your gastrointestinal tract work harder than it has to, says Paul Lachance, Ph.D., professor of food science at Rutgers University in New Brunswick, New Jersey. That means no raw vegetables or bran flakes, no french fries or cheesecake. Instead, go for toast with jelly, or a baked potato with fat-free sour cream or cottage cheese—whatever goes down easy.

And if you're taking drugs for your distress, extra precautions may be in order, says Lanzillotti. "Some antibiotics kill both the bad bacteria that make you sick and the good bacteria that allow your digestive system to function," she explains. "Eating yogurt with active cultures can help replenish these healthy bacteria." (Check the yogurt's label for active, live cultures.)

. . . black and blue and red all over. Whether you feel beat up (say, after falling from a ladder) or are beat up (the guy you stole the ladder from came looking for it), the right foods may help get you out of traction and back in action. In the case of a muscle tear or strain, go for a high-carbohydrate, moderate-protein diet, says Susan Kleiner, R.D., Ph.D., a high-performance nutritionist based in Seattle. That means plenty of beans, grains, fruits, and vegetables, says Dr. Kleiner. "Choose a colorful mix of orange and dark green, leafy vegetables and a variety of citrus fruits," she says. They'll provide antioxidants important for repairing the cellular damage that occurs in a muscle tear. "The antioxidant vit-

amin E may reduce some of the inflammation." Good sources of E include wheat germ and vegetable oils.

If you're dealing with a cut or a scrape, indulge in a few helpings of lean meat, says Thomas Alt, M.D., a cosmetic surgeon in Minneapolis who has studied nutrition's role in wound healing. "Meat is one of the best sources of the essential amino acids, which are the basic building blocks for healing," says Dr. Alt. "Without them, you won't heal as well or as rapidly as normal."

And if your injury is serious enough to keep you off your feet, start watching your calorie intake, warns Mel Williams, Ph.D., professor emeritus of exercise science at Old Dominion University in Norfolk, Virginia. "If you're used to exercising," he says, "you'll have to cut your normal caloric intake to avoid putting on weight."

. . . *dragging along.* If you're a modern-day Willy Loman, don't let business travel be the death of you. When you arrive at your destination, says Dr. Clark, skip the local steak house and the hotel bar, especially if you arrive at night in preparation for a morning meeting. Fat and booze will only make you sluggish. Instead, eat something small: salad, fruit, a baked potato, or a bowl of soup that isn't cream-based. If you're still groggy the next morning, wake yourself up with some lean protein—a glass of skim milk or some yogurt. Protein increases the brain chemical norepinephrine, Dr. Clark explains, which can make you more alert.

To keep jet lag at a minimum in the first place, think ahead, Dr. Clark says. "People overeat when they travel, often with high-fat airport food." So cut out the nachos and grab some fresh fruit instead.

. . . *putting in overtime.* The good part of shuffling out of the office at 9:00 P.M. is that it's easy to find your car in the parking lot. The bad part, of course, is that you probably feel chewed up and spit out. What you need is some relaxation. And what you eat—or avoid eating—can make a big difference. "The last thing you want when you're working late is caffeine or anything else that will prevent you from sleeping," says Heidi Shutrump, R.D., associate director of nutrition and dietetics at Ohio State University Medical Center Hospital in Chillicothe. "This means avoiding chocolate, caffeinated soft drinks, even iced tea."

Instead, when you finally make it home, curl up with some carbohydrates, such as bread, bagels, pretzels, or unsweetened cereal. Carbohydrates raise blood insulin levels, increasing the uptake of the amino acid tryptophan, which is then converted to serotonin—known to induce drowsiness. Tryptophan is found in high-protein foods, so add some peanut butter, a slice of turkey, or some low-fat cheese to the mix.

. . . *feeling like your head is in a vise.* If you think the only headaches associated with food come from trying to convince your golfing buddy to pick up the check, think again. "Your diet can help produce a migraine, but unfortunately it can't get rid of one," says Victor Herbert, M.D., director of the Nutrition Research Center at Mount Sinai Medical Center in New York City. So the best that food can do after you've had a migraine is to not wake the beast back up. Migraines are highly individualized, but certain foods—especially those high in a compound called tyramine—are known to induce them in some people. Key suspects: organ meats, such as kidneys; fermented products, such as yeasts and soy sauces; wine and beer; monosodium glutamate (MSG); hot dogs; certain aged cheeses; chocolate; and caffeine.

. . . *wishing you hadn't overindulged the night before.* Folk remedies for hangovers are more common than empty Pabst cans at a frat party. And, sadly, just about as useful. The best you can do, experts say, is drink plenty of water (since alcohol tends to dehydrate you) and weather the storm.

If you must do something, though, try a drink such as spicy V-8 vegetable juice or even a virgin Bloody Mary, says Dr. Lachance. "Too much alcohol can create free radicals," he says, "and tomato juice and vegetable juice are good sources of antioxidants." Also, says Dr. Lachance, spices can help dilate blood vessels, which could speed recovery by improving blood circulation to your throbbing head.

One final note: Stay away from acetaminophen (the painkiller found in Tylenol) before, during, or after a night of drinking. Acetaminophen with alcohol makes a dangerous combination that can lead to liver damage, says David Whitcomb, M.D., Ph.D., assistant professor of medicine at the University of Pittsburgh. "Doses up to two grams—about four Extra-Strength Tylenol—are probably okay," he says, "but I recommend playing it safe and skipping it altogether if you're drinking."

An Appetite for Sex

What you eat can make a big difference in how you make love.

Since the dawn of time, guys have been hunting for a natural aphrodisiac that, when ingested, would transform them into sexual dynamos. Most of what they've tried has been harmless but unpalatable, to say the least.

In China, you might be prescribed a meal of sea slugs, whose reputation for imparting potency comes from their tendency to swell when touched. In other cultures, a man might have eaten a beheaded male partridge, lunched on hippopotamus snout, or dipped a phallic object in oil, pepper, and nettle seed and inserted it where you would least like to—all to enhance sexual prowess.

Now, don't knock these options. Sex psychologists tell us that any food—no matter how outlandish or to which orifice it's applied—can have a placebo effect. It can boost your drive if you believe it will. But try this strategy (it's easier on your taste buds): Develop a palate for vitamins, minerals, and herbs that grease your sexual machinery. Begin your foreplay with some of these.

The Big One

Sure, other vitamins and minerals help. But zinc does the heavy lifting. It's linked to your fertility, potency, sex drive, and long-term sexual health. The mineral is critical to sperm production, and low zinc stores have been blamed for decreases in semen volume and testosterone levels, explains Sara Brewer, M.D., author of *Better Sex*.

"Each ejaculation can expend up to five milligrams of zinc, or one-third of your daily allowance," Dr. Brewer says. Luckily, zinc is easy to come by. Four ounces of lean beef provide half the daily requirement, and a single oyster gives you the whole shebang. Turkey, cereals, and beans are other good sources.

The Power of Celery

Forget about all those pheromone sprays that are supposed to attract women. Researchers looking for a real turn-on tonic have focused on the potent male hormone androsterone, which is also found in celery. They believe androsterone is released through perspiration after eating. Your partner may not actually smell it on you, but because androsterone is thought to attract females, don't be surprised if she snuggles up real close. Even if you don't get lucky, keep in mind that you're eating a low-calorie, fiber-rich food that helps clean your teeth and freshen your breath. Not a bad deal either way.

Ease Prostate Pain

An ailing prostate can reduce your ability to have erections, putting a severe damper on your sex life. Prostatitis, a deep, sometimes painful and debilitating inflammation of the gland, can be eased by foods such as nuts, seeds, and whole grains—especially rye products. They contain plant hormones, oils, and other agents that decrease swelling, congestion, and inflammation of the prostate, says Dr. Brewer. Pumpkin seeds in particular contain oils that ease the discomfort and pelvic pressure associated with enlargement of the prostate (benign prostatic hyperplasia, or BPH), she adds.

A diet with an Asian bent can help, too. Dr. Brewer says that soy products, rice, and Chinese cabbage can reduce the effect of dihydrotestosterone, a testosterone by-product that has been linked to BPH.

A Jolt from Java

Your morning cup of coffee might be doing more than perking you up. It might be turning you on. Men and women who have at least one cup of joe a day are nearly twice as likely to describe themselves as sexually active, according to one study. And guys who indulge report fewer problems with erections.

Jeanne Shaw, Ph.D., an Atlanta-based certified sex therapist and clinical psychologist, chalks up coffee's erotic potential to the java jolt. "If you feel sluggish and the caffeine wakes you, then you're going to say, 'Oh, I'm horny,' instead of roll over and go to sleep," she explains. Coffee in bed in the mornings is the idea, but practice moderation (with the coffee, that is). Once you move beyond one or two cups a day, caffeine can leave you agitated and edgy.

Boost Your Serotonin

If you're short on desire and have paltry ejaculations and a piddling sperm count, low serotonin levels may be the problem. Your brain produces this essential sex chemical when you eat carbohydrates combined with foods containing the amino acid tryptophan, which is found in a variety of meat and dairy products.

Stress depletes your serotonin supply, and that may be why tryptophan, a sleep inducer, is part of the equation. When you eat tryptophan and carbohydrates together, you calm down long enough for your body to replenish the serotonin and boost your desire. Try $3^1/_2$ ounces of fish, poultry, or lean beef with bread or pasta.

Follow the Germans

Ginkgo biloba doesn't roll easily off the tongue. But researchers have been talking up the herb's ability to increase blood flow and produce better erections. In a recent German study, 20 men with severe impotence took 80 milligram capsules three times a day for nine months. Every participant reported spontaneous erections and marked increase in hardness.

Hard Germans aside, ginkgo's punch hasn't been proven yet in the United States. And, as Varro E. Tyler, Ph.D., distinguished professor emeritus of pharmacognosy and dean emeritus at Purdue University School of Pharmacy and

Pharmacal Sciences in West Lafayette, Indiana, says, "If your erection problems aren't from impaired blood flow but rather nerve damage or other problems, then ginkgo won't help." Check with your doctor before taking ginkgo biloba.

The Big Climax

Without calcium, there won't be any fireworks. "Your muscles—and that includes the ones that control your orgasm—need calcium to spasm and contract," says Dr. Brewer. Dairy products, fish (especially canned sardines), bread, and green vegetables are all high in calcium.

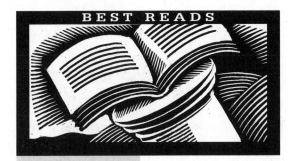

BEST READS

Getting What You Need from Food

Good nutrition is important to good health. No man would argue with that statement. But knowing it is important and following through on it are two very different things. This is why Donna Raskin and Brian Paul Kaufman explain how to tap into nature's nutrient storehouse in Vitamin Vitality: Use Nature's Power to Attain Optimal Health *(Rodale Press, 1997). In this excerpt, they've taken the major, and some minor, food groups and done a masterful job of laying out a plan for good nutrition. And, no, good nutrition does not entail popping a daily multivitamin and then eating as you please.*

Want to give less money to your doctor next year? Then give more money to your grocer. Economic research has revealed that if Americans ate more foods high in vitamins C and E and beta-carotene, our national health care costs would decrease by 25 percent—for cardiovascular disease alone. Cancer costs would drop by 16 to 30 percent, and cataract costs would plummet by 50 percent. It's an alchemist's dream: turning carrots to dollars.

"You can fulfill the Recommended Dietary Allowances for vitamins and minerals by following the Food Guide Pyramid," says Keith-Thomas Ayoob,

R.D., Ed.D., spokesman for the American Dietetic Association in Chicago, director of nutrition services at the Rose F. Kennedy Children's Evaluation and Rehabilitation Center, and assistant professor of pediatric medicine at Albert Einstein College of Medicine, both in New York City. "There are times when vitamin supplementation can be necessary and appropriate, but if you eat a proper diet, not only will you meet your nutrient needs but you'll probably exceed them."

That's because vitamins and minerals are only the tip of the iceberg, nutritionally speaking. No amount of supplementation can replace a good diet, nor can it fix the damage an unhealthy diet can do, in both the short and long term. In fact, trying to replace food with supplements can actually do more harm than good. Throughout the rest of this chapter, we'll discuss the variety of foods you need to eat every day—fruits and vegetables, whole grains, dairy products, meats, and fats, sweets, and oils. If that list sounds familiar, it should: It's on the official Food Guide Pyramid.

Fruits and Vegetables

Scientists have discovered that plant foods—fruits and vegetables—seem to be as important for what we don't know about them as for what we do. "A natural food is much more than the sum of its known nutrients," says Barbara Klein, Ph.D., professor of food science and human nutrition at the University of Illinois in Urbana-Champaign. "We know a lot about vitamins and minerals, but we don't know a lot about the other compounds that are present in plants. Our knowledge is not sufficient to warrant taking supplements and not eating well."

In fact, researchers have found that vegetables and fruits contain chemicals, dubbed phytochemicals, that help protect against cancer and other diseases. Among the handful of phytochemicals that have been isolated so far are capsaicin (found in peppers), flavonoids (berries, citrus fruits, and yams), allylic sulfide (onions and garlic), and indole-3-carbinol (cauliflower and cabbage).

Like vitamins and minerals, phytochemicals lose some of their protective powers when they're isolated from the food they come in.

For example, just a few years ago, researchers found that men with cancer had less beta-carotene in their blood than those without cancer. At first, it seemed that beta-carotene alone could block the development of cancer, but when researchers looked further into the issue, they found something else entirely.

"It turned out that taking beta-carotene supplements actually had an adverse effect, because when you isolate beta-carotene down to a pill, something important that appears in the food is removed. But we're still not completely sure about what it is," says Christopher Gardner, Ph.D., a nutrition researcher at Stanford University's Center for Research in Disease Prevention. Researchers are still learning how various chemicals work together to offer protection against disease. And their discoveries spark a sense of awe.

Nature packages foods in a miraculous way. For instance, while a mineral pill might contain more iron than a tomato, the tomato has vitamin C, which aids the body's absorption of that iron.

Likewise, the tomato will have other nutrients that can help your health. For instance, a study found that a carotenoid called lycopene has a more protective effect against prostate cancer than both vitamin A and beta-carotene. Lycopene is most commonly found in tomatoes and tomato-based foods, such as tomato sauce—a food, not a vitamin or mineral supplement. So, you'd have to take at least three supplements—vitamin C, iron, and lycopene—to equal just the known protective nutrients found in tomatoes and tomato products.

Even nutritionists who endorse supplementation agree that people taking vitamin and mineral tablets should do so in addition to a low-fat diet that features the recommended servings of fruits and vegetables. "A vitamin pill can't compensate for a diet that's loaded with fat or low in fruits and vegetables because there are thousands of plant compounds that may help reduce the risk of cancer and heart disease," says Bonnie Liebman, a licensed nutritionist and director of nutrition for the Center for Science in the Public Interest in Washington, D.C.

Federal surveys have consistently shown, however, that 60 percent of what Americans eat comes from animal-based foods, with the remaining 40 percent coming from plant sources. The ratio should be precisely the opposite, experts say.

Whole Grains

Talk to any nutritionist and he'll sing the praises of plants, but not just fruits and vegetables. The next group of foods to add to your shopping cart is whole grains.

"Whole wheat, oats, barley, rye, millet, brown rice, and corn are all whole grains," Dr. Klein says. "During processing, they have as little removed as possible to make them palatable." In other words, while the wheat no longer has those fuzzy things on the top, all that's taken off during processing is the hull. What's left (after processing) is the grain with the bran or the germ attached.

So, while oatmeal is a whole grain, traditional spaghetti isn't. (In fact, spaghetti, as we know it, contains all of the starch but little of the vitamins and minerals in the grain.) Rye bread contains whole grains, but white bread doesn't. Wheatena is a whole grain, but farina isn't. The more refined the flour, the less nutritious the food, Dr. Klein says.

Dairy Products

Guys don't drink enough milk, and that's bad because it's an extremely nutrient-dense food. (Sorry, but it's not true that you get extra fiber by drinking it straight from the carton.) In fact, all the vitamins as well as six minerals have been detected in cow milk. Of course, the most obvious nutrient identified with milk is calcium.

Two glasses (eight ounces each) of milk will provide about 60 percent of the Daily Value for calcium. About 95 percent of the milk supply in the United States is fortified with vitamin D, which helps the body absorb the calcium found in the milk. However, even though it's great to get calcium through milk, it's only worth it, calorically speaking, if you're drinking low-fat or skim milk. Whole milk is just too high in fat.

The ways in which milk is made into other dairy products also affects the food's level of calcium. For instance, one serving of Cheddar cheese has more than twice the calcium of a serving of cottage cheese. The drawback is that it also has four times the calories. However, it is still more nutrient-smart to consume a small amount of Cheddar.

Meat

Unless you're following a vegetarian diet, low-fat meats can still have an honored place on your plate—though probably not quite as large—because many of the vitamins and minerals in meat are more bioavailable than those in plant food. That means that your body absorbs them better.

"It's not an issue of never eating meat," Liebman says. "It's about how often you eat it. Your diet should be largely plant-based." A plant-based diet can cut your risk of cancer, heart disease, stroke, and diabetes, she adds.

Surveys show that only half of all Americans eat fruit every day and more than 20 percent consume no milk products. But 25 percent of all Americans eat fried potatoes on any given day. "The problem is that a meat-and-potatoes diet usually means that a man isn't eating fruits and vegetables," Liebman says. "If a guy wants his steak, he should think of the salad as the main course and the meat as a side dish."

Or, think of meat as what you eat when you go out to dinner on the weekends rather than your everyday evening meal. If you have meat for lunch and dinner, cut back to once a day, Liebman advises.

Fats

Hopefully, there's hardly any room left in your stomach. But if there is, you get to have a little treat. And most people choose fat-laden treats.

The Food Guide Pyramid recommends that you eat fat "sparingly," says Dr. Klein, which means that if you eat any animal products, such as meats, you don't need to add much fat to anything during the day. "That source alone probably fills your recommended intake," she says.

So put down the butter knife. If you must, lean toward oils rather than margarine or butter. "We have a lot of hidden fat in our diets, particularly with fast food," Dr. Klein says. "It's not the hamburger that's killing us. It's the special sauce, to say nothing of the french fries."

Aim for two tablespoons or less a day of oils (preferably, those high in monounsaturates, such as olive oil), which translates to a serving of salad dressing. "If you have a choice, don't use fat," Dr. Klein says.

Smart Eating

If you focus on getting all your vitamins and minerals, not to mention your carotenoids and phytochemicals, you'll have a full plate as well as a full belly. There might not be a lot of room left for nonnutritious items.

When it comes to food, Dr. Klein says, variety is indeed the spice of life. "There's no single food or group of foods that by itself is perfect," she says. "We have many nutritional needs that we know of and some that we don't know. Eating a balanced diet means you should eat a wide variety of foods." So while there's tons of proof that fruits and vegetables can help prevent cancer, they're not the only foods that provide vitamins and minerals.

"Remember that you can eat a pizza or hamburger for breakfast and still have a balanced diet," says Dr. Klein. "You just want to make sure that there's a large distribution among the kinds of food you eat."

In fact, you could take a tip from the Japanese. Their government recommends that its citizens eat 30 "foodstuffs" each day, which roughly corresponds to the highest number of recommended servings in the Food Guide Pyramid.

And don't think that all this eating means that you'll never take supplements. In fact, just the opposite is true. Studies have shown that people who take supplements eat more servings of fruits and vegetables than those who don't eat well. And you know what other group you'll join? Those with higher personal incomes and more education. They, too, eat better and take more supplements.

The Kings of Outdoor Grilling

From great guns and Mack trucks, to WD-40, bass fishing, fireworks, Westerns, and sports, The von Hoffmann Bros.' Big Damn Book of Sheer Manliness *(General Publishing Group, 1998) dishes up a wonderful mix of the "crazy, manly stuff men desire." Todd von Hoffmann, Brant von Hoffmann, Colby Allerton, and the other wiseguys behind this book conceived it as a "rallying cry for every guy who could use a reminder that his favorite pastimes are simply more fun than ever." Amen. In this excerpt, the authors reveal the fascinating histories behind the top dogs in backyard grilling.*

George Stephen of Illinois is the man behind the mighty Weber. Backyard brick barbecues were all the rage at the beginning of the 1950s, but experience has taught a lesson to suburban chefs—the big grills were impressive to look at, but a pain in the ass to work on. The fire was difficult to control, wind was a problem, and they became critter condos when neglected.

George wanted some way to elevate the fire and cover the food. He tried to improve the design of his own brick grill without success. Inspiration came to him at the office. He had a job with the Weber Brothers Metal Works and took a keen interest in the marine buoys they manufactured for Chicago Harbor. Two metal halves were joined to create a watertight, hollow sphere. With a tripod stand, this was just the shape he needed, by Jiminy, and by July 1952, he was selling George's Barbecue Kettle.

He formed a barbecue division of Weber Brothers in 1955 and the next year sent out his first catalogue. The year 1957 brought the marketing windfall of the century—the Russkies sent a Weber-shaped satellite into orbit. George's grill had a nickname, "sputnik"

The superior quality of the new kettle was unquestioned, but the price, back then about five times that of other backyard cooking devices, established it as a symbol of the kilty crowd. Today, Weber is the number one barbecue supplier in the world, and George's invention is a comparative bargain. In the process, it has become deeply ingrained in American culture. While toasting marshmallows with a pal, I remember discussing the merits of the "controlled burn" approach. His reply: "You can always tell someone who's grown up around a Weber."

The One-Match Fluid-Free BBQ Fire

Lighter fluid might have been fun to play around with when we were kids, but it really has no business at a BBQ. (If you can tell when the guy two doors down is pouring it on, why would you want anything that stinky anywhere near your own food?) Maybe people are dependent on the stuff, or maybe they like squirting it into the fire for effect. But for a better tasting, less dangerous experience in outdoor cooking, the following simple steps will help kick the can—for good.

- Put on an apron (guys should always BBQ with an apron—dressing the part keeps a cook focused and less likely to burn something—chef hats might be pushing it unless you're working with a team), and get a pair of those bargain variety leather-palm work gloves. This is a BBQ outfit—keep it together. And remember: Don't use those gloves for oil changes or taking out the trash.
- Remove the upper and lower grills and make sure that any vents on the bottom of the kettle are left open.
- Tightly twist up newspaper logs, two full sheets at a time, and place them slightly apart in the bottom of the kettle. Fill just the space under the lower grill (four or five logs will probably do it). Replace the lower grill on top of the paper logs.
- Now pour in fresh charcoal briquets and pile them up in the center.
- Reaching below the grill, strike a stick match and light four corners of the newspaper. This can be kind of a smoky stage as the paper burns—but not for long. Smoke will follow you around a BBQ kettle. (This used to be shrugged off as a myth, but it seems to me that some research institute spent a few million and discovered that smoke actually will billow into your face no matter where you stand in relationship to the kettle.)
- Next replace the upper grill, let it warm up, and then take a stab at cleaning it. A seasoned grill will remain black, of course, but make a good show of it and be sure the guests are watching.
- Now go get a beer.

In about 10 minutes, the briquets should be red enough so that you can spread them out. In another 10 minutes, or maybe less, they'll be ashed over—and ready to go.

Kingsford Original Charcoal Briquets

Is there a single living soul in these United States who has not cooked with—or eaten a meal grilled on—Kingsford Charcoal Briquets? With the possible exception of maybe a couple of French tourists, we think not. The name Kingsford has become synonymous with the great American afternoon BBQ, but it may surprise the reader to discover the original name behind this classic product: Ford, as in Henry Ford. The folks at Kingsford consider Henry Ford to be the baron of the backyard BBQ. Why?

The Ford dynasty was built on ingenuity, great products that a modest income could handle, and a bold embrace of automation. But it was also built on prudence. Mr. Ford was not a man to tolerate waste—he didn't waste time and he didn't waste materials.

At the turn of the century, production of the Model T was cranking right along and car ownership ceased to be the exclusive domain of the rich. North of Motor City, Ford operated a sawmill that punched out the wooden framing. What should catch Ford's eye but the huge piles of discarded scrap—surely there must be some use for all that material.

Together with Charles Kingsford, Ford came up with the idea of chipping the lumber waste and compressing the bits, scorching these into char, grinding them into a powder and compressing them into the now familiar pillow-shaped briquets. The bags were labeled Ford Charcoal and marketed through his automobile agencies. The name was later changed to Kingsford, still the number one seller in the country.

Kingsford offers the following BBQ tips in their literature.

- Apply vegetable oil or nonstick cooking spray to the grill to prevent food from sticking and pulling apart.
- Don't start grilling too soon—the coals should be at least 70 percent ashed over to sufficiently burn off any solvent.
- Soak wooden shish kebab skewers in water for 20 minutes to keep them from burning.
- Let the grid warm over the fire to ease cleaning. A stiff wire grill brush or crumpled ball of foil works best.
- Use tongs or spatulas. Forks allow juices to escape and dry out the meat.
- Add sauces toward the end of cooking to avoid burning.

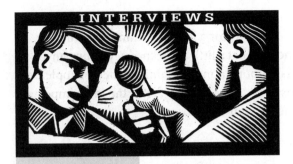

Top Experts on
Multivitamins

For many of us, the premise is irresistible: Swallow this vitamin pill, it will make everything better. A day's worth of dietary shortcomings can vanish in a single gulp. One little capsule can shield us from ill health. Our energy will return, our hair will sprout, we'll be able to hypnotize women with our voices.

That's hard to swallow. If only it were that easy. Walk into a drugstore today, and you're faced with a mind-numbing array of choices: an alphabet soup of vitamins and a mother lode of minerals, available individually and in every possible combination. It's tempting to grab the closest bottle and head for the cashier.

But this is one decision you don't want to make in the dark. We'll admit, even we were confused about all the options out there—and we're health writers, for cryin' out loud. That's why we culled all the information we could find on vitamins and minerals and interviewed the experts.

Do I really need a multivitamin?

While women of childbearing age have a host of jazzed-up nutrient needs, men generally don't. And men as a group risk fewer deficiencies than women do, simply because we eat more, according to Jeffrey Blumberg, Ph.D., professor of nutrition at Tufts University in Medford, Massachusetts. "If you're consuming 3,000 calories a day—even if you're diet is pretty lousy—you'll still consume lots of vitamins and minerals," he says.

"Food is really where it's at, in terms of health protection," says Suzanne Hendrich, Ph.D., professor of food science and human nutrition at Iowa State University at Ames. "There's more to food than just vitamins and minerals—things like fiber and phytochemicals."

And the fact is, you may already be taking a multivitamin without knowing it. "If you're eating fortified cereal every morning, such as Total or Life, you don't need a supplement," says Paul Lachance, Ph.D., professor of food science at Rutgers University in New Brunswick, New Jersey. In essence, experts say, Total is just a multivitamin in cereal form. Many energy bars also contain 100 percent of the Recommended Dietary Allowance (RDA) for a lot of vitamins and minerals.

That said, Dr. Hendrich concedes that a little insurance never hurt anybody. And even Dr. Blumberg admits he pops a multivitamin/mineral supplement every day. The conclusion seems to be that a healthy diet is the most important part of your game plan; vitamins are your backups.

What should I look for?

By definition, all nutrients are essential. But here are a handful that guys might be lacking in their diets, according to Dr. Blumberg: vitamins B_6, B_{12}, C, and E; folic acid; and the minerals selenium and chromium. He also suggests choosing a multi that gets at least some of its vitamin A as beta-carotene. "Beta-carotene is converted to vitamin A in the body, but it also has health benefits independent of vitamin A," he says, "particularly in cancer prevention." Also, check for these:

- **A reasonably short ingredients list.** "Things like PABA, inositol, bee pollen, and lecithin haven't been shown to be essential to human diets," says Marilyn Bush, a clinical nurse specialist and instructor of nutritional pharmacology at the University of Mississippi in Oxford. "Sometimes, ingredients are added simply to boost the price and make the product appear more complete."
- **Bushels of antioxidants.** "We're learning a lot about free-radical formation and its relationship to heart disease and cancer," says Dr. Lachance. "So we're talking about the big killers, and many people are low on these antioxidants." Look for 250 milligrams of vitamin C, 200 milligrams of E, 3 milligrams (5,000 international units) of A as beta-carotene, and as much as 100 micrograms of selenium. If your multi has ballpark levels of these nutrients, you're covered.
- **No gimmicks.** For example, Dr. Blumberg says, there's no need for time-release supplements. "Humans weren't designed to maintain a steady supply of vitamin C, or any other nutrient, throughout the day," he says. "There's no advantage in that."
- **An expiration date.** "They're still not universal," Dr. Blumberg says. "If one multi has an expiration date and one doesn't, which do you think I'd buy?"

Are name brands better than store brands?

A bottle of Centrum multis goes for $6.54 for 60 tablets at our local drugstore, while the same quantity of a store brand costs three bucks. Is that extra

$3.54 worth it? Not necessarily. A generic brand that you trust is generally as good as the more expensive brand name. The reason: A lot of the brand names and the store names are made by the same manufacturer. In any case, the FDA doesn't monitor multis with an iron grip, if you'll forgive the expression; it'll be a few years until standardized labels like those found on food products will be mandatory. And Dr. Blumberg says that soon, a nongovernment group called United States Pharmacopeia (USP) will put its seal of approval on multis that it deems acceptable. "But until that's universal and required, you can't know for sure that you're getting a quality product," he says. "The bottom line is, go with someone you trust."

Are "natural" vitamins better somehow?

Nah. In most cases, your body can't tell the difference between a vitamin or mineral from food and one from a test tube. "Essentially, you get the same chemical structure," says Leon Ellenbogen, Ph.D., who works in nutritional sciences at Whitehall-Robins, maker of Centrum.

What's more, supplements labeled "natural" aren't necessarily safer, according to Dr. Hendrich. "Some of those 'natural' sources have higher levels of contaminants such as lead, compared with the more carefully refined ingredients used in the manufacturing process," she says.

Do I need a "men's" multi?

Most of the current crop of men's multis boast that they have no iron, so the real questions here is, "Should I avoid taking extra iron?" While some experts say the RDA of 18 milligrams of supplemental iron is okay for men, most agree that that amount is overkill at best—and potentially dangerous at worst.

"Iron is a good example of why men shouldn't be taking a women's supplement," says Dr. Lachance. "Men need to be damn careful with iron. If you're not anemic, you don't need it." Dr. Lachance concedes that men who are strict vegetarians may need a bit of supplemental iron—but just a bit. "Eighteen milligrams is a lot of iron," he says. "And actually, that's the women's requirement. For men, it's 10 milligrams daily."

The bottom line: Look for a multi with 10 milligrams of iron. If you eat meat, forget it. You're getting plenty of iron.

Should I take "megadoses" of certain vitamins or minerals?

No. Super-high levels of one nutrient may throw others out of balance, says Dr. Hendrich, and it's too easy to overdose with tablets of individual vitamins and minerals—which is why she recommends taking a multivitamin rather than a shelf-full of single tablets. "Very large doses of iron or zinc or selenium or manganese could carry some risks, from liver disease to neurological problems," she says. What's considered a "megadose"? For Dr. Hendrich, 10 times the RDA for most vitamins is the absolute upper limit; for minerals, it's 5 times the RDA. "In general, minerals have much greater toxic potential than vitamins," she explains. "But in any case, staying close to the RDA is definitely a good idea."

Dr. Blumberg agrees that the vitamins aisle is no place to experiment: "It's important to note—five times the RDA for vitamin E, and it's perfectly safe. Five times the RDA for vitamin A, and you're risking toxicity." If you want to pop anything stronger than a balanced multivitamin/mineral supplement, consult your doctor first.

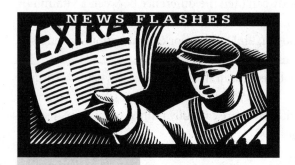

Olive Oil May Keep Heart Disease at Arm's Length

OXFORD, England—Olive oil may help prevent heart disease from gaining a foothold. Researchers at Oxford and the University of Surrey fed 60 men a diet rich in olive oil (higher in monounsaturated fats), while a control group ate a typical English diet (higher in saturated fats). After two months, the men who ate olive oil produced up to 20 percent less of the "sticky" molecules that glue white blood cells to artery walls—one of the first steps in atherosclerosis.

Garlic Named Again as a Disease Fighter

NEW YORK CITY—A compound in aged garlic fights prostate cancer, according to laboratory experiments. The compound, S-allylmercaptocysteine (SAMC), increases the breakdown of testosterone, which in turn slows tumor growth. "In this study, cancer cell growth was slowed by as much as 70 percent," says John T. Pinto, Ph.D., director of the nutrition research laboratory at Memorial Sloan-Kettering Cancer Center in New York City. Researchers can't say whether fresh garlic is effective, but Dr. Pinto says that commercially available aged-garlic tablets contain the same compound. "I take them myself," he says.

Too Many Vitamin E Pills May Be Counterproductive

BERKELEY, Calif.—Popping that capsule of vitamin E every morning may not offer all the protection against cancer and heart disease that you think. Taking vitamin E supplements may deplete the body of other forms of the antioxidant, studies have found. Dosages of alpha-tocopherol (the main type found in supplements) can lower your body's levels of a second form of the vitamin called gamma-tocopherol. One study suggests that both forms of vitamin E may be needed to maximize the nutrient's disease-fighting effects. People taking more than 100 international units of vitamin E daily should tap more dietary sources, says study leader Stephan Christen, Ph.D., researcher at the University of California at Berkeley. Olive oil, shellfish, and legumes such as peanuts and sesame seeds are rich in vitamin E.

Oat-Bran Bread Keeps Diabetes under Control

EDMONTON, Alberta—Eating bread made with oat bran can help control non-insulin-dependent diabetes. A preliminary study from the University of Alberta found that men who ate meals including high-fiber bread made with oat-bran concentrate had lower glucose levels and blood cholesterol than when they ate meals with plain white bread. The researchers say this is the first long-term evidence that oat bran can control glucose levels. Excess glucose has been associated with heart disease, blindness, and kidney failure.

Just Tasting Fat Raises Level of Heart-Harming Substance

WEST LAFAYETTE, Ind.—Just one Buffalo wing won't hurt you, right? Not so fast. Merely tasting fatty foods can raise the amount of fat in your blood. People who chewed and spit out full-fat cream cheese on crackers almost doubled their levels of potentially heart-harming triglycerides, compared with people who tasted fat-free cream cheese, according to Richard Mattes, Ph.D., associate professor of foods and nutrition at Purdue University. Dr. Mattes thinks that chemical sensors in the nose and mouth may detect the fat and trigger an increase in triglycerides.

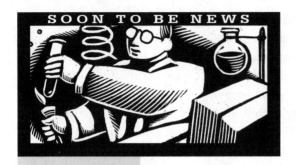

Aloe for Lunch?

Most people probably know that aloe is soothing to the skin, but one study suggests that eating aloe vera may help prevent disease. Researchers at the University of Texas Health Science Center at San Antonio found that rats regularly fed a formula with 1 percent aloe vera gel were less likely to develop kidney disease, blood clots, and cancer than a control group. "Even though 1 percent is a very high dose of aloe vera, we observed no adverse effects," says Byung Pal Yu, Ph.D., the study leader.

Researchers plan to test aloe's protective properties on humans once they identify all of its active ingredients.

Potatoes Prevent Parkinson's?

Parkinson's disease is a debilitating neurological disorder that can cause uncontrollable tremors and muscle weakness. A German study of 342 patients with this disease suggests that eating raw vegetables and potatoes may reduce your risk of developing Parkinson's. Conversely, researchers found that sweets and raw meat were common fare for a majority of Parkinson's patients.

These are preliminary results; future studies are in the pipeline.

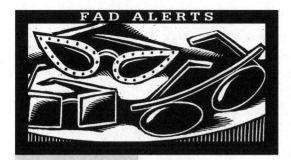

Lycopene Supplements

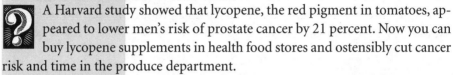

A Harvard study showed that lycopene, the red pigment in tomatoes, appeared to lower men's risk of prostate cancer by 21 percent. Now you can buy lycopene supplements in health food stores and ostensibly cut cancer risk and time in the produce department.

If only it were that simple. "First of all, we're not 100 percent sure that it's the lycopene that prevents cancer," says Edward Giovannucci, M.D., Sc.D., lead author of the Harvard study. "It might be an entirely different nutrient in the tomato." Further, like its cousin beta-carotene, there are several forms of lycopene. Researchers don't know which—if any—fight prostate cancer, and supplements likely lack several of the lycopene forms, says Dr. Giovannucci. "We do know, however, that the body can't benefit from lycopene unless it's cooked or accompanied by fats." That's why pizza and spaghetti sauce are better sources of lycopene than raw tomatoes—and much better sources than supplements.

Energy Bars

Those high-carbohydrate energy bars may help power you through a workout, but no better than some cheaper foods will. Researchers at Ball State University in Muncie, Indiana, found that a bagel offers the same exercise performance benefits as those popular energy bars. They fed three groups of cyclists brand-name energy bars or plain bagels and found no difference in performance levels during an intense cycling test. You can buy several bagels for the cost of one energy bar, and you'll get the same results, says David Pearson, Ph.D., lead researcher and exercise physiologist.

Coffee Colas

There are many ill-advised combinations: peanut butter and mayonnaise. Gasoline and a lit match. *The Sonny and Cher Comedy Hour.* Now we can add coffee and soda to the list. We slugged down several of the new coffee-colas and can confidently report that it's a marriage God never intended. Adding coffee to a regular 12-ounce can of cola can nearly double its 40 milligrams of caffeine. But considering the spine-curdling taste, even air-traffic controllers don't need caffeine this badly.

If you want to make the same faces we did while drinking the stuff, start with the frighteningly sweet Cafe Cola, which is actually the least offensive of the bunch. It has 75 milligrams of caffeine and 140 calories in every 12-ounce can. The gritty Bibicaffe espresso soda (25 milligrams of caffeine, 154 calories) and Big Head coffee cola (52 milligrams of caffeine, 175 calories) might appeal to Starbuck's habitués, but not us. And recently Pepsi—not one to back down from a challenge—unleashed Pepsi Kona (56 milligrams of caffeine, 150 calories). But we're not entirely sure that it's a new coffee-cola product. It may just be a badly skunked batch of ordinary Pepsi.

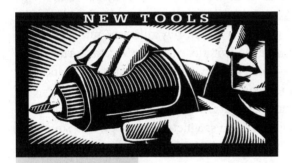

Exotic Indulgences

Mail-Order Meat

We keep hearing about new, healthy, and exotic meats, but our local Safeway has yet to stock fresh ostrich. Too bad: Although three ounces of regular beef contain 16 grams of fat, ostrich meat—which is just as tasty for our money—has just 2 grams of fat. Not only is it healthier but ostrich also cooks in about half the time.

After much searching, we found a shop in New York City's Greenwich Village—Balducci's—that offers an amazing shop-from-home catalog full of sensible indulgences. In addition to hand-trimmed steaks, alligator filets, and plenty o' ostrich, Balducci's stocks burgers made of Belgian beef ($35 for 12 patties), which contains less fat and cholesterol than even turkey breasts. You can also order two high-protein, low-fat buffalo ribeye steaks for $22. Your meat is shipped frozen and will arrive within 48 hours (or on the day of your feast), in some cases preseasoned and ready to slap on the grill.

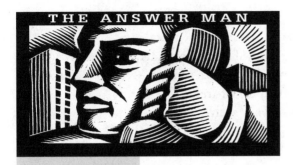

New Spread in Town

Have you heard of a new kind of margarine made with olive oil? Is it any better for me than butter or regular margarine?
—T. C., Chicago

Sold under the brand name Olivio, this spread stacks up well against full-fat butter and margarine, says Sonja Connor, R.D., research dietitian at Oregon Health Sciences University in Portland. It contains only one gram of artery-clogging saturated fat per tablespoon, compared with seven grams for butter and two grams for margarine. It's also low in trans fatty acids, a type of fat that has been linked to heart disease. Olivio gets 6 percent of its fat from trans fatty acids, compared with margarine's 7 to 30 percent—a pretty respectable figure, according to Connor.

What's more, most of Olivio's fat is monounsaturated, a type that some researchers think can lower harmful low-density lipoprotein cholesterol levels while raising the good high-density lipoprotein cholesterol levels. If you like its slightly stronger flavor, Olivio is a healthy choice, says Connor. If you don't, there are plenty of other reduced-fat spreads out there.

Foods That Will Wait for You

I'm a single guy who's frequently away on business. Still, I need something in the fridge when I get back or else I'll gorge on fast food. What long-lasting foods can I buy that'll survive sitting in the refrigerator for months?
—B. W., Stamford, Conn.

We hear you. Last time we got back from a road trip it looked like someone was growing a new strain of penicillin in the refrigerator. To avoid future wonder-drug discoveries, stick to this shopping list provided by Elaine Turner, R.D., Ph.D., assistant professor of food science and human nutrition at the University of Florida in Gainesville. All are healthy foods with a long shelf life.

- Whole-grain bread. Freeze it, then thaw a slice or two for each meal.
- Frozen low-fat dinners. We like the Lean Cuisine Cafe Classics Sirloin Beef Peppercorn and the Healthy Choice Beef Pepper Steak Oriental.

- Canned or frozen vegetables with no salt added. Add seasoning as you microwave.
- Single-serving canned fruit. Packed in juice or water, not heavy syrup.
- Frozen baked-chicken strips (in the frozen-meats section). Banquet and Tyson make chicken strips that are fat-free.
- Pasta and rice can be kept on your shelves for months.
- A jar of pasta sauce.
- For a healthy meal that's almost as easy as a frozen dinner, prepare the pasta and top with sauce, vegetables, and chicken, suggests Dr. Turner.

Kosher Everywhere

A lot of airlines offer kosher food, and now it's turning up all over my supermarket. Is kosher food healthier?
—M. G., Mount Kisco, N.Y.

Probably not. To be kosher, foods must be certified by a rabbi as meeting standard Jewish dietary law. Pork products, shellfish, and animals that have not been killed quickly and painlessly are forbidden. (In addition, consuming milk and meat at the same meal is a no-no.) "Kosher meat may be cleaner in the way it's slaughtered," says Lisa Young, R.D., nutrition instructor at New York University in New York City. "But it's incorrect to assume it will be leaner or more nutritious.

Also, kosher meat is salted, which you should be aware of if you're salt-sensitive." For the most part, Young says, people eat kosher food for religious reasons, not because it provides significant health benefits.

Anything but Fish

I don't like any type of seafood or fish. Basically, if it comes out of the water, and it's not water, I don't want any part of it. Is there any way I can get the health benefits of fish without having to eat it?
—P. B., Fairfax, Va.

Like skinless chicken and turkey breast, fish is a great low-fat protein source, says Mary Ellen Carmire, Ph.D., associate professor and chairperson of the department of food science and human nutrition at the University of Maine in Orono. But it offers at least one benefit you can't get from poultry: omega-3 fatty acids.

Found in fatty fish such as salmon and herring, omega-3's have been shown to help keep your blood more fluid, lowering your chances of heart attack or stroke. Studies also suggest they may be able to lower blood cholesterol. Some plants produce omega-3's, but unless you've figured out a use for flaxseed or canola-oil margarine, you might be hard-pressed to get these plant-based omega-3's into your diet.

An easier way to swallow your omega-3's is with fish-oil capsules, says Dr. Carmire. Available in most drugstores and health food stores, they're generally considered safe if you stick to the dosages on the label—usually one or two tablets with each meal for a total of 3,000 to 6,000 milligrams per day. But Dr. Carmire advises to check with your doctor first. Because omega-3's act as a blood thinner, they're not for everyone. They can be harmful in large doses.

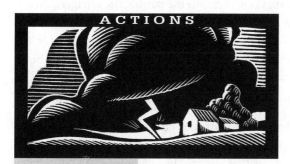

ACTIONS

After hygiene, your diet is the first thing to suffer neglect when you're over-worked and overwhelmed. Luckily, it takes only a few simple changes in your daily routine to improve your eating plan. We'll worry about your odor some other time.

1. Drink something green. Instead of having your usual two or three cups of joe, sacrifice at least one cup of coffee and drink green tea instead. "Coffee is highly acidic, so it can cause calcium to leach from your bones," says nutritionist Cheryl Hartsough, R.D., of the PGA National Resort and Spa in Palm Beach, Florida. Green tea has natural caffeine, but it also contains antioxidants, which may help reduce risk for disease, she says.

A study at the University of Kansas in Lawrence found that an antioxidant compound in green tea is 100 times more effective than vitamin C and 25 times better than vitamin E at preventing cell damage. Black tea—the kind most Americans drink—and oolong tea contain only about 40 percent of the compounds found in green tea, "probably because green tea is steamed immediately after it's picked, preserving the antioxidants," says study author Lester Mitscher, Ph.D., professor of medicinal chemistry. Another study found that other compounds in green tea slowed the growth of prostate cancer cells.

2. **Buy a blender.** No, not for margaritas (though that's not a bad idea). Use it to create healthful cocktails. For example: Mix skim milk, a banana or two, and some chunks of soft tofu. The milk contains vitamin D and magnesium, which can reduce your likelihood of heart disease. The bananas will thicken the drink and offer potassium, which is good for your heart, too. And by mixing in tofu, you'll benefit from a compound called genistein, which is thought to ward off prostate cancer.

3. **Eat a rainbow.** On your way home from work, stop at a vegetable stand or grocery store that's known for great produce and pick up at least five different colors of food. "That's a pretty easy way to make sure you're eating all the nutrients," says Hartsough.

4. **Take the junk to your job.** Look through the pantry, the refrigerator, the cupboards, between the mattress and box spring, underneath the crankcase of the car, and gather all the chips, cookies, snack cakes, and other junk food and throw 'em in a bag. Take it with you to the office. Force it on employees you aren't crazy about. There is a simple reason for this—other than revenge. "By removing the junk from your house, you'll be less likely to eat it when the cravings strike," says Hartsough.

5. **Trade in the T-bone.** For a meaty dinner entree, substitute portabella mushrooms for the steak. One portabella (roughly the size of a saucer) has less than one gram of fat, and when it's grilled, it tastes like a tender steak. Slice a few portabellas to half-inch thickness and brush them with a mixture of nonfat Italian dressing, thyme, and Worcestershire sauce. Grill for three to four minutes on each side over a medium-hot flame. Garnish with grilled onions and peppers. Then laugh at the neighbors as they cook hot dogs.

6. **Have a hearty soup for lunch.** "It takes 20 minutes for your brain to tell you that you're full, so when you eat food fast, you're bound to overeat," says Hartsough. Soup stays in your stomach longer, so it fills you up and slows your eating. (You'll only ruin your tie if you eat it fast.)

7. **Have a drink.** Just make it wine, not beer. Researchers at the University of North Carolina measured the circumference of the bellies of men who drank a beer a day as well as men who averaged a glass of wine a day, and a third group that didn't drink at all. They found that the wine-drinkers had the smallest guts; the beer-drinkers the largest. There may be a substance in wine that helps keep bellies trim. Yes, we know what you're thinking: It may not be the alcohol; it may be what I eat along with it. (It's hard to eat corn chips, after all, with a nice merlot.) But even if wine simply keeps us from shoveling other crap down our throats, that's okay, too.

8. **Fill up with fruit.** A study at the Brooke Army Medical Center in San Antonio found that eating pectin, a soluble fiber in the skin of fruits and vegetables, will make you feel full longer. Researchers gave 74 subjects orange juice, some of which had been spiked with up to 20 grams of pectin. The people who drank the juice with pectin felt significantly fuller than the other subjects, even four hours later. Researchers suggest that pectin may slow digestion and keep food in your stomach longer. So one apple before dinner could stop those fried chicken cravings.

9. **Keep your zinc up.** If you drink a lot of milk, make doubly sure your zinc intake is up to par. High levels of calcium may cut zinc absorption in half, say researchers at Tufts University in Medford, Massachusetts. When trial participants took a 600-milligram calcium supplement with a meal supplying 7.3 milligrams of zinc, zinc absorption was greatly decreased. A zinc deficiency may weaken the immune system and cut sex drive, potency, and long-term sexual health. Researchers don't know yet if extra calcium will reduce zinc levels in the body over the long haul. But to safeguard your health, study author Richard J. Wood, Ph.D., advises, "Eat plenty of foods rich in zinc, such as lean meat, or take a supplement containing about 8 milligrams of zinc."

10. **Lower cholesterol with a spoon.** A low-fat, high-fiber diet is a key part of any cholesterol-lowering plan, but here's a way to help the process along: Regular use of psyllium appears to lower cholesterol. In a six-month study of 248 patients at the University of Kentucky at Lexington, the bulking agent—found in products such as Metamucil and Perdiem—lowered total cholesterol levels 5 percent and harmful low-density lipoprotein cholesterol 7 percent in those who drank water and one heaping teaspoon of psyllium twice a day, says James Anderson, M.D., study leader and professor of medicine and clinical nutrition. "Take psyllium one hour before meals," he says. "You should see results in three to four weeks."

11. **Don't be a bottom feeder.** Fruit is good for you, so the best yogurt must be the kind with fruit in it, right? Not necessarily. For the most nutritious yogurt, skip the "fruit on the bottom" varieties, says Sheldon Margen, M.D., professor emeritus of public health at the University of California at Berkeley. The "fruit" may be mostly jam, which packs the equivalent of eight or nine teaspoons of sugar per cup—nearly as much as a can of soda. "Instead, choose plain fat-free yogurt or flavors such as lemon, which don't contain fruit, and add your own berries," says Dr. Margen. Fresh berries will provide a healthy dose of fiber as well.

12. **Heal the burn.** Before you abandon antacids, take note: Home remedies for heartburn, such as milk or peppermint, may come back to haunt you, says Fred Sutton Jr., M.D., a gastroenterologist at Baylor College of Medicine in Houston. "Milk or peppermint can provide temporary relief, but then they spur the production of more stomach acid," he says. For some people, it could lead to a return engagement with the very thing they're trying to avoid. Avoid problem foods that can cause heartburn, advises Dr. Sutton, and use an over-the-counter antacid when you feel an attack coming on.

13. **Soak your sirloin.** Researchers have found that marinating meat before grilling may cut cancer-causing agents by as much as 90 percent. Grilling can turn certain substances in meat into carcinogens, says research leader Mark Knize, a biomedical scientist at the Lawrence Livermore National Laboratory in Livermore, California. Marinating appears to stop this process in some mysterious fashion. His recipe? Olive oil, brown sugar, vinegar, lemon juice, garlic, salt, and mustard. "But lemon juice alone worked just as well."

14. **Make regular mineral deposits.** Research suggests that a full supply of magnesium can maximize exercise efficiency. When stationary cyclists were put on a low-magnesium diet (150 milligrams daily), they used up to 15 percent more oxygen, and their heart rates were 10 beats per minute faster, says Henry Lukaski, Ph.D., of the U.S. Department of Agriculture Human Nutrition Research Center in Grand Forks, North Dakota. Meeting your daily requirement of 350 milligrams of magnesium isn't hard. Eat more green vegetables and unprocessed grains, advises Dr. Lukaski.

15. **Look before you drink.** If you take allergy medication, be careful how you wash it down. Drinking grapefruit juice while taking allergy medication could increase your risk of heart attack. Grapefruit juice changes the chemical nature of terfenadine, an antihistamine used in allergy medicines such as Seldane. The altered form of terfenadine can cause an irregular heartbeat. Also, "ask your pharmacist if your allergy medication will interact with erythromycin, which has properties similar to grapefruit juice," advises David Spence, M.D., a clinical pharmacologist at the University of Western Ontario in London, Ontario.

16. **Go nuts for omega-3's.** You know that omega-3 fatty acids found in seafood may help lower the risk of heart disease and strokes. But you may not have known that walnuts are another rich source of omega-3 fatty acids. A handful (roughly ¼ cup) has more omega-3 fatty acids than three ounces of salmon. Of course, that handful also has a higher fat content (around 19 grams) than that piece of fish, so you can't down walnuts like popcorn. There's no Recommended Dietary Allowance for omega-3's, but toss a few walnuts into your cereal and you'll help protect your heart.

17. Trade fat for fiber. A National Cancer Institute study found that a low-fat, high-fiber diet may help protect you from prostate cancer. Men who followed a diet with lots of fiber and less than 20 percent fat for 10 weeks produced less testosterone—though well within the healthy range—than when they consumed high-fat (41 percent fat), low-fiber fare. Abnormally high testosterone levels may play a role in the development of prostate cancer, says study coauthor Christopher Longcope, M.D., so eating less fat and more fiber may be a simple way to safeguard your prostate.

18. Don't shun dairy. If you avoid dairy products because you're lactose-intolerant, you're courting trouble. Lactose-intolerant men still need calcium to fend off osteoporosis. Chew on a calcium-rich antacid (Tums, for instance), suggests Alan Buchman, M.D., a gastroenterologist at Baylor College of Medicine in Houston. Or you can slowly drink a cup of milk. Most lactose-intolerant men can handle that much. Yogurt and hard cheeses are also good calcium sources for men who have trouble digesting milk.

19. Down a stone-cold one. Your urinary tract may appreciate that fine Belgian brew as much as your palate. Drinking beer may help prevent kidney stones. A study of 632 men at the University of Washington School of Medicine in Seattle found that, compared to nonimbibers, beer-drinkers were 53 percent less likely to form kidney or bladder stones. One eight-ounce glass a week reduced the risk, but more didn't offer additional protection. Researchers aren't sure why beer wards off the stones, but John Krieger, M.D., professor of urology and study coauthor, notes that men in the United Kingdom, who quaff more pints than we do, also get fewer stones.

20. Prevent a big fat headache. Don't blame your screaming boss for that headache. Blame those cheese fries. Researchers at Loma Linda University School of Public Health in California found that a low-fat diet can shorten or prevent migraine headaches. Fifty-four migraine sufferers who cut their fat intake to less than 20 grams per day for two months reported fewer, less intense headaches, according to study leader Zuzana Bic, M.D., Dr. P.H. Researchers believe that fat may release a chemical into the brain that triggers headaches.

21. Yoplait it again. Next time your doctor prescribes antibiotics, reach for the yogurt. Antibiotics kill the "good" stomach bacteria that you need for healthy digestion, and a cup of yogurt can replenish these necessary germs. In one study of a group of patients taking antibiotics, half of the patients were given a mixture of *Lactobacillus acidophilus* and *Lactobacillus bulgaricus*, the beneficial bacteria found in yogurt. While 15 percent of people in a group that received no beneficial bacteria developed diarrhea, none of the bug-eaters had any such trouble. Yogurts labeled "live active culture" contain the beneficial bacteria.

22. **Have some fish for thought.** Feeling dim lately? Maybe it's all of those fat-free meals you're eating. At birth, our brains are made of up to 60 percent fat, the most prevalent being an omega-3 fatty acid called docosahexaenoic acid, or DHA (not to be confused with the hormone DHEA, or dehydroepiandrosterone). Researchers now believe that DHA may not only maintain the structural makeup of the brain's gray matter, but also fight memory loss, depression, and perhaps Alzheimer's disease.

Although we start out with a full tank of the good fats, our reserves are depleted over time, so you may need replenishment. "You can get DHA primarily from fish, red meats, eggs, and organ meats," says Barbara Levine, R.D., Ph.D., associate clinical professor of nutrition in medicine at New York Hospital–Cornell Medical Center in New York City. Fish is especially rich in DHA; a four-ounce serving of salmon, for instance, contains 850 milligrams of DHA. But if your diet doesn't include three ounces of fish or red meat a few times per week, says Dr. Levine, then you may want to take a DHA supplement. They're widely sold in health food stores; 100 milligrams per day is good insurance.

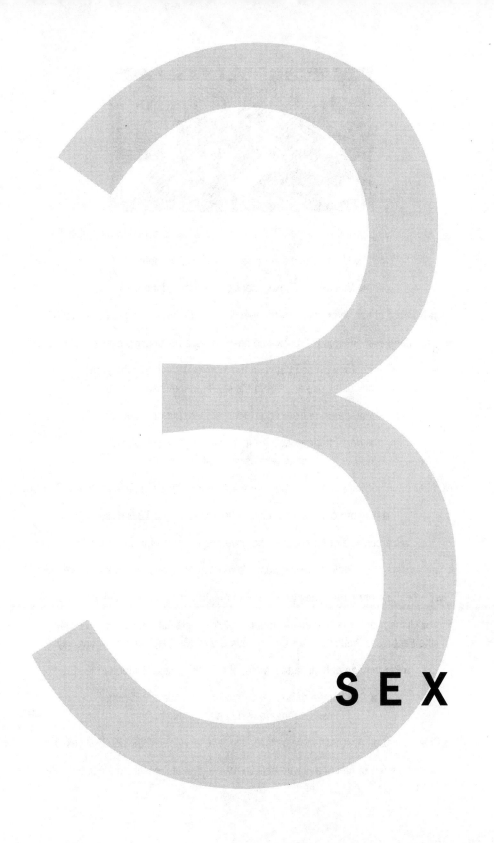

3

SEX

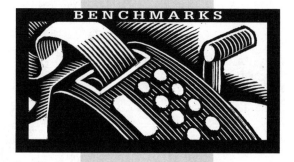

■ Total number of sex partners for a man, according to a worldwide study: 13

■ Minutes of a sexual session for single men: 21

■ Minutes of a sexual session for married men: 14

■ Number of sperm produced with every beat of the human male's heart: 1,500

■ Percentage of men ages 30 to 49 who have ended a relationship over the phone: 19

■ Percentage of men between the ages of 18 and 22 who admit
they didn't use a condom the last time they had sex: 48

■ Percentage of men who don't know how to put on a condom: 20

■ Percentage of college men who had sex with others
while in an "exclusive" relationship: 45

■ Number of unmarried people 65 and over who live with their romantic partners: 324,000

■ Number of American adults who use sex toys: 13.9 million

■ Percentage of Americans who have been celibate for one year: 18

■ Percentage of single men who admit to masturbating once a week or more: 48

■ Percentage of married men who admit to masturbating once a week or more: 44

■ Number of hours that employees from IBM, Apple, and AT&T spent viewing
the *Penthouse* Web site in a single month: 2,776 (347 eight-hour working days)

■ Percentage of heart attacks that occur during sexual intercourse: 1

■ Percentage of business travelers who admit to flirting
with strangers while on the road: 11

■ Chance that an American male believes that adultery doesn't include oral sex: 1 in 8

■ Percentage of Americans who believe marriages can benefit from adultery: 22

Get What You Want in Bed

How to Satisfy Her and Get Satisfaction for You

During the past decade, a revolution has taken place in the bedroom: Women are asking for what they want. Bookshelves are lined with rah-rah self-help tomes encouraging women to demand the pleasure they seek. While we applaud the courage of the fair sex to ask for what it desires, we feel left out. We take issue with the widespread assumption that men should just magically come on command with the slightest stimulation.

Why can't we have more? "Because we hesitate to ask," says Bernie Zilbergeld, Ph.D., an Oakland, California, psychologist and author of *The New Male Sexuality*. "Men are cheating themselves in bed by not making clear exactly what it is they want." And the sacrifice ends up hurting both partners. "I can't tell you how many women complain to me, 'I don't know what he likes; he won't tell me what turns him on,'" says Dr. Zilbergeld. Still, there's an art to making yourself heard. Ask for too much, and you're a drill sergeant; for too little, and you're still left hanging. Here's how to strike the right balance.

Lay the Groundwork

You may have heard that the best sex begins outside the bedroom. It's true. "A lot of sexual communication is best done in neutral territory where it's less likely to be mistaken for criticism," says Anthony Pietropinto, M.D., a New York City psychiatrist and author of *The Dream Girl*. Try these suggestions for tactful conversation.

Pick up the phone. Next time you're away on business, phone home and try popping that same question asked by thousands of hotel-bound guys every night: "So, what are you wearing?" When the only link between you and your partner is a collect call, you have no choice but to describe—in graphic detail—what you'd do to each other if you were there.

"This can be the perfect opportunity to slyly make your wishes known without the risk of insulting her," says Linda DeVillers, Ph.D., a sex therapist practicing in El Segundo, California, and author of *Love Skills*.

Head for the car. Even if you have a steady partner and she knows your body inside and out, you're bound to have new interests and changing needs. As you get older, for example, you'll need more direct stimulation to develop an erection.

The car is a perfect place for this kind of sexual clarification. "It's private, there are no distractions, and you can avoid constant eye contact during a potentially awkward discussion," says Dr. DeVillers. Be sure to keep your comments positive and focused on both your needs. Start with something like, "I'd like our sex to be the best it's ever been, and I have some new ideas we could try."

Tell her your dreams. You'd like to act out a fantasy or two you've been stewing over since the summer Olympics, but you're afraid she'll find it so kinky you'll wind up sleeping on the couch. Try passing it off as a dream, suggests Dr. Zilbergeld. After all, nobody can be held accountable for his subconscious thoughts. You can gauge her reaction and, if she's game, bring the dream to life.

Bedside Communication

While neutral talk is key, the signals you send in the throes of passion can make a tremendous difference. Here's how to nudge her into giving you maximum pleasure.

Be vocal. Moans, groans, sighs, and screams. They're standard cues you've probably been using to signal your pleasure for as long as you can remember. Use them more. "Women love to hear sounds of pleasure, and most men dramatically underdo them," says Dr. DeVillers. While a few well-placed sighs of pleasure may be all the encouragement she needs to fine-tune her technique, if she doesn't respond, turn up the volume.

Make suggestions. The key to offering effective sexual direction is to keep it short and simple, like harder, faster, slower, tighter, higher, firmer, lower. "Forget articulating your thoughts into complete sentences. One or two words at a time will get your point across without breaking the mood," says Dr. Zilbergeld.

Show her the way. There's no better way to teach than by demonstration. "Try wrapping your hands on top of hers and directing her touch in ways you find most pleasurable," suggests Dr. DeVillers. If she's going too slowly, speed her up. If she needs to squeeze harder, tighten her fingers.

One caution: Women hate having their heads pushed down during fellatio. If it's oral sex you're after, it's better to use words.

Talk dirty. If you have a request, try passing it off as dirty talk. "You don't want to sound like you're giving a command," says Dr. DeVillers. "Try starting with 'I'd love it if you'd. . . .' " If you have a term of endearment for your penis, use it.

Ask her what she wants. Of course, if you want her to help you, you need to reciprocate. That means doing all the things you know she likes, including that ridiculous fantasy about the cabana boy. Any fantasy where you play dumb and ask questions like "What next, Señorita?" offers the perfect opportunity to receive instructions along the way.

Another trick to try: Suggest she recount to you her all-time hottest love-making session—and then rise to the challenge.

View something together. Make a point to keep visual sexual fodder, like a sexy book or a video, handy. "Even a romantic, R-rated film can have plenty of erotic love scenes. When you find one you like, simply say, 'Wow, that really looks exciting. Why don't we try it that way?' " suggests Dr. Pietropinto.

Pour on the praise. It sounds obvious, but far too many of us get so caught up in the moment we forget to let her know when she's getting it right, says Dr. Zilbergeld. "You simply can't give too many compliments and appreciations." The best comments are both creative and plausible. "I'm still tingling with excitement from your touch" is far more memorable than "Boy, that felt good." To really reinforce a successful evening, compliment her again the next morning.

Trouble in Paradise

Avoid these seven sources of bad sex to maximize pleasure.

Thanks to tips from pals, glimpses of the nighttime soaps, and a history of dedicated movie-going, you're a master of the preliminaries. You wine; you dine. But getting that goddess from Accounting into bed is the easy part. Now it's show time. And nowhere is the fear of making a wrong move more intense than in the bedroom. "Many men who are fearless when confronting colleagues, scaling mountains, or handling a surly maître d' become paralyzed with anxiety at the thought of making a sexual mistake," says Linda DeVillers, Ph.D., a sex therapist practicing in El Segundo, California, and author of *Love Skills.* The cruel sexual irony: Fear of making a mistake is the fastest road to disaster between the sheets. Lucky for you, you have a regular Rand McNally's of lovemaking right here in your hands. Read it and never take an erotic wrong turn again.

Clawing the breasts. You watch as she slips the silk camisole over her head and then, of course, you grab, you clutch, you "cop a feel." Who can blame you?

Perhaps you continue, kneading as you would firm bread dough for several minutes. She's unimpressed.

What went wrong: Although most guys think of the breast as a homogenous bundle of erogenous material, it's actually composed of concentric zones of differing sensitivity. Think of the strings on a guitar. Hit them all at once and you have a cacophony. Pluck them one at a time and you have music.

Prevention: The key here is to build specifically and steadily to a nipple crescendo, says Dr. DeVillers. Start from the outermost rim and slowly spin inward. As your finger travels, you should notice the rim around her nipple (the areola) darken and the nipple itself stiffen. Place a finger on each side of the nipple, push down lightly and pull your fingers apart. Making the nipple taut in this way will heighten the tickling and licking you'll follow with.

Giving up on the clitoris. Oh, we know, you've heard it all before: The best lovers focus on the clitoris. So you dutifully reach down, pull back the hood that sheathes the supersensitive head, and stroke with the same vigor you'd use on your own member. Suddenly, you find that the tiny man in the canoe has, er, capsized. He's nowhere to be found. So you figure she's had enough and move on.

What went wrong: The clitoris is the trickster of the sexual world. Just as a woman's excitement peaks—but right before she climaxes—the tiny head beats a hasty retreat. The more direct your stimulation (and the more ecstasy it creates), the quicker the little guy makes his exit.

Prevention: Play peekaboo. Start by tempting the clitoral head out of hiding by touching it through the hood. "Using one or two fingers over the clitoral area, circle slowly in one direction, then the other," says Dr. DeVillers. As you feel the head (usually the size of a large pea) swell, gently pull back the hood. Now start vibrating your finger up and down (think of the vibrations of a butterfly's wing) and apply the finger gently to the head.

The kiss after oral sex. After doing your best manually with the clitoris, you decide (very wisely, we'd say) to enlist the aid of your tongue. You dart, you hum, you lunge—and, voilà, she has a rollicking orgasm. So you rise up to receive a well-deserved kiss.

What went wrong: Double standard #101: Women hate to taste their own vaginal secretions—even if they're on your mouth. "It's not that the scent of our own womanhood bothers us, but smelling ourselves is a reality check," says Anka Radakovich, author of *Sexplorations.*

Prevention: Personal style dictates here. You might bury your head in ecstasy in the nearby balled-up sheet. Or keep a glass of water (or, better, champagne) by the side of the bed and take a long, slow sip.

The rushed erection. You've tended her needs beautifully—at the expense of your own—and now that it's time for the real fun to begin, you're a little, well, limp. So you replay that fantasy with Gina, the cute waitress at the place down the street, and will an erection. Then, quickly so as not to lose it, you enter—and immediately go soft. Game over.

What went wrong: The vagina can be a very slippery place. Couple its lubrication with the condom you're probably wearing, and you have a recipe for flaccidity. There's simply not enough available friction to fuel an erection.

Prevention: Get what you need—and what you want. "Many men have difficulty asking their partners for the kinds of lovemaking techniques they prefer because of the antiquated notion that a 'real man' is not supposed to have any sexual needs other than for hot, frequent sex," says Patricia Love, Ed.D., a marriage and family therapist practicing in Austin, Texas, and author of *Hot Monogamy*. If you like receiving oral sex before intercourse, give, then ask to receive.

Mindless penetration. You've done your duties, now it's reward time. Without a second thought, you start pumping away. Curiously, her eyes wander to the ceiling—where they fix on that old water stain.

What went wrong: The moment the tip of your penis meets the lips of the vagina is one of grave significance for your partner. "This moment offers a tremendous opportunity for communication," says Dr. Love. Misspeak and she may opt out altogether.

Prevention: Tantalize her. Take your penis in hand and give her clitoris a long, luscious stroke. Then break away and kiss her deeply and passionately. (A recent poll of *Glamour* magazine readers found that women prefer being kissed during intercourse more than any other time.) As you kiss, stroke and slide your penis in slowly and surely.

Missing the target. You pump; she grinds. All is well in the world. That is, until she stops moving and moaning—sans orgasm—and looks to you to just get it over already.

What went wrong: Rare is the woman who can climax without attention to one of two spots. For roughly 70 percent, extra clitoral stimulation during intercourse is needed to push them over that glorious edge. For another 30 percent, penile stimulation directed specifically at the G-spot, the quarter-size area on the top wall of the vagina, can do the trick.

Prevention: If asking her which spot floats her boat is not your idea of dinner conversation, watch and learn, explains John D. Perry, Ph.D., coauthor of *The G-Spot*. Arrange things so she's on top early on. Then watch to see if she moves forward, rubbing her clitoris against the shaft of your penis; or backward, moving the head of your penis toward her G-spot.

If she's a forward leaner, when you're on top reach down and tickle her clitoris as you thrust. If she arches her back when on top, flex the muscles at the base of your penis next time you're in the missionary position. This sexy flex will angle your penis toward that top vaginal wall.

Another trick: Place a pillow under her lower back to give you better access to the spot. If she responds to your maneuvers, thrust harder and faster until you feel her vagina rhythmically contract in waves of pleasure.

Rolling over. Go ahead—you've earned it.

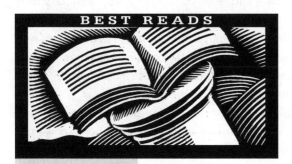

BEST READS

Overcoming Inhibitions

Getting into a rut: A common complaint of sexual partners who have been in the same relationship for years. But are all long-term relationships doomed to years of this result? The authors of Good Loving: Keys to a Lifetime of Passion, Pleasure, and Sex *(Rodale Press, 1998) certainly don't think so. Here, Donna Raskin and Larry Keller show how to put some zip back into your sex life. And, no, having an affair is not part of their prescription.*

Ever feel like punching a sex expert?

That's not recommended behavior, but if you're told "vary your sexual routine" one more time, you just may lose it. We hear you: You know there are other positions. You know there are other ways to do it. But it's not so simple. You want to try new things, but it's just that . . . well . . . you know. . . .

We know. We know that even in the closest relationships, there can be something holding you back from breaking out of that routine. Those same sex experts you're so mad at say such inhibitions are common and conquerable.

They're also understandable. There are at least three good reasons why you tend to trod the tried-and-true.

It's easier. Your sex habits can behave like water running downhill, finding the course of least resistance. That's one reason why a lot of couples seldom stray from the missionary position. "You know why man-on-top intercourse is the most popular?" asks Barry McCarthy, Ph.D., a Washington, D.C., psychologist for the Washington Psychological Center and author of *Male Sexual Awareness.* "Because it's easier."

It's more convenient. "The straight penis-vagina thing is really convenient for guys," says Gina Ogden, Ph.D., a sex therapist and author of *Women Who Love Sex.* "It's quick, it's efficient, it's right there, and it feels good. You don't even have to relate while you're doing it."

It's safer. As in emotionally safer. "Doing the same thing all the time is safe," says Daniel Beaver, director of the Relationship Counseling Center in Walnut Creek, California, and author of *Beyond the Marriage Fantasy* and *More Than Just Sex.* "Making things exciting by blazing a new trail is taking an emotional risk."

Birth of an Anxiety

Your inhibition has its childhood roots, of course, as you remember from Psychology 101. "If you weren't free to create, if you were told from the time your little ears could hear that you never were doing things right, you're going to lack confidence to pursue things," says Rachel Copelan, Ph.D., a psychologist and sexologist who wrote *100 Ways to Make Sex Sensational and 100 Percent Safe.*

But it's also a cultural thing. "You get horrible messages from the culture," says Kathleen Gill, Ph.D., a clinical psychologist, certified sex therapist, and adjunct professor of psychology at Harvard Medical School. "Like the idea that sex is dirty unless you save it for marriage. Even if you do save it for marriage, you still carry around with you the 'sex is dirty' part."

And it's a macho thing. "Men are supposed to know it all, and their bodies are supposed to always work," Dr. McCarthy says. "Inhibitions have to do with these unrealistic expectations."

That gets back to the position problem. Move out of the missionary, and you usually have to work with her to get things physically organized. This is a good thing, but your macho expectations may not see it that way. You don't want to lose control of the situation. "Penises tend to slip out of vaginas in many positions," says Dr. McCarthy. "Men tend to get anxious about that, so they just stay away from them."

But that's not a very good strategy for long-term sexual fulfillment in a relationship. Besides, anxiety comes with sex, says Dr. Gill. "Anxiety is motivating," she says. "We don't do anything in life without it." And that includes (please don't hit us for saying it) varying your sexual routine. What follows are strategies to help you identify and conquer whatever inhibitions might be lying around in your mind.

Manage your anxiety. The trick, Dr. Gill says, is to learn to tolerate a certain amount of anxiety. "Avoiding anxiety is not the point," she says. "Learning to live with it is." In other words, somewhere between paralyzing fear and total apathy is a level of anxiety that you can work with. Find that level. "And then manage it well enough so that you can confront what really turns you on," Dr. Gill says.

Accept yourself. Recognize that what turns you on is simply a source of sexual pleasure for you, not some kind of cosmic comment on your worth as a human being. You don't need to feel embarrassed or personally rejected if she doesn't happen to share that particular turn-on. "Rather than depending on validation from your mate for what you think, give that validation to yourself," says Louanne Cole Weston, Ph.D., a board-certified sex therapist; a marriage, family, and child counselor; and a sex columnist for the *San Francisco Examiner*.

Example: You'd just love it if at certain impassioned points of the process, the love chatter between the two of you turned X-rated. But you'd never bring it up because you're afraid she might think you're a foul-mouthed fool. Hence, nothing ever happens. "That's the kind of inhibition that keeps you from being real about sex," Dr. Gill says. "You have to be able to say, 'Hey, it may not be politically correct, but it really floats my boat.'"

Let go of something. One way to loosen the logjam, suggests sexologist Isadora Alman, who writes the syndicated sex and relationship advice column "Ask Isadora," is to find within you just one long-held sexual secret that you can somehow tell her about. "That doesn't mean sharing all your secrets," Alman says. "Just let go of something that has been keeping you from being closer to her."

A favorite one for women, Alman says, is "I always think that if you really knew me, you wouldn't love me." If she can get that out, you're more likely to say, "Of course I would, honey," than "You're probably right." So if you can manage to blurt out, say, "I'm worried I'll keep slipping out of you if we try it spoon-style," you'll probably discover that she won't immediately file for divorce. She might even say, "So what? It feels good when we get it back in."

Jettison excess baggage. You don't have to keep carrying society's sex-is-dirty messages around with you. Liberate yourself from inhibiting notions about sex that were forced upon you when you didn't know any better. "Do some self-examination," advises Dr. Gill. "Get conscious about what those messages are, and get rid of the ones that aren't serving you."

Helping Her Along

Now that you're overcoming your own inhibitions, you still have hers to think about. Last we looked, it took two to perform most sex acts.

Take oral sex, for example. Yeah, we know, you'd be glad to. But will she provide it just as gladly? The *Sex in America* survey conducted by the University of Chicago and the National Opinion Research Center found that while a not-so-surprising 83 percent of men consider it appealing to receive oral sex, only 57 percent of women consider giving it appealing. What's more, almost a third of women (32 percent) don't even like receiving oral sex. There's a discrepancy here.

You don't need statistics to tell you if she's uptight about pursuing new paths to pleasure. But why? Take all the social messages you got about the evil of sexuality and multiply it many-fold for her.

"It goes back to the virgin thing," says Dr. Copelan. "Girls are told not to let anybody touch them. They're taught early not to respond sexually."

That sort of programming can lead to body hang-ups. Next thing you know, years have gone by and she still won't consider making love with the lights on. "Women have the same kind of head noises about measuring up as men do," Dr. Ogden says. "But with them, it's more like 'I'm too fat' or 'I'm too thin.'"

And, just like you, women can be wary of what enjoying certain sex acts might say about who they are. "Some women might shy away from oral sex because of what it might uncover," Dr. Weston says. "It's not just that they might like it, but that they might even like it if you demand it in a demeaning way." Here are some suggestions for helping her confront and overcome her inhibitions.

Enlist in the battle. "Any woman can be helped," Dr. Copelan says. "You have to take charge and struggle to help her, if she wants you to." That means encouraging her to reveal her desires. How? Try asking. "You have to ask her what feels good, what she wants you to do," Dr. Copelan says.

Take it easy. Ask, but don't push too hard. "Have patience," Dr. Copelan says. "Don't overwhelm her with your desires and needs. Take your time." Remember, you have a lifetime (hers) of negative momentum to overcome. Go slowly. Start out a bit naughty and playful. Talk dirty. Get comfortable with your new sexual territory and lingo and keep experimenting.

Strike while the iron's hot. Ask her over coffee what she'd like you to do sexually, and she needs to answer in full, blushing sentences. Ask her if she likes what you're doing while you're doing it, and she can respond negatively or positively with a mere moan. "Do you like this?" is a lot more effective when the "this" is a real feeling instead of an abstract idea. "One of the best times to find out what your partner likes is during sex," says Timothy Perper, Ph.D., a Philadelphia biologist and independent sex researcher who wrote *Sex Signals: The Biology of Love.* "When you're in the throes, you can make personal requests of each other that at other times might horrify one of you."

Wash away the worries. One reason some women are shy about oral sex, according to Dr. Copelan, is because they think their sex organs are dirty. Or smelly. "There's a simple solution for that," she says. "Take a shower together. Take a bath together. Be clean together."

Be sexual friends. "The biggest secret to overcoming inhibitions is to think of each other as your intimate sexual friend," Dr. McCarthy says. "With a friend, you don't need to get defensive if something doesn't work."

The spirit should be camaraderie, not competition. Instead of judging each other, think of yourselves as partners in crime, of sorts. "When people back off from their adversarial ways, new solutions tend to rear their heads in funny, unpredictable ways," Dr. Weston says.

Understanding Sex Drive

Are women's sex drives weaker than men's? Many men would say yes, but some sex therapists disagree. They believe that women's libidos are different, not weaker. How to tap into that libido is something that men struggle with every day. In this excerpt from A Lifetime of Sex: The Ultimate Manual on Sex, Women, and Relationships for Every Stage of a Man's Life *by Stephen C. George and K. Winston Caine (Rodale Press, 1998), the authors delve into the physiological and mental factors that sexually drive both men and women. They touch upon why men's drives seem so much stronger, but more important for many men, they also describe how to recharge a flagging desire.*

What is it that sparks a man's hunger for sex? Don't try to count the ways. How can you count to infinity? The desire for sex is kindled by a complex mix of internal chemistry and external triggers as subtle as a smile, as blunt as a porno film. By the smell of a perfume or the sound of a song's lyrics. By touching another's body or our own. By a thought. A meal. A dream.

Just as the cause of sexual hunger varies with the wind, so does the amount of sexual appetite a person has at any given moment. While men and women may have a yearning for sex throughout their lifetimes, that hunger can vary enormously day by day, year by year, not unlike the wild undulations of a stock market. For some, sex drive can take a downturn from which they never recover. (Talk about a great depression.) Others, however, can look forward to being bullish in bed for a lifetime. One way to end up in the latter camp is to invest a little time in learning the intricacies of sex drive—yours and hers. It can pay big dividends.

First of all, know this: There is no typical or average sex drive or libido. "There is a very wide range," says Domeena Renshaw, M.D., director of Loyola

Sex Therapy Clinic at Loyola University in Chicago and author of *Seven Weeks to Better Sex.* "It's uniquely individual."

So men who have low libido needn't feel that they are inadequate. "If they're perfectly content, it shouldn't become a problem," Dr. Renshaw says. "It's a problem when in a committed relationship, the partner is discontented. Then we see them."

In the pages ahead, we'll cover the physiological factors first, then take up the role of the mind. Then we'll explore how the two mesh.

The Role of Hormones

Women might want to think twice the next time they make cracks about the male sex hormone testosterone when commenting on some guy's supercharged sex drive. That's because testosterone also revs up their own sex engines. It's just that all eight of our cylinders are pumped with this potent fuel. The women's motors get just a small amount. Testosterone and other hormones are the stuff that create "a vague unrest," says Ted McIlvenna, Ph.D., president of the Institute for Advanced Study of Human Sexuality in San Francisco. That unrest is your sex drive—a deep-rooted feeling that does not need erotic stimulation but upon which further sexual stimulation then builds. It is affected, for better or worse, by physical and emotional factors.

"It's testosterone that gives you the ability to sexually function," says Dr. McIlvenna. It does so by acting as a conduit between nerve cells and the brain and creating desire. Without desire, having an erection is like being given the keys to a Ferrari that has no gas.

Testosterone is produced in our testicles, and then flows into our bloodstream, where it is omnipresent. The amount of testosterone a man has in his blood varies not only throughout his life but also during the course of a day. When we win an argument or a tennis match, or when we have sexual thoughts or intercourse, our testosterone rises. Combine this testosterone with a mental stimulus, and the next thing you know, blood is rushing into our penises and—tah-dah!—we have erections. Preferably in the bedroom, not on the tennis court.

Oddly, testosterone also has a "loner profile" that, among other things, increases a guy's urge to masturbate rather than his desire for intercourse, says sex therapist Theresa Crenshaw, M.D., author of *The Alchemy of Love and Lust.* It's that quality in the hormone that also makes guys want to head to another room after intercourse, often to the chagrin of their partners, she says.

Of course, testosterone is much more than a sex hormone. It also is responsible for the following:

- Shaping our penises, scrotums, and testicles when we were embryos
- Promoting development of our muscle mass, bones, and cognitive skills
- Making us aggressive, assertive, confident—it's because of testosterone that we are more likely to get enraged by rude drivers or go to war
- Being a natural antidepressant—for both genders

A man's sex drive and his ability to get an erection or to ejaculate can be affected if he has a hormonal imbalance that causes a deficiency in his testosterone, says Dr. Renshaw. Tumors in the pituitary gland, for example, can cause an imbalance, as can radiation treatment for prostate cancer, says Dr. Renshaw. Fortunately, hormone imbalances are rare, particularly in younger men, and treatable.

But a guy with a normal testosterone level and a sex drive stuck in neutral will not benefit by infusions of more testosterone. In fact, it could harm him by interfering with his normal hormonal cycles. That's what happens when bodybuilders and athletes take anabolic steroids. These synthetic hormones, among other things, shrivel guys' testicles and destroy their fertility.

In truth, you probably don't want to have too much testosterone. A guy who does "is more self-centered, selfish, and has a personality profile not unlike a psychotic," writes Dr. Crenshaw.

A Pennsylvania State University study of hormone levels of more than 4,000 men seems to support her. The study found that men with high testosterone levels were less likely to get married. Those who did marry were more apt to have affairs, physically abuse their wives, and dump them because they could not get along with them.

The Role of the Mind

"People think sex drives are largely biological," says Al Cooper, Ph.D., clinical director of the San Jose Marital and Sexuality Centre in California. "They are mainly psychological events."

While acknowledging that testosterone is important to fueling one's sex drive, it's only one part of the equation, Dr. Cooper and other sex therapists stress. The other is that three-pound lump of gray matter inside our skulls.

It is our minds that convert a scent, a sight, even a sound into a desire for sex. Each person is triggered differently, based on preferences and attitudes that have accumulated since childhood. Some guys are aroused by legs, others by breasts, others by the sight of a bare back and long hair. This is not physiological; this is mental programming.

Are there commonalities among men? Certainly. Guys are justly famous—or infamous—for needing very little mental spark to ignite their sexual engines. And the top stimuli for men are visual—the sight of something arousing, usually an attractive female body. "Men are more tuned in to visual cues," says Dr. Cooper. "A man may not feel sexual toward his wife, but if he sees Pamela Lee on *Baywatch*, then he might feel very sexual toward her. The women won't get the same sort of charge out of looking at something." Skeptical? Just compare the sales of *Playboy* and *Playgirl* magazines, Dr. Cooper suggests.

In fact, our minds are so powerful that in some cases you can remove a man's testicles—where testosterone and sperm are produced—and he still will be interested in sex and become aroused, says licensed psychologist William R. Stayton, doctor of theology, professor of human sexuality at the University of Pennsylvania in Philadelphia and president of the American Association of Sex Educators, Counselors, and Therapists (AASECT). For that reason, proposals to castrate sex offenders are ludicrous, he says. "All that means is that they can't have children."

Conversely, a guy with a high level of testosterone might have little sexual desire if he has been taught to dislike sex, says Dr. Stayton. "You take three different men with the same testosterone levels, and they're going to respond three very different ways. A lot of it is going to come from how they were socialized."

Worry, stress, and depression can also impair one's sex drive as can illness, fatigue, and many drugs. Job pressures, mortgage woes, and anger at one's spouse or children are examples of the sorts of things that can run a man's libido off course, says Dudley Seth Danoff, M.D., senior attending urologist at Cedars-Sinai Medical Center in Los Angeles and author of *Superpotency*. "What happens between your ears definitely reflects what happens between your legs," he says.

"The old stereotype was the 365-day headache for women," says Dr. Renshaw. "But we've seen as many 'headaches' in the man as in the woman."

And yet some men who seek professional help don't really have deficient libidos, therapists say. Sometimes it's simply a matter of a guy's partner wanting sex more often than he does. Or a wife complains that her husband isn't interested in sex, but it turns out that he is routinely masturbating in secret. The problem is not with his sex drive but with his relationship.

"What I hear over and over is that it's less hassle doing it with yourself rather than going through the business of foreplay and everything else," Dr. Renshaw says. "It becomes another job to do."

How Hormones and the Mind Mesh

Like Astaire and Rogers or pigs and mud, your hormones and your mind are an inseparable duo. Each is dependent upon and connected to the other in the urge we call sex drive. Your testosterone is just sitting there in your blood minding its business when something—a touch, a fantasy, a smell—triggers the old arousal switch. Then the chemicals kick in. Testosterone and neurotransmitters such as dopamine create the urge to pursue pleasure. The brain then messages the penis ("Wake up, penis!") via the nervous system to prepare for an erection. Blood vessels expand and blood swooshes in. Congratulations. You have an erection.

To what extent our hormones or our minds influence our sexual behavior often depends on who is doing the interpreting. Men are often portrayed—probably accurately—as complaining that their partners have lower sex drives, while women say that men want sex too much, says Dr. Cooper.

Blame our brains, says Dr. Stayton. "Males are socialized that they are interested, ready at any time with anybody under any circumstances. Females are socialized much more that they're not sexual, that their interests and desires are going to come out of pleasing a man."

Unless the couple is married. Then the stereotype—again probably accurate—is of a husband who is shirking his marital duties in the bedroom, à la Al Bundy in the sitcom *Married with Children*, Dr. Cooper says. One reason for this discrepancy is that men want variety, women want romance, he adds.

Blame our hormones, says Dr. Crenshaw. Testosterone creates men's craving for sexual variety or novelty. Estrogen makes women want intimacy.

How Women Differ

You had better communicate well with your woman or be an awfully good mind reader in trying to determine when she's in the mood for sex. Because of their menstrual cycles, women's sex drive or desire is far more complex and varied than that of men, Dr. Crenshaw says. She contends that women experience four types of lust of varying intensity, depending on which of their hormones are ebbing and flowing. She identifies them as aggressive, passive, seductive, and resistant. Men, being the primitive brutes that we are, generally have just one type of lust—aggressive, she says.

The trick then for men is to figure out when, hormonally speaking, a woman is most apt to be in the mood for sex during her 28-day cycle. Dr. Crenshaw provides help there, too, by summarizing the results of nearly four dozen studies that have been done on this very subject. While each woman has a unique pattern of sexual desire, these studies show some commonalities. So grab a calendar and follow along (for our purposes, the start of menstruation is day one of a woman's cycle).

• Women generally report their most intense sex drive on days 6 and 7 after a period begins.

- A close second in terms of sex drive is just before a woman starts her period—days 25 through 28.
- A distant third is around the time of ovulation—when an egg is released from an ovary. This is days 13 through 15.
- Few women have strong sexual desire during their periods (the first few days of their 28-day cycle).
- Finally, the time of least sexual interest appears to be the second half of her cycle—the time between ovulation and the days immediately before the start of menstruation.

While testosterone is crucial to a woman's sex drive, estrogen is her most important hormone. This is her counterpart to testosterone in a man. Estrogen is responsible for:

- Shaping a female's primary sexual characteristics—the vagina, uterus, and ovaries—while she is still in her mother's womb
- Causing mood swings, budding breasts, rounder hips, and other dramatic changes during puberty
- Generating the need for intimacy during sex
- Promoting lubrication of the vagina and sustaining or improving tissue and texture of sex organs

Just as women have some testosterone, men have a little estrogen. But it does not have the impact on their sex drives that testosterone has on women's sex drives.

More men masturbate than women, and they do so more often. We also think about sex a lot more than women. So are women's sex drives weaker than our own raging beasts? No, say some sex therapists.

Women's libidos are just different. Disparities in sex drive are more prevalent within genders, not between them, says Barbara Levinson, R.N., Ph.D., a licensed marriage and family therapist and director of the Center for Healthy Sexuality in Houston. "Men are just more verbal about sex," she says.

Women actually have a greater capacity for sex than men, notes Shirley Zussman, Ed.D., a certified sex and marital therapist in private practice in New York City. Men's erections are more vulnerable to disease than women's sex organs, she says. Unlike men, women can have multiple orgasms. And women don't need to rest from an orgasm before resuming sex again.

Complicating matters more, the conventional wisdom has long been that while men reach their sexual peak in their late teens or early twenties, women don't reach theirs until they are in their thirties. No wonder men want to do it when women don't, and vice versa. Only not everybody buys it. "For me, that doesn't ring true anymore," Dr. Zussman says.

That perception about women may have come about in prior generations when there was more of a stigma attached to women being sexual when they were young and unmarried, Dr. Zussman believes. "I would say that young women between 15 and 20 probably have a high sexual drive. I think masturbation is much more common among young girls today, enabling them to learn much more about their bodies."

Decades of Dallying

One tip-off as to whether you will be amorous as you age is how horny you were as a kid. Studies have shown that both men and women who had a strong interest in sex at a young age were also more inclined to have a high level of interest in their later years, says Dr. Zussman.

That said, men and women both face hurdles to having a lifetime of sex, but most aren't insurmountable. With the onset of menopause, women suddenly and dramatically lose a large amount of one of their most vital hormones—estrogen. This can result in a number of physical and emotional symptoms—such as a dry, sensitive vagina—that can curtail their sex drive and that often make intercourse painful. Happily, there are treatments available. And for some women, menopause is a boon to their sex lives.

A man's decline in sex drive is so gradual that some continue to have active sex lives into their eighties and nineties, says Dr. Danoff, who estimates that he has seen more than 100,000 penises in his medical practice.

Indeed, while men gradually produce less testosterone as they age, most of us continue to manufacture this sex drive hormone, along with sperm and semen, until the end of our lives.

"One of the things we believe is that if a person stays sexually active through their early adult and middle years, their testosterone level is not going to go down as much," says Dr. Stayton. Use it or lose it? "Absolutely a truism," he says.

Actually, it's not diminishing testosterone per se that should concern men as they age, says Dr. McIlvenna. It's a decline in what he calls bioavailable-free testosterone that can affect men's sex drive. As we age, he says, more and more of our testosterone becomes bound to blood coagulates. That which doesn't is the good stuff that keeps us interested in sex.

For this reason, a doctor who rules out testosterone deficiency in a man with a flagging sex drive after reviewing his testosterone level may be in error unless the test includes a measurement of his unencumbered testosterone.

Certain medications and illnesses can also take their tolls on a man's sex drive as he gets older. But most of these can be corrected. As long as men and women remain interesting partners to each other, many will be able to continue to enjoy sex—albeit less often—into their later years.

"You don't stop having sex because you get old," Dr. Danoff advises. "You get old because you stop having sex."

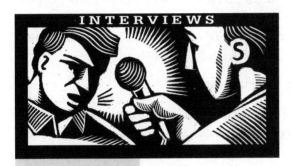

INTERVIEWS

David Courtwright on
A World without Women

We've always thought of women as wonderful, intelligent beings who enhance every facet of our lives. (At least, that's what they keep telling us.) But David Courtwright, Ph.D., professor of history at the University of North Florida in South Jacksonville, takes that appreciation to extremes. His book, Violent Land, *describes how trouble erupts wherever young men are left alone in large groups. (It does seem to explain Catholic boys' schools and the Dallas Cowboys.) We asked Courtwright to tell us why he believes single men are such self-destructive hell-raisers, and why marrying is perhaps the best thing a man can do for his health.*

It's bad enough we can't find a date. Now you tell us single guys are the scourge of society?

I researched the history of narcotics use in the United States and noticed that as many as 90 percent of nonmedical addicts—junkies, if you prefer—were young, single men. Looking further, this was true of many social problems—venereal disease, rioting, vandalism, murder, you name it. In every case, from Colonial Virginia to modern Los Angeles, most of the culprits were unattached men. My basic idea is simple: Wherever you have lots of young, single men, trouble is bound to follow. It's even worse when they're armed, intoxicated, irreligious, and homicidally sensitive about honor.

Why are young, single men so violent?

We all know that testosterone makes males more aggressive. But there's a genetic component, as well. In primitive societies, the best hunters and fighters had more mates, though they led shorter lives. But in the Darwinian scheme of things, life span isn't as important as passing on your genes.

Sounds like you're calling us savages.

Male aggression has its advantages. So do youth and bachelorhood. Look at the cowboys: They were dependable, competent workers. Their aggression helped carve out the country. But the cowboys killed each other in saloons and spread disease in brothels. Young men who work hard also play hard.

So why does it help to have a woman around?

Marriage often causes young men to cool their jets. Other things being equal, a married man with kids is going to think twice before he wades into the thick of a barroom brawl. A married man with kids, in fact, is less likely to be in the barroom in the first place. As a group, single men are at a statistical disadvantage. They're more likely to break the law, eat less nutritious food, pay higher insurance rates, and so on.

Surely not every woman will keep a guy out of trouble. Is there a certain type who tends to calm a guy down?

Religion makes a difference. A devout woman who draws her spouse into her church and devotional activities will discourage disorderly behavior. A Bonnie Parker type isn't going to be much help. Just ask Clyde Barrow.

What about all of those unhappily married guys we know?

Most men understand the advantages of marriage: companionship, regular meals, less risk of venereal disease. The one obvious disadvantage: Sooner or later, monogamy leads to a slowdown in the bed department. But sex isn't everything, even if our culture pretends otherwise. Married people consistently report that they are happier than unmarried people. And men who divorce typically remarry. They may give up on individual women, but not on marriage. It's a good deal.

Are you married?

You bet.

Gloria Horsley on
Managing Your In-Laws

You've finally found the perfect girl, but you wonder how her mom escaped that stake in Salem. If you want to avoid your own family trials, you might listen to Gloria Horsley, author of The In-Law Survival Manual. *Her clinical study on in-law relationships, the most complete since 1954, shows that not much has changed since the olden days—friction between in-laws is constant and timeless, kind of like* All in the Family *reruns. The good news: There are some effective strategies to make sure your home life isn't sitcom material.*

Any way to avoid problems with in-laws early in the marriage?

Before you get married, you should ask permission from your fiancée's parents. If they don't approve, try to find out why and work the problems out. This may seem old-fashioned, but research shows that 80 percent of the marriages that fail within the first year don't have parental approval. Another study showed that 70 percent of couples who divorced in the first year named in-law problems as a big factor.

Mothers-in-law are all-powerful beings capable of ruining your marital life. True or false?

True. Studies have shown that when couples have problems, they feel that mothers cause them 40 percent of the time. Naturally, you'll want to get in good with your mother-in-law. Help her in the kitchen; set the table for her. Guys never do this, and these are probably the best, easiest things a son-in-law can do. If you're a guy who likes to cook, show her a special dish you enjoy making. Find what her interest is and go with it. If she likes sports, sit down and watch a football game with her. I happen to like golf, and two of my sons-in-law go golfing with me.

Here's what not to do: Take on your wife's battles. I often hear a guy say he doesn't like the way his wife is treated by her parents. But they had those problems long before he came along, so he should stay out of them.

What if—no matter what you do—her mom still thinks you're a meathead?

If you've tried everything you can and she still hates you, it may be time to sic your wife on her. Have her warn that she won't be around as much if Mom-in-law continues to treat you the way she does. You'll be surprised at the results.

And if your mom thinks that your wife is a tramp?

Well, there are obviously things you love about your wife. Find ways to let your mom see those traits. Invite your family to your apartment for dinner so they can get to know her. It's also important to invite your siblings. People just want to be included so they know your new relationship is not going to cut them out of your life. If that doesn't work, get down to specifics. Find out who's leading the attack and why. You or she can talk to them about it, or you may find an ally in the family who can help.

You've found that women often idolize their fathers. Do we have any hope of measuring up?

Whatever you do, don't resent him or try to make him look bad in front of her. Remember, her father is very special to her. If you have a really great father-in-law who's done a lot, you need to respect that. Look at him more as a mentor than as a competitor, and ask him for advice on those things he does best. If you feel like you're competing, just think to yourself, "She married me, not him. I was chosen."

How can we keep screwball in-laws in line during Easter dinner?

Have dinner later, so these people aren't hanging around all day. Rather than inviting everybody over at one o'clock, say, invite them over at seven. If you have a guest who drinks, eat dinner right away, before they get the chance to become obnoxious.

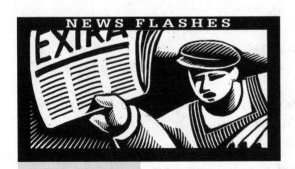

Determining Child's Sex May Be Possible

LIVERPOOL, England—If you want your firstborn child to be a son, look for a younger wife. Want a daughter? Better marry someone older. Does that sound silly? Not according to a study conducted at the University of Liverpool, which showed that husbands with wives 1 to 9 years older have more than twice as many daughters. Couples with wives 5 to 15 years younger had nearly twice as many sons. The researchers don't understand why the age difference between parents predicts the sex of the first child. However, they do know that during and immediately after World Wars I and II, women married older men and had more sons.

Sperm after a Vasectomy No Cause for Alarm

AMSTERDAM, Holland—Many men who undergo vasectomies are alarmed when tests detect nonswimming sperm in their semen weeks later. They should relax. Dutch researchers studied 395 such men and found that semen may contain nonmoving sperm for several months after a vasectomy, but they pose virtually no pregnancy risk. "If the sperm aren't moving, they won't fertilize the egg," says Arthur Wisot, M.D., executive director of the Center for Advanced Reproductive Care in Redondo Beach, California.

Global Sperm Counts Holding Steady

BALTIMORE—When researchers announced that worldwide sperm counts were on the wane, scientists pointed the finger at everything from polluted drinking water to an impending ice age. But now researchers from Johns Hopkins University, using sophisticated computers to collectively reanalyze the results of 61 studies, maintain that sperm counts have actually remained unchanged since the early 1970s. Why the discrepancy? The folks at Johns Hopkins say that the previous research didn't take into account natural geographic variations in fertility.

Women Still Want Sex as They Age

WATERTOWN, Mass.—During midlife, women want as much sex as men. After surveying more than 700 couples in their fifties, researchers from the New England Research Institutes found that both men and women say they want sex six times per month and are basically satisfied with their sex lives. One gender gap: Men reported having more desire and a more active sexual fantasy life than women.

Common Spermicide Does Not Protect against HIV

WASHINGTON, D.C.—In the 1980s, researchers discovered that the popular spermicide nonoxynol-9 could destroy the AIDS-causing HIV virus in test tubes. Since then, some couples have counted on the chemical for protection. Bad idea, say scientists from the National Institute of Allergy and Infectious Diseases. When they studied 940 Cameroonian prostitutes, they found that the risk of contracting HIV remained the same for women who used a latex condom and applied a spermicidal gel as for those who used condoms and applied gel sans spermicide.

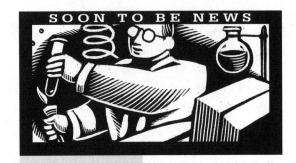

An End to Impotence?

Many men saw their impotence come to an end with the spectacular widespread introduction of Viagra (sildenafil) last year. But it was not a cure for everyone. Unfortunately, impotence is still out there. We may, however, see impotence vanquished once and for all in the coming decades. "Within a few years, we'll have drugs that promote regular nighttime erections to keep the penis oxygenated and healthy," predicts Irwin Goldstein, M.D., professor of urology at Boston University School of Medicine. "And by 2020, men will take a daily drug to prevent the gradual buildup of penile scar tissue. For severe situations, we'll use gene therapy to regrow damaged penile muscle."

Men who need only an occasional boost will be able to choose from a variety of easy-to-use oral drugs and medicated gels, adds Dr. Goldstein.

Here are several impotence slayers that are currently in various stages of development.

Topiglan. A company called MacroChem is combining the drug alprostadil, known to create erections when injected, with a formula that will help it be absorbed through the skin as a cream. In early trials, abut 70 percent of men who tried Topiglan responded, according to the company.

Alprox-TD. Another company, NexMed, is working on a similar cream that combines alprostadil with a compound that will make it available to the tissues of the penis. Alprox-TD has just completed initial safety trials and will be undergoing more research later this year.

Powderject. This innovative system will deliver a powdered form of alprostadil through the penile skin by using a special handheld device that accelerates the drug to supersonic speeds. The space-age technology recently completed its initial safety trials with only a 2 percent incidence of complications.

A company called Medi-Ject is planning a similar needle-free system but has not yet begun clinical testing.

Rub-On Testosterone?

An estimated 400,000 American men ages 18 to 59 suffer from testosterone deficiency, a condition that can foster low sex drive and obesity. Treatment options are limited to lifelong injections or transdermal patches, but a testosterone gel may soon be available. "It should be as effective as patches and cause very little skin irritation," says Ronald Swerdloff, M.D., an internist at Harbor–University of California, Los Angeles Medical Center. *The testosterone gel is in human trials and should be available by prescription within a year.*

Tanning Lotion a Cure for Impotence?

Men injected with chemicals (melanotropic peptides) developed to promote tanning and reduce skin cancer experienced an unusual side effect: stronger erections. Within a few years, a drug called Melanotan II may be used to treat impotence. In a small study done at the University of Arizona Health Sciences Center in Tucson, eight men with psychological impotence were injected with Melanotan II. Seven of them developed erections that lasted for about 30 minutes. *The drug, which could one day be available as a nasal spray, may foster erections by stimulating production of dopamine in the penis.*

A Helper for Viagra?

With all the hubbub surrounding the oral impotence drug, Viagra, information about another up-and-coming pill, Vasomax, has been scarce. We caught up with Raymond C. Rosen, Ph.D., professor of psychiatry at the University of Medicine and Dentistry of New Jersey–Robert Wood Johnson Medical School in Piscataway, who explained that one study has shown that 42 percent of men with erectile dysfunction who took Vasomax developed erections hard enough for intercourse. *While those numbers are not as impressive as Viagra's, it's possible that— pending Food and Drug Administration approval—the two pills could be used together to deliver a double punch against flimsy erections.*

Better Sex in the Future?

"Reach out and touch someone" could take on a whole new meaning if we're to believe the predictions of futurologist Kenneth Maxwell, Ph.D., an emeritus professor of biology at California State University at Long Beach. He foresees a system of computer-driven attachments that will make virtual sex intensely pleasurable, and telephone links that will ensure you and your partner can make love even when separated by thousands of miles. *Dr. Maxwell also predicts the production of sex toys able to provide stimulation beyond anything experienced "naturally," and looks forward to a more open society in which men and women can discuss sexual pleasures as freely as they would sports and weather.*

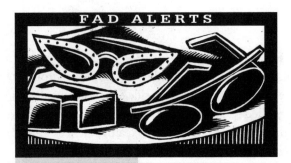

Female Condoms

 Despite its awkward look, the Reality condom (designed to be inserted in a woman's vagina) has long been a favorite of those engaging in anal sex, due to its strength and durability. A new study suggests that it may become the first choice for some couples having traditional intercourse as well. When study author David Quadagno, Ph.D., professor of biological sciences at Florida State University in Tallahassee, asked 66 women to test-drive Reality, more than half were enthusiastic about the results and almost a third continued to use it regularly. Best of all, 40 percent of their partners found it more comfortable than a standard male condom.

Love Pheromones

 At $99.50 for a sixth of an ounce, a "human pheromone" potion that you pour into your cologne to enhance your sex appeal ought to have women nibbling at you like piranha. Athena Pheromone 10x is marketed by Winnifred B. Cutler, Ph.D., a researcher who struck media gold in 1986 while working with George Preti, Ph.D., of the Monell Chemical Senses Center in Philadelphia. They discovered that a component in male underarm sweat could alter women's menstrual cycles. Dr. Cutler claims she later isolated the key pheromones, which supposedly affect sexual attractiveness.

But many don't buy it. "Absolutely nothing in that menstrual cycle research hinted at the existence of a human pheromone for attraction," says Dr. Preti.

Richard Doty, Ph.D., director of the Smell and Taste Center at the University of Pennsylvania in Philadelphia, agrees. "Believe me, there's no evidence for a bona fide attraction pheromone in humans," he says. "Save the $100 and learn how to be nice to people."

Dr. Cutler backs up her secret potion with a one-page abstract, which states that 17 men who dabbed themselves with Athena 10x found themselves in more intimate situations during an eight-week interval than 21 subjects who used a placebo. But Dr. Cutler won't provide the actual data. She maintains that it's being considered for publication by an unidentified journal, though her short abstract has already been reviewed by such groups as the American Society for Reproductive Medicine (ASRM).

"We did not see her full manuscript, and by no means does the Society endorse her product," counters Susan Klock, Ph.D., who was chairperson of the ASRM seminar at which Dr. Cutler spoke. "I have concerns about the claims she was making with such a limited study."

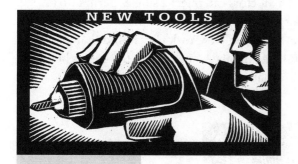

NEW TOOLS

An End to Herpes Outbreaks

Famvir

Of the 500,000 people newly infected with genital herpes every year, 80 percent go on to have regular outbreaks—as many as one a month. But a drug may actually help first-time herpes sufferers avoid recurrences. Herpes-infected mice that were immediately treated with famciclovir (Famvir), a Food and Drug Administration–approved herpes medication from SmithKline Beecham Pharmaceuticals, remained virus-free up to four months later, prompting a clinical trial in humans. "If the trial is successful, this will be an important breakthrough in the treatment of genital herpes," says Lawrence Stanberry, M.D., director of infectious diseases at Children's Hospital in Cincinnati. If you suspect you have genital herpes, ask your doctor about the Famvir trial.

Rub Away Warts

Aldara

An estimated 750,000 Americans contract genital warts (a human papillomavirus infection) every year, making it the most common sexually transmitted disease. Measures to remove the warts include acid treatments, laser surgery, and cryotherapy (which freezes them off). But now, a Food and Drug Administration–approved topical cream can clear up genital warts. Aldara, a prescription cream developed by 3M Pharmaceuticals, may help the body's immune system fight the warts, says Mary L. Owens, M.D., of 3M. A three-month regimen costs about $300.

Better Fertility Treatment

Intracytoplasmic Sperm Injection

For years, infertility specialists have been capitalizing on a single egg through in vitro fertilization techniques. Now they've found a way to make do with just one sperm—even if it's one that can't swim. Using a technique called intracytoplasmic sperm injection, doctors can inject a single sperm into an egg. In a study of 751 couples undergoing such a procedure, researchers from New York Hospital–Cornell Medical Center in New York City found that almost 40 percent went on to deliver a child. And only 2.6 percent of the babies born had any significant congenital malformation.

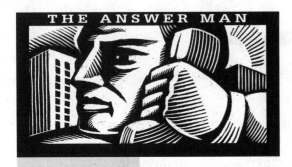

No Help for Potent Men

I've heard that the impotence pill, Viagra, can give much harder erections to men who aren't impotent. Can it? If so, send me a case.
—B. K., Charlotte, N.C.

The rumors that Viagra (sildenafil) can somehow improve a healthy erection are unfounded.

"Viagra is unquestionably the most exciting therapy for impotence that has been developed," says Harin Padma-Nathan, M.D., director of the Male Clinic and clinical associate professor of urology at the University of Southern California School of Medicine, both in Santa Monica. "But if you have normal erections, there is no room for improvement with this drug."

Viagra blocks an enzyme that causes erections to wilt, which helps impotent men become hard "naturally." If you still attain erections normally, your body chemistry doesn't need the extra help. Taking Viagra may only make your head throb; headaches were reported in about 15 percent of men who tested the drug.

"Viagra is only for men who have consistent inability to attain and maintain an erection adequate for sexual performance," Dr. Padma-Nathan emphasizes. If this description hits home, see your doctor. He can prescribe Viagra only if you have a genuine erectile problem.

Lousy Kisser

When we were breaking up, my girlfriend accused me of being a lousy kisser. She didn't offer any specifics, and now I'm self-conscious with dates. How can I figure out what my kissing is missing?
—S. W., Newport, R.I.

Hey, you were breaking up, so maybe your girlfriend wasn't being entirely fair; and short of kissing you ourselves, we can't tell you exactly what you're doing wrong. But there are a few mistakes that are pretty typical, says Patrizia DiLucchio, author of the "Sexpert" column on the Women's Wire Web site. "Some guys approach a kiss like it's an invasion," she says. "It's not erotic when somebody attempts to annex your tonsils with his tongue." Just keep your tongue in your mouth until your date wants it in hers. (Don't worry—she'll let you know.)

Another common complaint is that guys are only interested in kissing during the five minutes before they start removing a woman's clothing. If this sounds familiar, you'll enjoy kissing more if you try varying the speed (shorter and longer kisses) and pressure (softer and harder). And throw a few timid, tender kisses in with the brazen, forceful ones.

Once you've done the mouth thing, remember that there's plenty of other stuff you can kiss. Slide your lips down her body, stopping at her throat, her fingers, the nape of her neck . . . you get the idea. Expand your repertoire by occasionally sucking on her earlobe and neck. If she likes it, move on to soft biting, paying particular attention to any move that elicits happy noises. And avoid asking her for a performance evaluation. If you relax and let yourself enjoy it, your kissing will improve.

Testicular Lumps

For the last several years, I've had a protrusion on my right testicle that comes and goes. At its worst, it's nearly the size of a marble. My urologist said it's probably a damaged spermatic cord, and it's nothing to worry about. But now I am concerned it's interfering with ejaculation. Semen used to explode out of my penis, and now it just sort of oozes.
—B. L., Boulder, Colo.

"The lump you describe sounds most like an epididymal cyst, a harmless nodule that forms in the coiled tubes through which sperm pass on their way out of the testicle," says Marc Goldstein, M.D., director of the Center for Male Reproductive Medicine and Microsurgery at the New York Hospital–Cornell Medical Center in New York City. It could also be a spermatocele, a fluid-filled sac that sometimes develops adjacent to the sperm-carrying tubes; or a varicocele, which is essentially a varicose vein in the scrotum.

"None of these problems are too serious, but you should ask your urologist for a scrotal ultrasound exam to be safe," says Dr. Goldstein. This simple test uses inaudible sound waves to construct a computerized image of the testicle that your doctor can then use like an x-ray to identify the lump. He'll also be able to rule out testicular cancer, the most common cancer in men under 40.

As for the decline in ejaculation, that's more likely a natural consequence of aging than a side effect of testicular troubles.

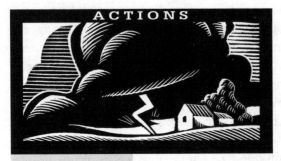

ACTIONS

If your sex life has become a bit of a bore . . . congratulations. It means you're in a long-term monogamous relationship. We commend you. But there are some easy ways to make your sex life more interesting, without taking a member of Congress to lunch. Here are 11 of them.

1. Get out of bed. If that good-night peck she gives you doesn't tilt your windmill anymore, there's a simple way to boost your arousal level: Try starting your foreplay while you're standing up. If you're like most men, blood flow to your penis will be strongest when you're in an upright position, according to Drogo K. Montague, M.D., director of the Center for Sexual Function at the Cleveland Clinic Foundation. That means your erection will make its presence known more quickly—and be stronger than usual.

2. **Use a third party.** "Everyone wants to spice up his sex life," says Marilyn Fithian, Ph.D., co-director and researcher at the Center for Marital and Sexual Studies in Long Beach, California. "The problem is that most of us are afraid of what our partners might say if we make a kinky suggestion." Her advice: Use a third party to introduce the concept. No, not those swinging next-door neighbors. Us. Instead of making the kinky suggestion yourself, just say you read it in *Men's Health Today 1999.* Here, we'll make it easy. Following are two simple phrases you can use to spark the topic. Use them; blame us.

- "Hey, honey, it says right in here in this book (point to this open page) that using sex toys during foreplay burns more calories than simply lying quietly in bed!"
- "Marge, dear, this (wave the book) claims that one thing all successful marriages have in common is light bondage (wave handcuffs). Isn't that interesting?"

3. **Look at her birth control pills.** Your partner's libido could by affected by the type of birth control pill she takes. After studying 364 college-age women, researchers found that those who were taking triphasic pills reported higher libido, more sexual fantasies, and greater pleasure from intercourse than those taking other types of oral contraceptives or no pills at all (common triphasics include Ortho-Novum 7/7/7 and Triphasil). Just don't start taking them yourself. This only works for women.

4. **Start rooting for the Bulls.** Whether as a player or a fan, competing and winning boosts testosterone production. Researchers at Georgia State University in Atlanta found this out after looking at the testosterone levels of 21 soccer fans before and after the World Cup Final. They found that the hormone levels shot up 28 percent in the winning team's fans and sank 27 percent in the losing team's sullen supporters.

5. **Shift positions.** If you're normally on top, it may be time to let her ride for awhile. This isn't just for the sake of variety. During prolonged man-on-top thrusting, you may experience "pelvic-steal syndrome," in which blood is shunted from the penis to the legs, resulting in leg cramps and, worse, weakened erections. Put her on top and you'll be more relaxed.

6. **Have dessert in bed.** "This never fails," says Dr. Fithian, who suggests this messy tip to her clients. Take a bunch of finger foods to bed and feed each other. Put down a top sheet beforehand, and avoid pomegranates.

7. **Try a new angle.** If your erections point south, it may be because of your ill-spent youth. An informal study conducted by Joseph Sparling, Ph.D., a retired researcher from the University of North Carolina in Chapel Hill, suggests that your erection's angle may result from where you "wore" your erections as a teenager. Of 110 subjects, the 46 men who'd kept their frequent teenage erections angled "up" were three times as likely to have upward-pointing erections today than were the guys who wedged Mr. Jones against their thighs. "Over time, this may have affected the suspensory ligaments and tissues that shape the erection," explains Dr. Sparling. To help things look up, always keep your spontaneous erections angled toward your stomach.

8. **Increase your strength.** You may be able to make your erections stronger by eating enough arginine, a protein building-block found in meat, beans, and fish. In a recent study, rats that received daily arginine supplements were found to have erections roughly 30 percent stronger than those that received none of the extra arginine. Researchers speculate that arginine relaxes smooth penile muscle, allowing more blood to flow into the penis and stiffening the erection.

9. **Needle for an answer.** If you are considering testosterone replacement therapy to boost your sex drive, consider requesting a needle biopsy of your prostate first. Testosterone therapy can stimulate prostate cancer. Urologists from Boston's Beth Israel Deaconess Hospital found that low testosterone levels can make tumors undetectable to your doctor's probing finger and give you a falsely low reading of your prostate-specific antigen (PSA) blood test. An increase in testosterone can cause these undiagnosed tumors to grow rapidly. So if prostate cancer runs in your family, or your previous PSA readings have ever been high, get that biopsy before you wear the patch.

10. **Go shopping.** The supermarket, depending on the time of day you "shop," offers many opportunities for meeting the opposite sex. Midmorning, expect married women. After school lets out—well, don't even think about it. Best time to meet professional women is right after work, and if you're looking for a waitress, try late, late in the evening. That's when their shifts end and they pick up the cat litter and bubble bath.

11. **Head to the local Videodrome.** Pick the right movie to attract the right female. Rules of thumb: Sharon Stone movies attract angry, unstable women. Tom Hanks movies attract sensitive, dependable women. Keanu Reeves movies attract horny undergraduate women as well as their older male professors. Oliver Stone movies don't attract women at all. Pass.

With movie in hand, approach her. Stop by her side, look down, and say: "Gee, I wonder if this is any good." "It's important that you say it to the film, not to the woman," says *Men's Health* magazine editor-at-large Denis Boyles, author of *A Man's Life: The Complete Instructions.* Then she thinks you're sincere, not scamming. And if all attempts at connecting with other human beings fail, you can just rent *Showgirls* and go home alone.

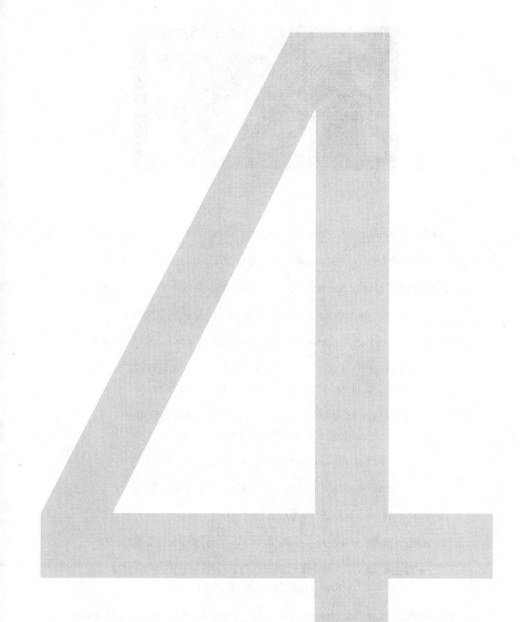

WEIGHT LOSS

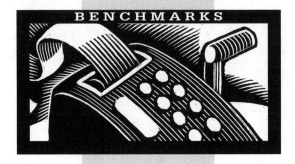

■ Number of men who underwent liposuction in a recent year: 20,192

■ Percentage of overweight or obese people who aren't dieting: 78

■ Weight increase of the average airline passenger since 1958: 20 pounds

■ Estimated annual cost of obesity in America: $100 billion

■ Medical expenses baby boomers could save by eating less fat: $68 billion annually

■ Percentage you can cut your diabetes risk if you shrink
your waist from 40 inches to 37 inches: 50

■ Number of Americans consuming low-calorie, sugar-free
foods and beverages: 144,000,000

■ Percentage of Americans on a diet in 1996: 24

■ Percentage of Americans on a diet in 1986: 37

■ Number of new reduced or low-fat products introduced in 1996: 2,076

■ Percentage of Americans who admit they need to lose weight: 60

■ Percentage of Americans who say their present diet is healthier
than it was three years ago: 71

■ Amount of money spent each year on diet products and services: $33 billion

■ Factor by which a parent's obesity increases a child's change of obesity: 2

■ Chances that an American's last family dinner was made entirely from scratch: 1 in 5

■ Percentage of Americans who engage in sports more than seven times a week: 1

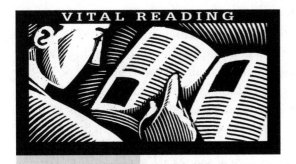

VITAL READING

Slim Down with Weights

Lose pounds by picking them up.

When it comes to weight loss, everybody has a theory, and almost nobody has the vaguest idea what he's talking about. The diet industry has hatched more schemes than any group since the Three Stooges. Today, anyone with a literary agent and a bad hairdo qualifies as a weight-loss expert, and the more complicated the diet, the more scientific people believe it is.

But losing weight has never been very complicated. (Hard, yes; complex, no). In fact, we can make it simpler than it ever has been: If you want to lose weight, lift weights.

Weight lifting may burn more calories than many aerobic activities, such as slow jogging and stationary cycling. Your body eats up about 8 to 10 calories per minute while lifting weights at a high intensity, compared with only about 7 calories a minute during a brisk walk or moderate cycling, according to Wayne Westcott, Ph.D., fitness research director at South Shore YMCA in Quincy, Massachusetts. "If you have only a limited time in a given week," he says, "concentrate on the weights. From a calorie-burning standpoint, you're better off spending your half-hour lifting weights than going for a jog."

Training with weights is also the only thing that has been proven to increase your metabolic rate so you burn more calories even when you're watching basketball. "That makes it the single most important activity you can do to maintain long-term weight loss," explains Everett Aaberg of the Cooper Fitness Center in Dallas.

In a recent study from Colorado State University in Fort Collins, researchers measured the afterburn (in other words, the rise in resting metabolic rate) associated with aerobic exercise and with an intense, 90-minute weight workout. After aerobic exercise, the resting metabolic rate returns to normal in about an hour, eating up an extra 15 to 50 calories, says Christopher Melby, Dr. P.H., one of the researchers who worked on the study. After the weight workout, though, researchers found that the subjects' metabolic rates remained elevated by 12 percent two hours later, and that they still averaged about 7 percent higher when measured the following morning—a full 15 hours postworkout!

Simply put, the more muscle you build, the more calories you burn, day and night, running or sitting. This is because lean muscle tissue is 17 to 25 times more metabolically active than fat, explains Dr. Westcott. So by adding just 2 or 3 pounds of muscle, he says, you'll force your body to burn at least an extra 70 to 100 calories every day. Consider that it takes a deficit of about 3,500 calories to lose a pound, and you're looking at losing roughly 10 pounds over the course of a year. And that's on top of the calories you burn from the actual exercise. Not bad.

Perhaps best of all, weights burn off pure body fat. Normally, when you diet, about 75 percent of the weight you lose is fat and 25 percent is muscle. Lifting weights while you diet shifts that ratio closer to 100 percent fat loss. "It's no longer just the calories expended during the exercise but also the hormonal changes that weight lifting sets off, helping you oxidize fat better while protecting your lean muscle tissue," says Dr. Melby.

Any weight routine will burn calories. But if you want to register some real numbers—the ones we're talking about here—you'll need to pump up the intensity. That's why we recommend a nonstop weight training routine that keeps your body burning calories at a rapid-fire pace. We've filled the normal downtime between weight exercises with intervals of aerobic training. The idea here is to keep your heart rate elevated throughout the workout, which is the key to an intense calorie burn.

But let us warn you. This is one killer workout. We advise that you start out with short aerobic intervals before going hog-wild. Work up slowly to our recommendations.

Now, a few more tricks to get the most out of this program.
- Concentrate on the larger muscle groups such as the chest, back, and buttocks before moving on to the smaller muscle groups.
- Alternate sets of upper- and lower-body exercises since this routine doesn't allow for any recovery time between sets. You'll have a more efficient workout if you do.
- Keep the aerobic sessions to no more than 90 seconds before going back to the weights. If you add more time to your aerobic intervals, you may not have enough energy to complete the program.
- Increase the repetitions; lighten the weights. You don't want to exhaust your muscles with heavy weight before you've had a chance to burn as many

calories as possible. Do 10 to 15 repetitions of each exercise using a weight that's a bit lighter than your usual 12-repetition maximum.

- Start with one circuit for your first week of workouts. After you've built up your stamina, then go for two.
- Use whatever activity you have available for the aerobic intervals. We offer a number of different aerobic possibilities, but if your gym is limited to just a few items, add the activities at hand.

Warmup. Never head for the weight bench without first getting your heart rate up, your blood pumping, and your muscles warm. Start by hopping on the stationary bike, pedaling moderately for a minute or two, then revving it up for five minutes. Ideally, you want to be at least on the verge of breaking a sweat by the time you get off. Without giving yourself a chance to catch your breath (or your heart rate time to slow down), move directly into the first exercise.

Squat (quadriceps, buttocks). Stand with your feet hip-width apart, holding a dumbbell in each hand. Keeping your back curved naturally and placing your weight over your heels, slowly bend your knees and lower your hips until your thighs are parallel to the floor. Then straighten up slowly. Keep your eyes focused straight ahead during the movement, with your toes pointed slightly outward. Do 12 to 15 repetitions.

Run. The second you finish your last squat, jump onto the treadmill and break into a fast run for 60 to 90 seconds. Or run in place, fast, for the same period of time.

Dumbbell bench press (chest). Lie on your back on a flat bench with your knees bent and your feet firmly on the floor. Hold one dumbbell on each side of your chest, a few inches above your shoulders, palms facing away from you. Slowly press the weights upward, extending your arms straight above your chest, but stopping before your elbows lock. As you push the weights up, rotate your wrists so your palms end up facing each other. Slowly lower the weights to the starting position. Repeat the movement 12 to 15 times. (For a good bench- and weight-free alternative, do a set of pushups.)

Jump. Get up from the bench and perform 50 rapid-fire jumping jacks (no breaks in between), or as many as you can do in 60 to 90 seconds.

Dumbbell side lunge (inner-thigh muscles and hamstrings). Hold a dumbbell in each hand and extend your arms out to your sides, with your palms facing down. Keep your feet close together, your back straight, and your head up. Step to the right as far as possible until your right thigh is almost parallel to the floor. Try to keep your left leg as straight as possible (although your left knee will naturally bend a bit). Return to the starting position. Alternate your right leg with your left. Perform 10 to 12 repetitions per side.

Climb. Drop the weights and head (quickly) for the nearest staircase or stair-climber. Run up and down a couple flights (or the machine equivalent) for 60 to 90 seconds.

Dumbbell row (back). With your left knee and hand on a weight bench and your right foot flat on the floor, grasp a dumbbell in your right hand so the weight dangles as your right arm hangs down. With your back straight and in line with the bench, lift the weight until it touches your armpit, then slowly lower it to the starting position. Do 8 to 12 repetitions, then switch sides.

Skip rope. Grab a jump rope and start moving. If you can't do 100 repetitions without a lot of tripping, stopping, and starting, then run in place for 60 to 90 seconds.

Lunge (hamstrings). Stand with your back and neck straight and your feet eight inches apart. Hold a dumbbell in each hand, with your palms facing toward your body. Keeping the dumbbells at your sides, take a large step forward with your right foot. As you do this, your left knee should almost touch the floor. The toes of your left foot should not leave the floor, and your right knee shouldn't extend beyond your right foot. Step back to the original position. Repeat the exercise with your left leg. Do 12 to 15 repetitions per side.

Bike. Hop on a stationary bike and really jam on those pedals for 60 to 90 seconds.

Military press (shoulders). Sit on a bench and hold a pair of dumbbells in front of your chest, elbows at your sides, with your palms facing away. Slowly lift the weights to shoulder height, then press them straight above your head, stopping just before your elbows lock. At the top of the movement, the weights should be shoulder-width apart. Lower them to shoulder height. Do 12 to 15 repetitions.

Run. Do a few quick laps around the gym. If you don't have the space, run in place, lifting your knees as high as you can.

Pullup (upper back, triceps). Grip a pullup bar with your hands about 18 to 20 inches apart. Your fingers should be facing toward you and wrapped tightly around the bar. Pull yourself up, and try to raise your chin above the bar. Then return slowly to the starting position. Do not swing while doing the exercise. Shoot for six to eight repetitions.

Jump. Whip off another 100 jumping jacks.

Barbell triceps extensions (triceps). Lie on your back on a bench with your head resting on the bench, your feet on the floor. Hold a barbell with your hands roughly six inches apart and your palms facing up. If possible, have a helper hand you the bar once you're on the bench. Press the bar to arms' length above your shoulders. This is the starting position. Now bend your elbows and lower the bar in a semicircular motion toward, but never touching, your forehead. Return to the starting position and repeat the movement 12 to 15 times.

Step. March quickly up and down a single step (or a step bench) for 60 to 90 seconds.

Calf raise (calves). Holding a dumbbell at your left side with your palm in, step up on a stable platform high enough so your heels hang off the edge and your weight is supported by the balls of your feet. (One of the steps from aerobics class will do.) Place your right hand against a wall or stationary object for support. Tuck your right foot behind your left heel. With both your head and back straight, rise up on the toes of your left foot. Hold the position for a moment, then return to the original position. Do 12 to 15 repetitions, then change to your right leg, with the dumbbell in your right hand.

Pedal. Hop on the bike for 60 to 90 seconds.

Crunch (abdominals). Lie on your back with your knees bent and suspended in the air and your feet crossed at the ankles. Rest your hands gently behind your head. Keeping your head tucked slightly, slowly curl your upper body toward your legs until your shoulder blades are four to six inches off the floor. Hold this position for a couple seconds. Do 15 of these crunches. Then do 15 bringing your right elbow toward your left knee, followed by 15 bringing your left elbow toward your right knee.

Unlock the Secret to Weight Control

Melt fat and feel great all day with these tips.

We're eating less and getting fatter.

The statistics are in: According to the Centers for Disease Control and Prevention, 32 percent of American men are schlepping around potbellies, an all-time high. Government researchers blame Western sit-on-duff syndrome, but there's another, less obvious reason: our obsession with low-fat, high-carbohydrate eating.

It might go against a lot of nutritional information you've heard before, but the fact is that the high-starch, low-fat, low-fiber diet we've been hooked on since the 1980s is the biggest nutritional fraud ever foisted on the American public. We continue to shovel down pasta, bagels, and other processed carbohydrates, many without a lick of fat, and we continue to grow fatter. Worse, we're also stuffing our kids full of these potentially fattening "health foods." Children in the 1990s consume, on average, 20 percent less food than kids did in the 1960s. But, like us, they're fatter.

But while everyone is screaming about the obesity epidemic in this country, there's one factor that many forget: Four billion people around the world perfectly control their weight. In central China, you'd be hard-pressed to find anyone with a body fat percentage higher than that of a marathoner. A Cornell University study showed that even sedentary Chinese office workers weighed 20 pounds less than their American counterparts—though they ate 30 percent more calories!

The difference? The Chinese know how to eat. They innately practice perfect weight control (how do you think their population grew so large?), through foods passed down to them over the millennia and with ingredients that control their moods and their waistlines.

With a little planning and resolve, you can do the same. Here are some tips that will turn on the natural fat-burning engines in your body and keep your spirits and mental energies high.

Keep your hormones in check. The most likely reason that you are overweight is not too many calories but too much insulin. Insulin, the hormone that regulates blood sugar levels, is up to 30 times more effective at turning extra calories into fat than it is at turning them into muscle. The key to staying slim is to control your insulin levels. When you eat foods high in sugar or starch, your blood sugar (glucose) level surges. Your body reacts by raising your insulin level; insulin then turns all the extra glucose into fat, which quickly migrates to your gut. That's why the combination of fat and starch—such as steak and potatoes—is so incredibly fattening.

Pitch the bagels. If you're exercising and eating a low-fat diet but you're still not losing weight, maybe it's time to wipe bagels, Cream of Wheat, instant rice, and soft pretzels off your grocery list. These refined carbohydrates—although filling for the moment—cause a surge in blood glucose and, consequently, insulin. What's worse, after the insulin surge abates, you're famished. You'll quickly crave another high-glucose meal.

Check out some oatmeal. Replace high-glucose starches with low-glucose carbohydrates, which don't cause an insulin gush. Fruits, vegetables, beans, and especially grainy cereals are absorbed slowly into your bloodstream, and they'll make you feel full. They're perfect foods—no insulin surge, no overeating.

Forget you ever heard of "carbo loading." Stuffing yourself with starchy grains for sustained energy gained popularity in the 1980s. Now most Americans carbo-load every day. It has helped make our youth the fattest generation ever. If you regularly run marathons, you may burn off the truckloads of fat that a high-calorie, high-carbohydrate diet produces. If you don't, you won't.

Ease off on the sugar. The U.S. Department of Agriculture estimates that the average American consumes almost a cup of sugar a day. The starches you eat are already being broken down into sugar, so don't add any to your cereal, and watch the spoonfuls you toss in coffee. More sugar means more glucose, which means more insulin, which means tighter pants.

Rein in the pasta. Pasta isn't a bad food, but a diet that includes too much of it can quickly cause our glucose and insulin levels—and weight—to rise. If you're hooked on that nightly bowl of capellini, try eating whole-wheat pasta, which has some fiber and won't go down as fast as white-flour pastas.

Feed your head. Most of the time, we aren't seeking a sugar high when we eat that afternoon bagel or chocolate bar. We're seeking a serotonin high. Serotonin is one of the most important chemicals among the brain's mood neurotransmitters. It causes a calm, sated, "feeling-groovy" effect. Quickly digested foods such as white-flour breads, bagels, muffins, and snack foods cause your serotonin levels to rise in minutes. They're the dietary equivalent of jet fuel. But the inevitable crash quickly sets you on the prowl for another feeding.

Conversely, slowly digested carbs, such as whole-wheat bread, oatmeal, soybeans, or bran cereal, will stop your blood sugar from diving and consequently measure out your serotonin rush over several hours. Keep some high-fiber foods in your office to nosh on at stressful moments.

Charge your body. Another neurotransmitter you can influence through diet is dopamine. It creates mental energy, vigilance, and alertness. As your brain's dopamine neurons light up, you can feel yourself becoming more positive, growing more buoyant, even cheerful. The best way to keep dopamine levels high is to eat low-fat, high-protein foods. They're rich in the amino acid tyrosine, the key building block of dopamine. Soy products are especially good. Cheeses are also densely packed with tyrosine—two ounces of skim mozzarella provides more tyrosine (794 milligrams) than two ounces of beef, chicken, or fish.

Seek out hard stuff. Hard foods make hard bodies. This is one of the most effective strategies for weight loss. Food that is hard to chew and slow to be digested will kill your hunger, cut your glucose load, and turn off the hormones that make you fat. Think bulgur, fiber, hard beans.

In fact, inhale beans. Hard beans of any type—pinto, soy, tepary, mung—are true superfoods. They're high in fiber, low in fat, and packed with protein.

Don't go hungry. How do dictators get prisoners to talk? They starve them. Depriving yourself of calories will make you depressed, mentally worthless, and eventually fatter. Researchers have found that dieting wrecks reaction time and mental calculations, and can cause sleep disorders and loss of libido. So eat regularly to stay sharp—and prevent bingeing. Regular meals will stabilize your insulin, maintain your energy levels, and help you lose fat—if you build them around high-fiber, low-calorie foods.

Eat bulky food. Quench your appetite with roughage. For instance, four pounds of cucumbers would leave you feeling ready to explode, yet you would have eaten only 324 calories. An entire plate of vegetables is very satisfying and less than 200 calories. Add high-bulk foods to every meal—zucchini or broccoli, spinach, cantaloupe, or peaches—and pounds will begin to drop off.

Lose Weight Fast

Running the right workouts is a great way to burn fat.

Running to lose weight makes perfect sense. After all, aren't runners some of the leanest athletes on the planet? This was my brother's logic when he decided to drop some excess poundage a while back. But after two months of regular dates with the track, trail, and treadmill, he was deeply discouraged.

"I haven't lost a pound," he told me. "How can this be?"

"Four words," I said. "Bill . . . Clinton . . . runs . . . too."

My brother's problem—and a problem for many people who turn to running to lose weight—is that it's not as simple as it looks. Sure, an easy quarter-mile run to the Golden Arches is a better workout than nothing at all; but as our First Jogger has already proven, it isn't nearly enough to burn off the calories you consume when you get there. If you want to lose serious weight, you have to do some serious workouts.

Now, I'm not going to tell you to run yourself into the ground, but you are going to have to stress your body. And unless you're utterly couch-bound, that's going to take more than a leisurely 20-minute jog. If you're running to lose body fat, you have to make sure your workouts produce a caloric deficit—that you're burning up more calories than you're taking in each day. The harder you run, the more calories you burn per minute. The longer you run, the more total calories you burn per workout. Combine the two, and you'll maximize your weight loss.

Of course, if you're new to running—or if your last run was during the Carter administration—you'll need to ease into this program with a combination of walking and running, preferably with your doctor's okay. Once you're able to run continuously for 30 minutes or so at a moderate pace, you should be ready to try one of the following workouts.

That said, getting up to speed is well worth the effort. You do the math. To lose one pound, you need to burn roughly 3,500 calories (and not replace them with an entire sausage-and-pepperoni pie). To compensate for your caloric deficit, your body is forced to burn a pound of stored fat. For the average 170-pound man, running 30 minutes at a good clip (seven minutes per mile) burns about 540 calories. If he keeps at it every other day for two weeks, there goes a pound of fat. Twenty weeks: 10 pounds. And if he occasionally runs longer or faster, he'll lose even more weight.

Of course, running isn't the only way to burn calories. It's just the fastest and most efficient way. Even an easy run burns 383 calories in 30 minutes. Compare that with 30 minutes of easy swimming (306 calories) or easy cycling (230) or walking (a mere 134). Add up that 153-calorie-per-day gap between running and cycling, and, in a month or two, you're looking at the difference between down-sizing your waist measurement or giving in to elastic-waist chinos to accommo-date the paunch you couldn't lose.

The running workouts that follow are the best at burning calories and helping you burn fat. Do two or three a week. On the other days, run easy for 20 to 30 minutes or spend the time cycling, lifting weights, or playing sports. You'll lose weight if you combine these special workouts with a sensible eating program.

Tempo run. When you're pressed for time and have just 20 to 30 minutes to run, pick up the pace. "The faster you run in those 30 minutes, the more fat you'll burn because your total energy cost is up," says Ken Sparks, Ph.D., an exercise physiologist at Cleveland State University and coauthor of *The Runners Book of Training Secrets.*

Run 20 to 30 minutes at a pace that makes you breathe hard but doesn't ex-haust you—the effort should feel fast but controlled. This is known as a tempo run, a time-efficient way to burn as many calories as possible in a short workout. Just remember to jog five minutes to warm up, and jog five minutes afterward to cool down.

The skinny: A 30-minute tempo run can burn more than 450 calories for a 170-pound man.

Speedwork. Ever wonder why sprinters are so lean? For one thing, speed burns, baby. Fast running creates a calorie-burning fire in your belly that stays stoked long after you've showered and your date is on your arm.

When you're pressed for time, a short, fast run will stoke your calorie-burning furnace much more than a slow run in the same amount of time. In fact, scientists at the University of Texas have found that fast running burns up to one-third more fat per minute than slow running.

Try this: After a five-minute warmup jog, run one to three minutes at 85 to 95 percent effort (very fast but not all-out). Then walk or jog the same amount of time to recover. Do 5 to 10 of these fast intervals in a session, then finish with a five-minute cooldown run. Speedwork also produces an afterburn effect. That is, you keep burning calories at a high level even after you've stopped running. And running fast suppresses your appetite for an hour or two, so you'll eat less and burn more.

The skinny: A speed workout that includes eight of these 2-minute intervals at 90 percent effort burns 386 calories in only 32 minutes. Add a 5-minute warmup and cooldown, include the afterburn, and a 170-pound man will use up about 500 calories in 42 minutes.

Long run. When you have a little more time to spend, a long, slow, running workout is a great way to recharge your batteries and keep your weight-loss program on track. When weight loss is the goal, run steadily at a pace where you can carry on a conversation for at least 45 minutes, or even longer if you can—60 to 90 minutes would be optimal.

If you're out of shape and have trouble sustaining a run for 45 minutes, you can still burn a boatload of calories with a long, slow workout. Just run at an easy pace for as long as you can, and slow down to a brisk walk when you need to catch your breath. Walk until you've recovered, then speed up to a slow jog. Even if you do more walking than jogging on your first few runs, you'll gradually build up enough endurance to run for 45 minutes straight.

The skinny: A 90-minute run for a 170-pound man can burn more than 1,000 calories.

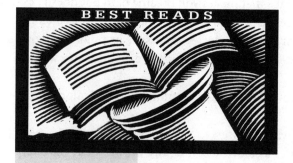

BEST READS

Developing Willpower

Losing weight is all about choices: Choosing the chicken sandwich over the burger, the fresh fruit over the pecan pie, one glass of wine instead of three. Sounds simple, but if it was, we'd all be walking around with the midsections we had when we were 18. In this excerpt from Break the Weight-Loss Barrier *(Prentice Hall, 1997), authors Jim Meschino and Barry Simon show you how to develop the willpower that is necessary to make the right choices. Their advice won't give you willpower overnight, but it will empower you to make the best choices for the rest of your life.*

Probably the most underrated technique to change how we feel and think is to act differently—to make a conscious decision to change. Nowhere is this technique more successful than in a wellness program. Exercising, eating healthful foods, and taking vitamin supplements build a sense of confidence, well-being, and certainty. By actively choosing small tasks, we avoid two of the typical health promotion failure situations:

- Blindly accepting someone else's health plan—either the latest diet, prepared foods, or weight-loss clinic.
- The passive sense of helplessness that there is nothing we can do to help ourselves.

Both of these situations fail to develop our willpower—our own ability to direct, not impose, a way of life on ourselves.

Two things can develop your willpower: 15-minute commitments and action.

15 Minutes at a Time

Forever is a long time, but you can manage 15 minutes! When you decide to make a final and absolute change, each failure will make you feel resentful, angry, and disappointed.

Instead, make a 15-minute commitment. Every time you successfully complete a commitment, you build the foundation of your success story. You will also feel differently about yourself. Once you gain a sense of trust, you can move to a 30-minute, hour-long, or morning, afternoon, or daily commitment. Move slowly. Each successful commitment block is a powerful moment of building your willpower.

Lights, Camera, Action

Your ability to direct your actions is like a muscle. The more you use it, the stronger it becomes. By taking even small steps, you show yourself that you can succeed. Doing something—anything—proves that you can be in control if you choose to. Small things such as walking away from a buffet or rushing to an exercise class increase your sense of dedication and commitment.

Often the act of doing something that a part of you doesn't want to do also frees up your inner energy. Committing yourself to action can shift you from a passive, helpless mindset to a motivated, enthusiastic one. This higher-energy mental state fuels future successful actions. Remember, no action is too small to help you move from despair.

Indecision can be more painful than actually choosing. Try this experiment when you have an urge that is filled with indecision: simply go with the clearest action. For example, if you are caught between a desire for a treat and what you should do on your health plan, simply take a deep breath and pick up the treat. Let it settle into your hand and see how you feel about it. Examine it, take a deep breath, and see how you feel. Don't rush to eat, but experience it. Decide on your next action.

One of the most powerful will-builders is to do something you don't want to do and to do it every day. For example, if you don't feel like exercising, exercise. Set a reasonable goal, even if it means compromising your typical workout, but get out there and see what happens. Use this technique next time you encounter a task that you dislike, one for which your automatic response is, "I'll do it later." Instead of feeling burdened or forced, feel free because you chose to do the activity.

Commit yourself to completing one chosen task every day. Note how you feel about yourself before and after you do it. Checking how you predict you'll feel and how you actually feel are important parts of gaining a more successful, confident you. You may find that your feelings are more positive and more energetic. For example: "Before the workout I felt tired, run down, not interested, and could barely get up the four steps of the change room. Not short of breath, just short of enthusiasm." Afterwards: "I have a burst of energy. Great!" By acknowledging your achievements, you will also boost your self-confidence. The fastest, most effective way to overcome negative feelings is to commit yourself to doing something. Make it a reasonable goal. Don't wait to feel energized every day or to feel enthusiastic. Do something, and your enthusiasm and energy will follow.

The program in *Break the Weight-Loss Barrier* provides you with many choices. As you go through the program, decide what you can commit yourself to doing and make a 15-minute plan. Take the approach that any new action, any change in the way that you are, is a positive event. The accumulation of these small, realistic events will build your positive self-image and direct your successful journey to health and fitness.

Sensible Weight Loss

Despite all of the gimmicks on the market that would have you believe otherwise, losing weight is not complicated. Eat sensibly and exercise, and any extra pounds should come off with time. But there is more to it than that. Donna Raskin and Brian Paul Kaufman provide some helpful tips to make sure your weight loss is permanent in this excerpt from Vitamin Vitality: Use Nature's Power to Attain Optimal Health *(Rodale Press, 1997).*

Remember crash diets? They were fine if you were a crash-test dummy. But for flesh-and-blood men, they didn't work.

The pattern went like this: You'd eat nothing but the occasional grapefruit or dollop of cottage cheese. You'd walk around for a few days feeling weak, deprived, and crabby. Then you'd quit the diet in frustration and dive into a three-day pizza and ice cream binge. In the long run, you didn't lose weight . . . you lost friends.

Even if you had the willpower to stick to a deprivation diet long enough to lose a few pounds, you'd be making a big mistake. Your bodily systems will not function without the nutrients that come with regular, sensible eating, nutrition experts say. This leads us to a weight-loss rule you'll love: Make sure that you get enough to eat.

Very low calorie diets are out—way out. Modern man has evolved to a more satisfying way of eating to lose or maintain weight. "Men need more calories than women, in general, to get all the nutrients they need. A man must make sure that he consumes enough while on a weight-loss program," says Gail Frank, R.D., Dr. P.H., professor of nutrition at California State University, Long Beach, and nutritional epidemiologist. So eating moderately, in a nutritionally balanced way, is the key to successful weight loss, she says. Besides, if you eat enough food to prevent feeling deprived, it will be easier to keep up your healthier eating habits over the long haul.

Here are some tips to help you lose the pounds you want without losing vital nutrients.

Make every calorie count. Vitamins and minerals do not help you lose weight faster, but they are important in your weight-loss program. "Vitamins and minerals help in the metabolism of fat, carbohydrate, and protein. If you aren't getting enough of these nutrients because of your weight-loss plan, you run the very real risk of interfering with these functions," says Dr. Frank. Many vitamins and minerals help each other get absorbed better, too. So to make every calorie count, don't just fill your gut—choose foods that are packed with these nutrients.

Do the math. So how many calories do you have to consume in order to get enough nutrients and still lose weight? There's a formula that you can use to determine the lowest number of calories you should allow, says Leslie Bonci, R.D., nutritionist at the University of Pittsburgh Medical Center and dietitian for the NFL's Pittsburgh Steelers and University of Pittsburgh athletics department. "Men should multiply their weight in pounds by 11," she says. That means that a 180-pound man should consume at least 1,980 calories a day. You can usually take in about 200 calories above this number and still lose weight, says Bonci, who also is a spokesperson for the American Dietetic Association (ADA). Height, activity level, and various health conditions also play a factor, so if you are looking for an exact caloric plan, it's best to be evaluated by a dietitian.

Diversify your assets. Make variety your dietary motto. "There are so many low-fat and fat-free choices of vegetables, fruits, and grains available in today's supermarkets, it's easier than ever to keep your vitamin and mineral sources interesting and diverse," says Bonci. If getting variety into your regular meals is hard for you to arrange, eat lots of different fruits and vegetables as snacks throughout the day. Then you can eat smaller portions of your usual fare at mealtime.

Ponder a multi-pill. If you're restricting the calories you consume to lose weight, you may want to consider taking a multivitamin/mineral supplement, but only as an addition to a nutritious diet. "They are called supplements and not substitutes for a reason. Relying on supplements to take care of your micronutrient needs is like putting an adhesive bandage on a gaping wound," says Bonci. It won't replace eating the complex arrangements of nutrients found in healthy foods. A supplement can, however, act as nutritional insurance in case you accidentally fall short of any of your essential nutrients from one day to the next.

Accelerate the process. It all seems like a frustrating catch-22: You want to lose weight, but to prevent wrecking your body in the process you have to keep up your nutrient consumption, which means eating. This means more calories, which get stored as body fat if they aren't burned up.

If you want to accelerate the weight-loss process, then shave off those excess calories by stepping up your physical activity. "You can achieve your weight-loss goals and nutritional goals at the same time and obtain other health benefits by incorporating exercise into your moderate-calorie weight-management plan," says Dr. Frank. Exercising will increase the amount of calories your body burns throughout the day, not just when you are working out. A very low calorie diet won't do that for you.

Contrary to one popular myth, exercise has no effect on vitamin or mineral absorption in men. "Exercise does affect how the body uses fat, protein, and carbohydrate; but it does not affect the body's use of vitamins and minerals," says Anne Dubner, R.D., a dietitian in Houston who has worked with the NFL's Houston Oilers and is a spokesperson for the ADA.

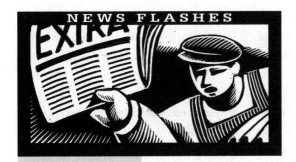

Small Weight Loss Brings Big Drop in Blood Pressure

JACKSON, Miss.—If you have high blood pressure, dropping just a few pounds can yield far-reaching benefits. In a study of 102 people with severe high blood pressure, researchers at the University of Mississippi Medical Center found that people with high blood pressure who lost an average of seven pounds reduced their need for medication for more than two years. The patients maintained their weight loss only for 6 to 12 months, but the benefits were sustained for as long as 30 months. Maintaining a healthy blood pressure with less medication could mean fewer side effects, so ask your doctor about reducing your drug regimen after you lose weight.

Low-Fat Diet Can Reduce Muscle-Friendly Testosterone

UNIVERSITY PARK, Pa.—Lowering your fat intake is generally a good thing. It helps you lose the love handles, corral the cholesterol levels, and win knowing glances from those women in Bally's commercials. But Pennsylvania State University researchers have found that extremely low fat diets can reduce testosterone—almost to preadolescent levels. If you want to build more strength and muscle mass, you may want to keep just a little lard in your diet. The researchers monitored the diets and hormone levels of a group of resistance trainers for 17 days. "The subjects with the lowest fat intakes had the lowest testosterone levels," says researcher Jeff Volek, R.D.

How low is low? "You start seeing real changes when the fat intake drops to about 10 percent," he says. It's worse if you're overtraining, because you're already sapping your testosterone levels. Adopt a draconian no-fat diet and you compound the problem. This can ultimately hamper your immune system, endurance capacity, and ability to build muscle. Eat healthfully, but try to keep your fat levels between 20 and 30 percent of your diet, says Volek.

Exercise Sheds Less Fat as Men Age

ST. LOUIS—As they age, men burn less fat during strenuous exercise. Researchers at Washington University School of Medicine discovered this clue to why men become flabbier over the years. In a study, older men and younger men rode stationary bicycles for one hour, and though both groups burned roughly equal calories, researchers found that the gray-haired cyclists mainly metabolized carbohydrates for energy as the younger men oxidized fat. Men in their fifties and sixties may have to work out longer to stay trim, but sticking to a regular exercise schedule throughout your life will help maintain a higher fat-burning ratio.

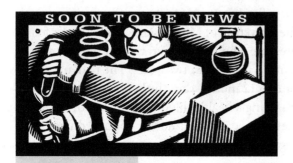

Weight Loss from the Survival Instinct?

Experts at the Scripps Research Institute and Salk Institute in La Jolla, California, have discovered a brain hormone that suppresses appetite in humans and animals. Urocortin is usually released during fight-or-flight situations so hunger pangs won't get in the way of survival. Tests are being conducted to determine the effects of urocortin injections in rats.

Pharmaceutical companies are hoping this will pave the way toward safe and effective appetite-suppressant drugs.

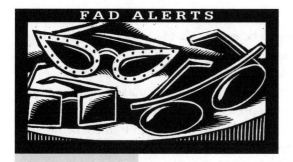

Body Fat Monitors

 We all own bathroom scales, but they won't show how fit we are (neither will a gut-sucking squint at the bathroom mirror). The best measure is your percentage of body fat, but it's not as if you can measure that every morning, right? Well, the people who make the Tanita TBF-515 Body Fat Monitor Scale say you can. Simply step on the device as you would an ordinary bathroom scale; it shoots an undetectable electrical signal through you, then displays a body fat reading along with your weight.

The fancy name for this is "bioelectrical impedance," which measures the different ways that fat and muscle resist electricity. The method is used in many clinics, and it has a margin of error of about 2.5 to 4 percent, notes John Porcari, Ph.D., of the department of exercise and sports science at the University of Wisconsin in La Crosse. That's pretty darn close, especially considering our waistlines. But Dr. Porcari points out that underwater weighing can pin down the blubber number within 1.5 to 2 percent, so don't take bioelectrical impedance as gospel. The readings can be skewed by hydration levels, too. "If you sweat a lot or drink a lot of water, it may throw off your body fat measurement," he says.

Weight Control Shield

 The Weight Control Shield is just about the lamest lose-weight-fast gizmo we've ever seen. It's an orthodontically fitted mouthpiece that covers the taste buds on the roof of your mouth, so you can't enjoy the taste of food. "That's a better way to lose weight than dieting, exercising, and all those kinds of things," says company president Terry Weber. Sure, Terry, except that "those kinds of things" don't cost $300 to $500 or require a couple of dentist trips.

"This is one of the most screwball ideas I've ever heard," says John Renner, M.D., president of the Consumer Health Information Resource Center in Independence, Missouri. "Taste is only a small part of appetite control, so I doubt this will have any effect." Guys—if you really want a cheap and easy way to remove the taste from food, have dinner at the in-laws'.

Chromium Picolinate

Most guys don't have iron deficiencies. That is, until they screw around with chromium picolinate. A preliminary study at the U.S. Department of Agriculture Human Nutrition Research Center in Grand Forks, North Dakota, found that men taking 200 micrograms of the popular supplement—believing that it lowers body fat while preserving muscle—had iron deficiencies within two months. "The chromium picolinate binds with transferrin, the substance that transports iron in the blood," says Henry Lukaski, Ph.D., director of the research team. "This may cause iron to be knocked out of the body."

That brings us to the other problem: The supplement is worthless. "Chromium picolinate has absolutely no effect on reducing body fat or building muscle," says research chemist David Milne, Ph.D., also of the Human Nutrition Research Center. "It's a complete waste of money. The manufacturers say to exercise regularly, eat healthfully, and take chromium picolinate. They're right about the first two."

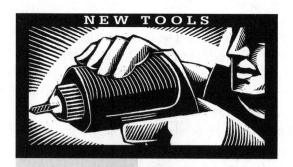

Safer Weight-Loss Drug

Meridia

When fenfluramine (a key ingredient in the diet drug fen-phen) was implicated in heart-valve problems last year, drug companies hunted for alternatives. A new, safer anti-obesity drug, Meridia, was recently approved by the Food and Drug Administration. Meridia (sibutramine hydrochloride monohydrate) enhances the effect of serotonin, a brain chemical that affects hunger. "Unlike fenfluramine, this new drug doesn't appear to pose dangers to the heart, although it can raise blood pressure," says Allan Geliebter, Ph.D., of St. Luke's–Roosevelt Hospital Center in New York City. Like fen-phen, it's only for seriously obese people and those with weight-related diseases such as diabetes. "Unless you change your lifestyle, the weight lost with Meridia will likely be regained," adds Dr. Geliebter.

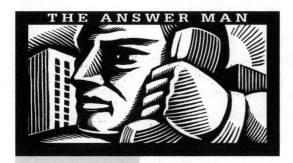

THE ANSWER MAN

Can't Go Wrong with Fruit

I'm trying to lose weight, and I've recently switched to fruit as my regular snack. A co-worker told me that grapes are among the highest-calorie fruits due to their high sugar content, and I've heard that bananas should be avoided because they're too starchy. So what should I eat?
—A. L., Charlottesville, Va.

"Grapes and bananas may have more calories than other fruits, but they're still far better than most other snacks," says Elaine Turner, R.D., Ph.D., assistant professor of food science and human nutrition at the University of Florida in Gainesville. For example, a can of soda and a bag of chips contain roughly 300 calories, 10 to 12 grams of fat, and hardly any nutrients. A handful of grapes and bottled water, on the other hand, ring up only about 100 calories, and quite a few vitamins and minerals. Just this one change, made daily over the course of a year, could be worth almost 20 pounds of weight loss, says Dr. Turner.

As far as fruits go, citrus fruits and melons contain the fewest calories because of their high water content. But we recommend eating a variety. "The bottom line," says Turner, "is that all fruits are nutritious and virtually fat-free."

Separating Fact from Myth

I've read that exercising twice a day for 15 minutes can help me lose flab. But I've also heard that the body doesn't start burning fat until you've been working out for more than 20 minutes. Will two 15-minute workouts help?
—L. K., St. Louis

The idea that it takes 20 minutes to start burning fat is a myth, says Alan Mikesky, Ph.D., director of the human performance and biomechanics laboratory at Indiana University–Purdue University at Indianapolis. Of the calories you burn during the first 20 minutes of exercise, a greater proportion may come from stored carbohydrate than from fat. However, the difference isn't significant.

Studies suggest that in low-intensity exercise, about 47 percent of the calories burned during the first 20 minutes come from fat and 53 percent come from carbohydrates. After 20 minutes, those percentages are reversed.

If losing fat is your goal, just focus on burning as many calories as possible. Whether those calories come from fat or carbohydrate isn't that important since both are burned for energy and excess calories in either form end up as excess fat on your body. "Assuming intensity level is equal, you'll burn as many calories with two 15-minute workouts as with one of 30 minutes," Dr. Mikesky says.

Home Testing

Is there a way I can figure out my body-fat percentage without going someplace to have it tested?
—A. G., Fort Collins, Colo.

You can get a rough estimate by giving yourself a skin-fold test, says G. Michael Steelman, M.D., chairman of the board of the American Society of Bariatric Physicians in Englewood, Colorado. This won't be anywhere near as accurate as having the measurement taken by a professional, he emphasizes, but it will give you an idea of whether your body-fat percentage is higher than it should be. Here's what to do.

• Find a millimeter ruler, and take off your shirt.
• Pinch a diagonal fold of skin at your chest, halfway between your shoulder crease and nipple. Measure the thickness of the fold in millimeters.
• Pinch a vertical fold of skin at the front of your thigh, halfway between your hip and knee, and measure that one, too.
• Pinch a vertical fold of skin at your abdomen, about an inch to the side of your belly button, and measure that.
• Add all three measurements together and see the chart below.

"A measurement of more than 20 percent could indicate an elevated health risk," says Dr. Steelman. "Check with your doctor and use a more sophisticated method to verify those results. Underwater weighing and bioelectrical impedance, which uses a mild electrical current to determine lean-to-fat ratio, are two of the more accurate methods that may be used."

Total (mm)	Body Fat (%)
8–19	2–4
20–34	5–9
35–67	10–20
68–85	21–24
86–100	25–28

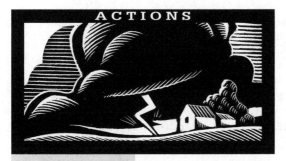

Despite an endless parade of products that promise quick ways to drop pounds without sacrificing an extravagant lifestyle, the best way to shed excess weight remains lifestyle modification. There's no need to be scared off by that phrase. It's actually a simple process. A little change here, a little change there, and before you know it, the pounds will be falling off. Here are some tips to achieve daily changes that will lead to a lifetime of manageable weight control.

1. Include some fat in your diet. If your new crash diet entails eating nothing but fat-free foods, rethink your strategy. Study subjects who replaced 20 percent of their fat intake with fat substitutes (such as Olestra) were not only ravenous by day's end but they also stuffed down almost twice their normal quota of fat-laden foods the next day. That's because fake fat fools your taste buds, not your stomach. "Real fat slows down digestion, but fat substitutes don't," explains Stanley Segall, Ph.D., professor of nutrition at Drexel University in Philadelphia. The result: You're hungry sooner after eating. "If you try to eliminate every morsel of fat from your diet, you may end up craving high-fat foods," says Dr. Segall. A low-fat diet is smart, but trying to subsist on Kate Moss rations will have you hunting cheeseburgers at 2:00 A.M.

2. Go fish. Slim down without cutting back by eating a salmon steak instead of that burger. A preliminary study suggests that substituting fish oil for other dietary fat may improve the body's handling of fat. When subjects consumed five grams of fish oil in place of six grams of other fat for three weeks, they lost nearly two pounds of fat, or three times more than their non-fish-consuming counterparts.

3. Stop and smell the fruit. In a study by the Smell and Taste Treatment and Research Foundation in Chicago, more than 3,000 overweight subjects were given aromatic inhalers laden with the scents of bananas, apples, and peppermint. The subjects were told to take a whiff whenever they felt hungry, but otherwise to eat and exercise as they always did. After six months, they lost an average of five pounds.

4. **Aim for three grams or less.** "If you're looking at food labels, one rule of thumb is that if it has three grams of fat or less per serving, that would be acceptable," says Wayne C. Miller, Ph.D., assistant professor of kinesiology at Indiana University in Bloomington. "Not that you're never going to have anything that has more fat in it, but that's a good rule to follow."

5. **Don't let size fool you.** Even if you're strict about following the three-gram rule, "you can get into trouble with quantities," says Paul R. Thomas, Ed.D., a staff scientist with the Food and Nutrition Board of the National Academy of Sciences in Washington, D.C. Suppose you're eating low-fat ice cream and the single serving size is a half-cup. Don't routinely scarf down a pint at one time and then wonder why you haven't lost weight.

6. **Add spice to your life.** Spicy condiments such as hot peppers, horseradish, and chili powder serve double duty in the fight against fat. They fill you up more quickly and they speed up your metabolic rate. So if you're looking for something quick and easy to spice up that drab grilled chicken breast, forget the salt and try this: Stir a small amount of chili powder, cumin, and chopped cucumber and green onions into nonfat sour cream or plain yogurt.

7. **Take it easy.** The best way to lose weight is to do it slowly, says John P. Foreyt, Ph.D., director of the Nutrition Research Clinic at Baylor College of Medicine in Houston and coauthor of *Living without Dieting.*

"Whatever you weigh today, you can lose about 10 percent without a whole lot of difficulty," says Dr. Foreyt. "A 200-pound man can drop to about 180 and then maintain that reasonably well. If you get much lower than that, it becomes harder."

According to C. Everett Koop, M.D., the former U.S. Surgeon General, whose Shape Up America campaign encourages people to lose weight and be more physically active, weight loss should be taken about 10 pounds at a time. "If you come down from 220 to 210 and you hold it there for about six months, then it's pretty easy to do the next 10," he says. "It's pretty difficult to lose 10 pounds and then start right over next week and say 'I'm going to lose 10 more.'"

8. **Pack it.** It's hard to eat healthy meals when you're dependent on the company cafeteria or the fast-food joint down the road. To take control of your noontime meal, make lunch a B.Y.O. affair. Bringing a sandwich, some fruit, and maybe pretzels or low-fat yogurt can save you from putting on the pounds.

9. **Run with it.** Dried fruits such as raisins, dates, and apricots are perfect for the man on the move. "They're concentrated in calories, and they're loaded with vitamins and minerals," says Chris Rosenbloom, Ph.D., associate professor in the department of nutrition and dietetics at Georgia State University and nutrition consultant for the Georgia Tech Athletic Association, both in Atlanta. "I always encourage people to keep some in their desk drawers or, for students, in their backpacks."

10. **Forget the fries.** A burger and fries. They go together like Abbott and Costello. But for your health's sake, it would be better if they were more like Dean Martin and Jerry Lewis—ex-partners.

"A large order of fries is almost like having two sandwiches," says Bonnie Liebman, a licensed nutritionist and director of nutrition for the Center for Science in the Public Interest in Washington, D.C. "We think of it as a side dish, but it's really as fatty and caloric as a main dish. Large fries have 450 calories, compared with 420 in a Quarter Pounder at McDonald's. And the fries have 22 grams of fat, compared with 20 in the Quarter Pounder."

11. **Travel light.** Airports aren't exactly bastions of healthy eating, but when there's nothing else to nosh on, you can at least limit the damage. "The hot dog, burger, and nacho kiosks are really bad choices—all of that food is very high in fat," says Patti Tveit Milligan, a nutrition columnist for *Selling* magazine, a publication devoted to men who travel for a living. "You're better off getting just a snack until you can have a decent meal."

Milligan recommends assuaging the beast within with a more-or-less healthful snack—a bagel, say, or a soft pretzel with mustard. "A lot of the cafeterias have a bowl of fruit at the end of the line. That's a good choice. And if you go into some of the newsstands, you might even find a bag of dried fruit snacks.

12. **Break bread before bed.** While no one recommends cracking a loaf of French bread every night at bedtime, there are advantages to having a healthful late-night snack.

Your body starts processing carbohydrates—such as rice, potatoes, and bread—immediately so they don't hang around all night. Furthermore, they help speed tryptophan, a sleep-inducing amino acid, to the brain, says Judith J. Wurtman, Ph.D., a clinical researcher at the Massachusetts Institute of Technology in Cambridge and coauthor of *The Serotonin Solution*. In other words, they'll fill you up and help you sleep.

"Diets that don't contain enough carbohydrates usually turn people into insomniacs," Dr. Wurtman adds.

13. **Maximize opportunity.** Exercise doesn't happen only on the track or in the gym. Every day, there are dozens of little opportunities—going shopping, walking to your car, or just going from the basement to the fourth floor—that help us burn a little more flab, says Kelly Brownell, Ph.D., co-director of the Yale University Eating and Weight Disorders Clinic.

For starters, lose the remote control, get out of your chair, and actually walk over to the TV to change the channels. It's not a marathon, exactly, but it helps. So will getting out of the car and opening the garage door by hand; walking the shopping malls instead of ordering by mail; taking stairs instead of elevators; walking at lunch instead of having an hour-long meal. All these small efforts add up to decent workouts, and workouts subtract pounds. When you're in a race, every step you take counts.

5

DISEASE-
PROOF

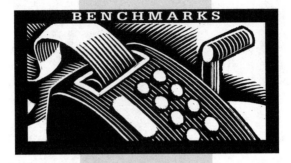

■ Number of hours truckers sleep per day, according to a recent study: 5.2

■ Approximate number of poisons contained in secondhand smoke: 200

■ Approximate number of carcinogens contained in secondhand smoke: 43

■ Age of a Wisconsin man who recently got married: 103

■ Age of the Wisconsin man's bride: 84

■ How much more concerned women are about
gym cleanliness than men are: 4 times

■ Number of Americans killed in 1997 by the plague: 2

■ Annual deaths in the United States attributed to the flu: 20,000

■ Number of years by which an American president is likely
to fall short of his life expectancy: 3

■ Percentage of cancer deaths that might be prevented through dietary changes: 33.3

■ Percentage of people who are not aware that they have diabetes: 50

■ Percentage of Americans who don't know that dust is a health hazard: 50

■ Percentage of Americans who report washing their hands
after going to the bathroom: 90

■ Average number of years right-handed men might outlive lefties: 10

■ Number of years a child born in 1996 is expected to outlive one born in 1900: 29

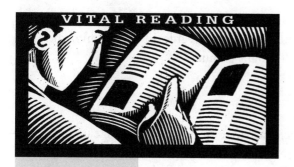

Years of Good Sex

Simple changes you make today can improve your erections tomorrow.

We're not going to kid you: An American man's odds of keeping erections strong and hard into his golden years aren't good. Almost one out of five men over 40 rarely gets an erection hard enough for penetration, and half have some trouble staying hard, according to a landmark 1994 study of more than 1,200 Massachusetts men. And when researchers from Harvard quizzed men in their eighties about their sex lives, only 26 percent reported having an erection in the past 30 days.

Although we refer to such statistics as "odds," luck is rarely a factor. Nor can we lay the blame on simple aging. "For the vast majority of men, the ability to maintain hard erections into their eighties is under their own control," says Irwin Goldstein, M.D., professor of urology at Boston University School of Medicine. The minority of men who escape impotence are those who understand the logic of the penis and put that logic into practice—morning, noon, and night.

Logic first: The penis is composed of two inflatable cylinders. When your brain registers pleasure, valves in the arteries leading to those cylinders open and blood rushes in. At the same time, small muscles embedded in the cylinders relax, allowing the tissue to expand. Then valves in the veins that drain the penis snap shut. The result: a hard, fully blood-filled erection.

System failure can occur at any step. If the arteries leading into the penis are clogged, insufficient blood may make it in. If the tissue and muscle that compose the cylinders have fallen out of use, they may be stiff and unwilling to expand. If the valves controlling outflow have become damaged, blood may leak out.

What allows these maladies to take hold? Usually it's a combination of poor diet, lack of exercise, and, perhaps most important, penile disuse. "Erections are good for erections. If a man's penis isn't regularly recharged with oxygen-rich blood, permanent damage to blood vessels or muscles may result," says Dr. Goldstein.

By facilitating daily erections and making other simple lifestyle changes today, you can dramatically reduce the risk of erectile difficulty tomorrow. With that in mind, here's a penis health "daily planner."

Morning

Wake up early. It's no coincidence that the erection you wake up with is the hardest of the day. The phenomenon, known as "pee hard," occurs when a full bladder presses against the veins that drain the penis, trapping extra blood. Though nature calls such erections, a little fantasy or stimulation can turn that accidental happening into a rise-and-shine to remember.

While young men spend an average of two to three hours a night in full penile erection, once a man hits his forties and fifties, that period tends to diminish. This decline can have serious consequences if not made up for at other times of the day. "In the flaccid state, the penis receives less than 0.1 percent of the blood circulating through the body," says Dr. Goldstein. "That's lower than virtually every other organ. The only time the penis gets a lot of blood and oxygen is during erections." Use it—more often as you get older—or lose it.

Bonus points: Extend the duration and the intensity of the erection by bringing it into the shower and using the water to clean and stimulate.

Reach for the C. Down one glass of fruit juice or gobble up a grapefruit half. Recent research has found that men who consume extra vitamin C have wider, more relaxed arteries. In one study, researchers tracked down men whose arteries were capable of expanding only 2 percent. Then they gave them large amounts of supplemental vitamin C—more than 33 times the Recommended Dietary Allowance. After just one dose, the subjects' arteries widened by almost 10 percent. And the wider an artery, the more blood it can carry along the erection highway.

"When it comes to healthy erections, the bottom line is that anything that's good for your arteries is good for your penis," says Michael P. O'Leary, M.D., associate professor of surgery at Harvard Medical School and director of the Center for Male Sexual Function at Brigham and Women's Hospital.

Bonus points: Squeeze your own OJ. Fresh squeezed delivers 29 percent more C than the stuff made from concentrate.

Opt for oatmeal. Pair your citrus with a steaming bowl of oats. Simply adding a bowl of oatmeal to your current diet may decrease harmful low-density lipoprotein (LDL) cholesterol levels by as much as 10 percent, according to one study of men with high cholesterol. And less LDL can translate into big erection benefits: Every one-point increase in total cholesterol makes you 1½ times more likely to have erectile difficulty.

Bonus points: Add a teaspoon of cinnamon. Test-tube studies show that cinnamon triples the body's ability to break down sugar. And the better your body takes care of breaking down sugars, the less likely you are to develop erection-dampening diabetes.

Ditch the coffee and go for tea instead. Substitute rich black tea for your usual morning joe. Unlike coffee, tea contains natural substances called flavonoids, which diffuse the ability of LDL cholesterol to stick to arteries. And cholesterol that doesn't stick won't impede blood flow to the penis.

Bonus points: Keep the tea bag soaking for five full minutes for maximum flavonoid effect.

Noon

Pick up the pace. Whether it's a walk in the park or a few laps in the pool, try to do something that elevates your heart rate for at least 20 minutes. Exercise boosts levels of high-density lipoprotein (HDL) cholesterol, which helps whisk artery-clogging LDL cholesterol out of the body. In one study, the probability of developing impotence soared from 6 to 25 percent as HDL levels dropped from 90 to 30 milligrams per deciliter. In separate research, scientists found that for each 6.2 miles jogged per week, HDL levels climbed 3 milligrams per deciliter.

And exercise can have a more direct effect on your sex life as well. In one study, men who exercised aerobically three times a week had sex more, masturbated more, and had more frequent orgasms than their couch-potato counterparts.

In another study of 751 volunteers, researchers found that regular exercisers reached orgasm during masturbation and intercourse faster than nonexercisers.

Bonus points: Skip the bike—unless it has a soft seat. Hard, narrow bicycle seats reduce blood flow through the penile arteries by 66 percent and can eventually contribute to impotence, according to Dr. Goldstein.

Have Charlie for lunch. Toss some water-packed tuna with a little low-fat mayonnaise for a healthy salad you can make into a sandwich or pair with greens. Fish is a great source of arginine, an amino acid that is an important component of nitric oxide, a gas produced in the penis that relaxes the penile muscles, allowing even more blood to flow into the penis. Arginine has also been shown (at least in mice) to reduce artery-clogging deposits by 50 percent. "Until we know the optimal supplemental dose of arginine, I'd recommend getting it from foods such as fish and beans," says John P. Cooke, M.D., Ph.D., director of vascular medicine at Stanford University School of Medicine.

Bonus points: Drop by a seafood restaurant for a grilled salmon steak and stock up on heart-healthy omega-3 fatty acids, which researchers believe help to widen and protect arteries.

Mid-Afternoon

Take time for a fantasy. Take 5 to 10 minutes, stare into space (or at your latest report, if you think your boss may wander by), and imagine an erotic scenario. Let your mind take you—and your penis—wherever it will. Each lusty daydream, however brief, sends an influx of blood into the penis, helping to keep it well-nourished even when it's languishing under those Dockers. And Australian researchers have found that men who had undergone a "sexual fantasy training program" had enhanced arousal during sex.

Grab some nuts. Skip the chocolate candy bar and grab a handful of mixed nuts. Not only are nuts portable and mess-free but they're also loaded with vitamin E, which has been shown to prevent damage to erectile tissue in some men. Vitamin E is such a potent penis-protector that doctors recommend vitamin supplements of 400 to 800 international units to men with bent or injured penises.

Bonus points: Make that a handful of roasted soy nuts and you'll increase the benefits. Soy has been linked to lowering cholesterol levels as well as reducing the incidence of prostate problems. "It's not prostate disease itself that causes impotence as much as the treatments that are often used to combat it," explains Dr. O'Leary.

Evening

Flex your penile muscles. On the drive home, try squeezing and releasing your pubococcygeal (PC) muscles (the ones at the base of your penis that control your urine flow). Aim for five sets of 10 rapid squeeze-releases. Strong PC muscles can drive more blood into your penis and help keep it there. In one Belgian study of 178 impotent men, 43 reported being cured after an intensive, four-month-long PC "rehabilitation program."

Bonus points: Next time you're making love, flex your PC muscles just as your arousal builds to put the brakes on your climax and enjoy the benefits of a continued erection.

Drink a glass of wine with dinner. Pair your low-fat cuisine with a glass or two of good wine. The same flavonoids found in tea are also present in dark beer and wine.

Bonus points: Opt for a dry red, such as petite sirah or pinot noir, for maximum blood-pumping effect.

Lay it on the line. If something that's going on in your household is bothering you, make your feelings known in a direct, calm manner. When researchers studied men with erectile problems, they found that many were loath to assert themselves. "In terms of impotence, breaking out of a passive mode and taking control of one's situation is key," says Stanley Ducharme, Ph.D., professor of rehabilitation at Boston University School of Medicine. Different from aggression, which involves an angry venting, assertion is characterized by a calm, reasonable statement of what's bothering you.

Bonus points: Express your grievances calmly enough, and what started as a fight could turn into an erection-bolstering reunion.

Night

Turn off the tube. Sure, you might miss Letterman, but you'll end up getting more sex and more sleep. Your penis depends on nocturnal erections to supply oxygenated blood to the penis as you sleep. "Fatigue is probably the most common cause of sexual distress," says Michael A. Perelman, Ph.D., assistant professor of psychology at New York Hospital–Cornell Medical Center in New York City. For most men, nine hours a night gives the mind and the penis ample time to recover and rejuvenate.

Bonus points: Avoid sleeping medications and alcohol right before bed. Both inhibit the amount of deep sleep during which nighttime erections occur.

Ask for a back rub. Take that extra time you have in bed to give and receive a back rub with your partner. Just two 15-minute massage sessions a week have been linked with markedly lower levels of stress, anxiety, and depression, all of which can leave erections limp. That's because massage lowers levels of cortisol, a stress hormone believed to inhibit sexual response in some men. Mentally relaxed men have roughly half the rate of impotence of their overstressed counterparts.

Bonus points: Add a scented massage oil, which heightens the sensation and increases the odds that a "penis workout" will be forthcoming.

Disconnect the phone. Turn on your answering machine and turn off your bedside phone. Being interrupted during sex is not only annoying, it can be dangerous, especially if she's on top (and can't resist reaching for the receiver). "Between three million and four million American men are impotent today because of injuries they sustained to their penises during masturbation or intercourse," says Dr. Goldstein. Any sudden movement during penetration—especially the twisting motion she needs to reach the nightstand—could result in penile fracture, which occurs when the blood-filled penis cylinders rupture.

Bonus points: Turn on the lights. Extra visual stimulation causes more oxygen-rich blood to flow into the penis.

Reach for the lubricant. No nightstand should be without a bottle of high-quality lubricant. Use a dab on your fingers before working your magic. Thrusting without enough lubrication may lead to Peyronie's disease, a painful curvature of the penis. When the penis meets even slight resistance, tiny tears develop along the blood-filled cylinders. As those tears turn into scars, the penis can be thrown off-kilter. Lube keeps things slipping and sliding safely.

Bonus points: Have a spray bottle filled with water handy. When the lube starts to dry out, refresh it—and your partner—with a spritz.

Treat Your Teeth Right

Check out this lifetime guide to care for your choppers.

Examine your life and you'll probably find some things you wouldn't mind losing—a few pounds, a few stressors, that brown Naugahyde La-Z-Boy you bought during the Ford administration. But unless you're bucking for a role in a remake of *Deliverance*, losing your teeth is probably not on your list. After all, men without teeth are like, well, women without teeth. And we all know how attractive they are.

Staying sharp in the teeth department takes some work, however. You have to be vigilant throughout your life if you want to avoid looking like a jack-o'-lantern. Here's a rundown of dental problems that can plague you at various ages and what you can do about them.

Cavities

If you were a kid during the past few decades, fluoride and vigilant parents gave you a chance of surviving your teens with no cavities. But don't be cocky—the bad habits that sometimes go along with being young and newly independent make you particularly susceptible to tooth decay in your twenties. Here's what you need to do about it.

Ditch the sinful lifestyle. No one knows exactly why, but smoking, drinking alcohol, and chewing tobacco will definitely make you more cavity prone, says

Linda Niessen, D.M.D., a professor in the department of public health sciences at Baylor College of Dentistry in Houston. Those Coke-and-Twinkies breakfasts don't help either—the killer sugar/starch combo sits on your teeth all day, creating a welcome mat for decay-causing bacteria and plaque.

Try to brush after every meal. "One of the big mistakes people make is associating the quantity of sugar in food with cavities," says Carole Palmer, R.D., Ed.D., cohead of the division of nutrition and preventive dentistry at Tufts University School of Dental Medicine in Boston. "In reality, it has to do with the amount of time that sugars—even in small amounts—are in contact with your teeth." To lessen your risk, brush and floss at least twice a day, preferably after every meal. If the path to the men's room leads you past the boss's office, and you're just too embarrassed to be seen carrying your toothbrush after lunch, you can do two other things:

• Swish before you swallow. "When you eat a cookie, there are a lot of crumbs left sitting around in your mouth, and the bacteria are going to go into a full feeding frenzy," says Dr. Palmer. "If you drink water and you swish before you swallow, you'll wash away at least some of the fodder."

• Chew gum. Your body's best defense against cavities is saliva, and there's no better way of stimulating spit than by chewing gum. Sugarless is best.

Launch a counterattack. If you already have some small degree of decay (dental x-rays should reveal it), ask your dentist if either of these will help.

• Bombard your teeth with minerals. Toothpaste with fluoride can remineralize the enamel on your teeth, essentially stopping early decay in its tracks, says Joel M. Boriskin, D.D.S., associate professor at the University of California, San Francisco, School of Dentistry.

• Paint your teeth with plastic. If you don't have any other cavities, a sealant can be painted on the chewing surfaces of your teeth to snuff out the decay and protect against further attacks.

Periodontal Disease

The big risk once you hit middle age is periodontal disease, an infection that is caused by an accumulation of bacteria and plaque. In its first stage, gingivitis, it causes inflammation of the gums. When it progresses and begins to destroy the bone—periodontitis—teeth loosen and either fall out or have to be pulled. "The greatest cause of tooth loss in adults is gum disease, and it's all preventable," says Richard H. Price, D.M.D., a clinical instructor at Boston University School of Dentistry.

Periodontal disease can be treated—remedies range from scraping away part of the tooth to gum surgery. All are costly and painful, and often, the only solution is to yank out your teeth.

Be vigilant. Now is the time to be obsessive about oral hygiene—and that means thoroughly brushing and flossing your teeth no less than twice a day. Here's a test: The next time you brush, time yourself. "It should take you three minutes to brush your teeth," says Dr. Niessen. "Most people spend 30 to 40 seconds."

Try a new toothpaste. Crest and Colgate both offer toothpastes that help control bacteria and plaque.

Take the test. Dr. Niessen says a new blood test costing about $200 can indicate whether you're genetically predisposed toward periodontal disease. Ask your dentist about it.

Be on the lookout for changes. In the beginning, periodontal disease will make your gums bleed and your breath bad. Charming. If your gums are inflamed and bleed frequently when you brush, be sure to visit a dentist as soon as you can.

Staining and Yellowing

"As we grow older, teeth darken," says Dr. Price. Enamel loses its luster; stains proliferate. "It's not unhealthy, it's just the way it goes."

Don't throw your money away. Dr. Boriskin says once your teeth start to change color, nothing you try on your own—including tooth whiteners from the drugstore—is likely to be very effective. But yellowing and staining can be bleached out by your dentist. For $250 to $500, you're fitted with a customized tray of bleaching solution to make sure all the little nooks and crannies in your teeth are treated.

Oral Cancer

It can happen at any time, but because of the cumulative effects of smoking and alcohol, oral cancer is most prevalent in the 45-and-up age group.

Kick the habit. Stick this in your pipe and smoke it: Tobacco puts you at a greater risk for both periodontal disease and oral cancer.

Take a peek. "The great thing about your mouth, unlike your lungs, is that you can see it," says Dr. Niessen. "You brush your teeth every morning. While you're doing that, check your gums, tongue, cheeks, and lips to see if you have any sores that aren't healing or anything else that looks funny."

Cavities Redux

Your roots are showing. Maybe it's periodontal disease. Maybe it's just normal wear and tear. Whatever the reason, your gums have receded, exposing the soft roots to decay-causing bacteria and plaque. What's more, old fillings are weakening and cracking, leaving some cozy niches where bacteria can thrive, says Dr. Price. That's right, cavities. Again.

Keep brushing and flossing. No sense stopping now—they're still one of your most effective defenses.

Rinse with fluoride. Fluoride protects the surface of your teeth from decay. You'll need even more if your saliva glands are malfunctioning—a dry mouth is a common side effect of lots of medications, including antihistamines, antianxiety, and blood pressure drugs.

Finish off your meal with Cheddar cheese. Cheese stimulates saliva flow, and Cheddar actually counteracts the acid released by bacteria.

Lay off the candy. Sucking on candy or mints all day deposits a constant coating of sugar on your teeth, says Dr. Palmer. The same goes for sipping soda, sweetened coffee, even fruit juice.

Sensitivity

With the roots hanging out there unprotected, their soft coverings can wear away and expose microscopic nerve endings. Here's what you can do.

Switch your toothpaste. A number of manufacturers make toothpastes specifically for sensitive teeth. (They cover the exposed nerve endings and prevent air from getting at them.) Try one, but be patient, says Dr. Price. You may go through several different brands before you find one that works for you. If none help, ask your dentist about bondings and sealants that can give you relief.

Sneaky Health Problems

Get these unexpected health problems before they get you.

To paraphrase John Lennon, life is what happens while you're making other plans. And—unfortunately for John—he was more right than he knew.

Weird things happen all the time. Tires blow out, lightning strikes, trains crash, and there's little we can do to prevent it. But we can help prevent some of the unexpected (and not-so-rare) health problems that strike many of our fellow men. You already know about the importance of exercise, eating right, and getting regular checkups. But you might not know about these very simple steps that could save you a lot of pain—and maybe even save your life.

Move around the cabin. Airplane seats are starting to gain a nasty reputation for causing thromboses, or blood clots. It's no wonder: Sitting through *Mr. Holland's Opus* and a four-hour snooze will make blood pool in your legs. Blood that doesn't move can coagulate. Then as you start walking again, clots can travel to the arteries that supply blood to your lungs. That's bad. According to a three-year study at Heathrow Airport, blood clots caused 11 sudden deaths among long-distance travelers. And that's in one airport.

"No one keeps statistics," says Stanley Mohler, M.D., director of aerospace medicine at Wright State University School of Medicine in Dayton, Ohio. "But clots probably occur at airports around the world every day." It happened to Dan Quayle in 1994, so it's not a Chicken Little worry. Take precautions: Drink a lot of nonalcoholic liquids. Dehydration caused by dry airplane air can cause blood platelets to clump. And of course, keep moving.

"Stroll around the cabin at least once, preferably twice, an hour," says Dr. Mohler. An easy trick: Poke your head into first class and take drink orders. Then sit down. See how they're doing in 20 minutes. If you keep moving at about the same rate you do at work, your capillaries should stay unplugged.

Take a tablespoon of psyllium every day. Eating powder made from psyllium plant seeds may sound a little strange, but it's one of the best ways to guard against diverticulitis. This painful condition occurs when weak spots in your intestinal lining bulge from bowel pressure, like an inner tube ballooning through a hole in a tire. Particles collect in the pouches and cause infection. A recent study from the Hospital des Diaconesses in Paris found diverticulitis is 10 times as common as it was a century ago. The main reason: We're eating more processed foods.

Of course, more fiber is the answer. "The high-fiber diet of the South African Bantu allows them the lowest incidence of diverticulitis in the world," says Edward Goldberg, M.D., professor of gastroenterology at Lenox Hill Hospital in New York City. Great advice, but who eats their recommended 25 grams of fiber daily? Who even wants to think about it?

Psyllium is extremely high in fiber and painless to eat. "A small daily serving can help prevent pouching of the intestinal lining," says Dr. Goldberg. So pick up some psyllium powder at any health food store and throw a tablespoon in your cereal or soup. It'll keep you in the clear.

Limit your leg extensions. Major League catchers and middle-age men often have one thing in common: wrecked knees. Weak leg muscles and a shoddy foot-strike (from an orthopedic problem) can slowly pull the kneecap out of line. This causes the cartilage grinding that eventually leads to a painful condition called patellofemoral syndrome. "You'll probably feel it first as a sharp pain under your kneecap as you're climbing the stairs," says Allan Levy, M.D., team physician for the NFL's New York Giants.

If you've felt a twinge or two in the knees, the way to stave off further pain is to strengthen the muscles around the knee joint, says Dr. Levy. Do seated leg extensions—but only the top six to eight inches of the exercise. Simply mount a leg extension machine, put the pin on a light weight, and straighten your legs. Bend your knees slightly, and then press the pad back to the top. Ten repetitions three times a week should do it. "If you go through the bottom part of the exercise, you'll grind your kneecap more," warns Dr. Levy. Drugstore orthotic inserts may also help correct the way your foot lands, but talk to your doctor. Knee grinding also can speed up osteoarthritis.

Keep your neck straight. If you picked up a nasty neck crick after a day in the gym, it probably wasn't from that 180-pound shoulder press you foolishly attempted. It was most likely a sloppy set of crunches, says Stephen Hochschuler, M.D., chairman of the Texas Back Institute in Plano. Pulling your head can stress your neck joints, which makes supporting your 12-pound brain box painful. Keep your hands on your chest and don't tuck your chin during situps, warns Dr. Hochschuler. "Imagine you're holding a softball between your chin and chest," he advises.

Neck pain can be caused by bicycling as well. The problem can be a low seat or low handlebars, either of which can force you to arch your neck. Head to a local bike shop for proper adjustments.

Swear off high-protein diets. Bodybuilders, dinosaurs, and other clumsy carnivores who eat too much protein can end up walking funny. It's not from going barefoot; it's from gout. Gout is a common male disorder that causes pain in the knuckle of your big toe and other joints. Though it's hereditary, it can be spurred by high blood pressure and diabetes. It was called the "rich-man's disease" because it often results from a diet of red meat, fish, pâté, and alcohol. These high-protein foods create uric-acid crystals, which become wedged in your lowest joints—typically, your knees, wrists, and toes. After awhile, the gritty crystals cause painful inflammation. "The pain is so great that some people can't stand to have bedsheets resting on their toes," says David Goldfarb, M.D., co-director of the kidney stone prevention and treatment program at New York University Medical Center.

Gout usually hits men older than 60, but you can nip it now. Keep your protein intake less than 20 percent of your diet and take a blood test for uric acid during your next physical. High levels don't necessarily guarantee you'll develop gout, but they're fair warning to change your diet. If joint pain has already struck, ask your doctor about antiarthritic drugs.

Swallow an antihistamine. We've all felt pressure in our ears while flying or scuba diving. Few of us, however, know that it can damage our hearing. Hold your nose, close your mouth, and gently blow. If your ears don't "pop" within a few seconds, you may suffer from eustachian-tube dysfunction, according to Christopher Linstrom, M.D., chief of otology at the New York Eye and Ear Infirmary in New York City. That means the valves that clear ear pressure are blocked, and sudden changes in pressure could actually injure your delicate inner ear.

According to researchers at the Gentofte University Hospital in Denmark, an estimated 5 percent of adult flyers (and 25 percent of children) suffer from such ear problems. Luckily, they're preventable.

"Tube dysfunction is often associated with allergies," says Dr. Linstrom. "Antihistamines that bring down sinus swelling usually open the tubes." Taking an antihistamine prior to flying or diving (choose one that won't cause drowsiness) may allow you to equalize faster. If the problem is chronic, an otologist can insert a tube in your ear that'll relieve the pressure.

Nip colon cancer in the bud. If you're older than 40, ask your doctor to test for hidden blood in your stool during your exam. It may seem like a lot to ask of the guy for his measly $175 per hour, but this simple screening test can decrease your risk of colon cancer, says Cary Schneebaum, M.D., a gastroenterologist at Beth Israel Hospital in New York City.

Blood in the bowels usually means two things: hemorrhoids or polyps, growths on the wall of the colon that may become cancerous. In a study at Oregon Health Sciences University in Portland, of 297 patients with rectal bleeding, 26 had polyps and 13 had colon cancer. Colon cancer almost always starts as polyps, so removing them early can prevent it. Case closed.

Heed the other warnings between exams, says Dr. Schneebaum. Head to your doctor if you have persistent abdominal cramps, constant diarrhea or constipation, or—of course—if you see red in your stool.

Stretch before you play. Elton Strauss, M.D., chief of the orthopedic trauma and adult reconstructive surgery service at Mount Sinai Hospital Center in New York City, sees many weekend golfers with agonizing lower-back pain because they didn't follow a very simple warmup plan before teeing off. The twisting motion of a golf swing (or a botched layup) can strain the muscles that attach the pelvis to the thigh, says Dr. Strauss. "You'll know when you've done it," he says. "The pain centers right under the belt line over the gluteal region." That is, a pain in the butt.

A little stretching can save you months of discomfort, warns Dr. Strauss. Walk at a fast clip to warm up, then touch your toes with your knees bent to flex your spine. Finish by gently twisting your body with your hands on your hips. In five minutes, you're ready to drive.

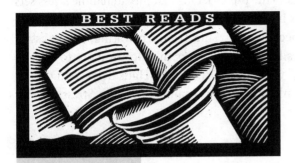

Stress and Disease

Wouldn't it be great if you could significantly reduce your chances of getting a wide variety of diseases and ailments just by eliminating one thing from your life? Well, you can. And that one thing is stress. The authors of Stress Blasters: Quick and Simple Steps to Take Control and Perform under Pressure *(Rodale Press, 1997), Brian Chichester and Perry Garfinkel, do an excellent job in this excerpt of simply explaining the complex physiological damage that stress does to your body. But they don't stop there. Once you understand how stress hurts, they help you fight back to control it.*

Remember way back to the days of old vinyl records? (That was sometime after the saber-toothed tigers had disappeared. What if you had left "Rock around the Clock" on the phonograph with the arm off so that the record played over and over again? Eventually, you'd have worn the grooves of that 45 down so far that even Bill Haley and His Comets would have lost their shake, rattle, and roll.

That's how the constant repetition of the fight-or-flight response acts on you when those stress hormones keep rockin' round your body clock day and night.

Reed C. Moskowitz, M.D., clinical assistant professor of psychiatry and director of the Stress Disorders Medical Services program at New York University in New York City and author of *Your Healing Mind*, uses a similar analogy. "Stress is like having one foot on the accelerator of a car, with the other foot on the brake," he says. "We wind up stripping our gears. The chronic buildup of stress takes an enormous toll on our bodies in terms of wear and tear."

Those stressors come with increasing frequency as our lives merge into the fast lane. And because we live in relatively civilized times, we have fewer ways to burn off that hormonal buildup. We can't punch our bosses (unless we're trust-fund babies). We can't run over the cars that cut us off (unless we're shooting a chase scene from a Sylvester Stallone action flick). We can't kill the saber-toothed tiger (because evolution beat us to the punch). Our inability to handle stress sets off a chain reaction that results in increased vulnerability to disease.

"Each period of stress, especially if it results from frustrating, unsuccessful struggles, leaves some irreversible chemical scars that accumulate to constitute the signs of tissue aging," wrote endocrinologist Hans Selye, M.D., who was the first to establish the link between stress and disease, in *Stress without Distress*.

The High Cost of Stress

As many as 90 percent of office visits to primary care physicians are connected to stress, some experts estimate.

Dr. Moskowitz's partial list of stress-related illnesses includes alcoholism, anorexia, arthritis, asthma, back pain, bulimia, chronic fatigue, colitis, compulsive overeating, depression, dermatitis, drug abuse, heart disease, high blood pressure, high cholesterol, infertility, irritable bowel syndrome, migraine headaches, multiple chemical sensitivities, obesity, panic disorder, phobias, severe allergies, sexual dysfunction, tension headaches, and possibly ulcers.

Long before illness sets in, stress can cause these physical symptoms involving the voluntary muscular system or the automatic nervous system: belching, bloating, blushing, chest pain, cold and sweaty hands, colds, constipation, decreased sexual desire, diarrhea, dizziness, dry mouth, ear ringing, faintness, frequent or lingering chills, frowning, gas, goose pimples, heartburn, heart palpitations, hives, jaw pain, light-headedness, muscle tension and aches, neck pain, night sweats, painful cold hands and feet, rashes, sound and light sensitivity, stammering, stuttering, swallowing difficulty, teeth grinding or temporomandibular disorder, trembling hands and lips, and widening pupils.

And that's just the body. Here's the toll that stress takes on the mind: anger, anxiety, apathy, concentration problems, confusion, crying, depression, difficulty learning new information, disorganization, emotionally drained feeling, fatigue, fear of closeness, forgetfulness, frustration, hopelessness, indecisiveness, insomnia, irritability, loneliness, low energy, low self-esteem, moodiness, nervousness, nightmares, obsessions, oversleeping, poor judgment, rapid thinking, recurring negative thoughts, self-doubt, tension, trapped feeling, and suicidal thoughts.

Seeking Immunity

One of the effects of the stress response is that it cuts off any body function that doesn't directly relate to repelling the perceived threat, which makes sense—provided the threat is real. Why grow fingernails when you're about to have your hand bitten off? Why fight nasty cancer cells when a Mack truck is about to make you one with a cement wall?

Similarly, when your body is reacting to stress, digestion gets interrupted and reproductive urges decrease. The same is true for your immune system, which defends against infections and illness.

Here's why. Main parts of your immune system include your thymus, bone marrow, lymph nodes, lymphatic vessels, lymph (one of the three main fluids that circulate through the body), liver, and spleen. All have nerve fibers that communicate with the brain. Since there is a direct link between your immune system and your mind, psychological stress can greatly affect your body's ability to fight disease.

The thymus is the big cheese of the immune system. It produces, among other regulating hormones, white blood cells known as T lymphocytes—the good guys that promote cell immunity. The lymph group helps, too. The nodes filter the lymph and contain B lymphocytes, which promote production of antibodies when you're exposed to bacteria and virus. The liver, another player, is where lymph is produced. It contains large cells that do a full frontal attack on foreign substances that invade our bodies. The spleen destroys old blood cells and also produces lymphocytes.

Hopefully you're still with us here, because here's the kicker. This whole interconnected immune system operates more efficiently under the parasympathetic nervous system, which controls body functions during rest and sleep. But stress arouses the sympathetic nervous system, which basically knocks out the parasympathetic system. As more and more hormones such as epinephrine, norepinephrine, and cortisol are released, they trigger chemical changes that decrease the number of white blood cells in the blood, thereby decreasing your level of immunity.

Naturally, the guys in the white coats have a big word for this whole process. It's called immunosuppression.

Making the Connection

Most of us have learned the hard way about the connection between stress and disease. It's the headache when we're under the gun or the cold that we catch when we're frazzled. But there is more than just anecdotal evidence that the two are linked. Studies have scientifically corroborated that stress can lead to or exacerbate the following physical problems. And thanks to the field of psychoneuroimmunology, it has been shown that mental stress can cause physical distress.

Heart disease. For a long time, there was just anecdotal evidence that stress caused heart attacks. But since the 1970s, there has been a growing body of research that shows a direct link between stress and high blood pressure, cholesterol, clogging of the arteries, hypertension, diabetes, and other conditions.

For example, a long-term Harvard University study found that men who experienced symptoms of anxiety—fear of strange people, nervousness, the jitters, cold sweats (all signs that have been related to stress)—were as much as four times more likely to suffer sudden cardiac death than those without those symptoms. The study ranked anxiety right up there with smoking, excessive drinking, high sodium intake, and lack of exercise as risk factors in heart disease. The Montreal Heart Institute found that heart attack survivors suffering from depression have three to four times the risk of dying within six months as nondepressed survivors. Depression is another indicator of stress. Similarly, in another study, emotional distress has been related to mortality in patients with coronary heart disease. In still another study, New Yorkers working in high-strain jobs—such as air traffic controllers and bus drivers—had higher blood pressure.

Why is the heart such a vulnerable victim of stress? Simple, says Robert Sapolsky, Ph.D., professor of biological sciences and neuroscience at Stanford University and author of *Why Zebras Don't Get Ulcers: A Guide to Stress, Stress-Related Diseases, and Coping.* "The cardiovascular stress response basically consists of making the heart and blood vessels work harder for a while, and if you do that on a regular basis, they will wear out, just like any pump or hose you buy."

Back pain. The muscles of your back are particularly vulnerable to the constant contraction and relaxation that the stress response puts them through, says Willibald Nagler, M.D., physiatrist in chief at New York Hospital–Cornell Medical Center in New York City. That's especially true of the lower back because "so many parts of all the nerves to the lower extremities come through the lower spine," Dr. Nagler says. "The lumbar (lower) spine is a fine-tuned organization of bones that demands a lot of adjustment every time we sit or stand."

The best way to avoid back pain caused by stress is to "stay limber by doing stretching exercises every day when you're not under stress," suggests Dr. Nagler. "Well-stretched muscles can tolerate a lot more pain than stiff ones. Also, move around a lot. Don't sit in one place." For back pain and muscle spasms, he recommends ice packs, not heat. "Ice decreases the sensory nerves' ability to conduct painful stimuli."

Headaches. "We still really don't know exactly why stress causes headaches," says Seymour Diamond, M.D., director of the Diamond Headache Clinic in Chicago and author of *The Hormone Headache*. What is known, he says, is that stress hormones make the muscles of the neck and scalp tighten. There's a reflex swelling of blood vessels in those areas that cause the pain we commonly call headache, whether episodic or migraine. Episodic, or tension, headaches are caused by bosses yelling, children crying, and other garden-variety daily tensions.

"We're all living hectic, computer-controlled lives, which can certainly increase the number of episodic headaches that we're getting," he says. For common tension headaches, he recommends aspirin, "probably one of the greatest discoveries ever made," he says. Migraines, on the other hand, are related more to psychological problems, he notes, and often can be treated with counseling, relaxation exercises, and prescription drugs. "Migraines can be an inherited disorder related to neurological manifestations in the brain," he adds. Interestingly, migraines don't usually occur during times of stress, but a while after.

Colds. Several important studies have shown that psychological stress increases susceptibility to cold viruses. Besides depleting the immune system's ability to fight viruses, stress also makes us breathe more rapidly, sometimes twice the normal rate, says Georgia Witkin, Ph.D., assistant clinical professor of psychiatry and director of the Stress Program at Mount Sinai Medical Center in New York City and author of *The Male Stress Syndrome*. This hyperventilation dries up the mucous membranes in the respiratory system. They become more irritable and less protected against bacteria and viruses. Cortisol levels are down, and inflammations are up. Temperature regulation goes on the blink. Achoo!

"The way you handle a stress cold is the same as any cold," says Jeffrey Jahre, M.D., clinical associate professor at Temple University in Philadelphia and chief of infectious diseases at St. Luke's Hospital in Bethlehem, Pennsylvania. "Eat nourishing food, drink plenty of fluids, and get rest. These are the pillars of good health. You basically should change some of the things that may have made you more susceptible in the first place."

Indigestion. When the stress button gets pushed, Dr. Witkin explains, the rhythmic, smooth muscle contractions (called peristalsis) that push food through the intestinal system slow down, probably because digestion takes a backseat to basic survival needs. Also, gastric glands diminish their output, making absorption of food more difficult. The release of glucocorticoids indirectly increases the amount of stomach acid, which, in turn, leads to heartburn and worse gastrointestinal problems.

Belly Fat and Health

In the late nineteenth century, a belly on a man was considered a status symbol. It meant that he had the economic resources to attain and maintain it. If they knew then what doctors know now, we doubt they'd intentionally be sporting those bellies. In this excerpt from Banish Your Belly: The Ultimate Guide for Achieving a Lean, Strong Body—Now *(Rodale Press, 1997), author Kenton Robinson points out some very scary statistics about men with large girths and what you can do to attain the modern-day status symbol of no belly.*

Brian Wallace likes to tell the story of the guy in Utah who weighed 400 pounds.

"His blood pressure was 220 over 180, which is incredibly high; his blood sugar was 487, again, incredibly high; he actually was vision-impaired—blind—because of diabetes, which he didn't even know he had.

"Then he put himself on an exercise program, a pretty intense program. In eight months, he had lost 200 pounds, his blood pressure was down to normal range, he was off all medications, his blood sugars were down to 67, and he could see."

For Brian Wallace, Ph.D., chairman of sport fitness at the U.S. Sports Academy in Daphne, Alabama, the guy from Utah is a perfect, if extreme, example of the kind of price we pay when we let our bellies take over our lives.

"It's as much a commentary on the negative effects of a sedentary lifestyle as it is on the benefits of exercise," Dr. Wallace says. "I think it's just amazing what people will let themselves do to themselves."

By the same token, it's a commentary on what you can do when you put your mind to it. Within 10 months of going on his exercise program, says Dr. Wallace, the guy from Utah was running in a marathon.

The Risks of Being Round

You might say that every one of us makes a bargain with his body, and regardless of which deal we make, we all pay a price. It's just a matter of which price you pay and whether you pay now or later. If you want to be svelte and healthy, you pay now with the sweat and effort needed to maintain your machine. If you choose instead to sit on your butt and cultivate a belly, you pay later with a plague of illnesses and an early grave.

If this seems like a strong statement, you should know that while excessive belly fat does not unconditionally guarantee that you will suffer a host of maladies and cut short your life span, it is, without question, a large step in a direction that you don't want to go.

Henry Kahn, M.D., an internist and associate professor of family and preventive medicine at Emory University School of Medicine in Atlanta, studied heart attack victims in six Atlanta hospitals. He found that a man may be the same in most respects to his next-door neighbor, but it was the guy with the bigger belly who ended up with a heart attack.

Asleep at the Wheel

Experts agree that the fatter you are, the more likely you are to suffer from high cholesterol and high blood pressure levels, both of which can lead to heart attack or stroke. In addition, there is ample evidence that the more ample your belly, the more likely you are to become a victim of diabetes, heart disease, sleep apnea, gout, and cancer of the prostate and colon.

This is serious business here. And the equation is fairly straightforward: The heavier you get around the middle, the more serious your risk of chronic disease.

It's difficult to find a part of your life that is not affected to some extent by being overweight. For example, if you are really heavy, you also tend to be more tired most of the time—not only because it is extra work to move all that extra you around but also because one common affliction of the overweight is sleep apnea, a condition in which you stop breathing for short periods many times during the night. The overall result? You wake up repeatedly during the night and therefore feel like a zombie most of the day.

Fatigue, no less than heart disease, can be a killer. In one study, researchers at the Stanford University Sleep Disorders and Research Center found that fat truck-drivers are more likely to suffer breathing problems when they sleep and so are more likely to zone out at the wheel and run you over. As a matter of fact, the researchers showed that fat truck-drivers have more than twice as many accidents per mile as thin ones.

Think about that the next time some huge guy in a semi climbs your tail.

Mr. Unhappy

In addition to being linked to a mass of physical problems, obesity has been tied to a variety of psychological problems as well. Put simply, fat people are more likely to be unhappy—and to suffer such things as depression and anxiety—than their thinner peers.

Here's the kicker: Anger, depression, heart disease, high blood pressure, and diabetes have all been linked with a higher probability of impotence.

The explanation is not far to find: Fat bellies tend to be accompanied by cholesterol-clogged arteries (atherosclerosis). Cholesterol doesn't just plug up the arteries running to your heart; it plugs up the ones running to your penis as well. In other words, the more you line your belly and your arteries with fat, the harder it is for your heart—or your penis—to keep on pumping.

Reversal of Fortunes

Fortunately, there is a lot of evidence that a reduction in belly fat can alleviate a lot of health problems. You don't even have to lose all your belly to make significant improvements to your health. Even a 10 percent reduction in body fat can reduce the severity of high blood pressure, high cholesterol, and diabetes.

Studies show, for example, that symptoms of diabetes may improve within days of beginning a weight-loss program. Many of those who stick with the program can actually improve to the point where they don't need medication.

And there is overwhelming evidence that losing excess weight reduces blood pressure. In fact, patients who are obese can often bring their blood pressures down to normal by losing only half their excess weight.

Losing weight has beneficial effects on cholesterol as well. One, it helps reduce the amount of "bad" cholesterol that's flowing through your veins while increasing levels of "good" cholesterol. And two, the process of losing weight—as long as it involves an intense exercise like playing tennis or basketball or running faster than five miles per hour—can cause further decreases in total cholesterol.

Fat Ain't Fate

Your belly is not your destiny. We said earlier that every man makes a bargain with his body. Not only can you renegotiate it, but, like the 400-pound guy from Utah, you can turn back the clock.

So if you have yourself something of a belly already, and even some of the related health problems, don't despair. There are more than a few ways to shed your past and redesign yourself. For starters, here are a few simple recommendations.

Start safe. Since men with high levels of abdominal fat are at increased risk for so many serious conditions, it's important to get checked out by a doctor at least once a year, says David Levitsky, Ph.D., professor of nutritional sciences and psychology at Cornell University in Ithaca, New York. Catching weight-related health problems early gives you a much better chance of preventing them from getting serious later on.

Take a walk. Even small changes in your habits can make a big difference in your health. Doctors recommend that you try to do a minimum of 30 minutes of moderate-intensity physical activity a day. This means taking a brisk (three to four miles per hour) walk or doing something that requires a similar level of exertion, like biking or even vigorous yard work.

Even if this 30 minutes is broken up into smaller chunks of time during the course of the day—10 minutes in the morning, say, followed by 20 minutes after supper—the benefits will still accrue, says Dr. Levitsky, who gets his exercise by riding a bike to work, a 15-minute ride each way.

Watch your mouth. In particular, start tuning in to how much fat and salt you put in your mouth every day. You want to minimize fat because, well, it makes you fat. As for salt, most of us eat a lot more in a day than we really need, according to the U.S. Departments of Agriculture and Health and Human Services. And there is plenty of evidence linking a high salt intake to high blood pressure.

One easy way to curtail fat and salt? Eat more fresh fruits and vegetables.

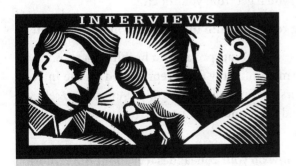

Tom Ferguson on
The Internet and Good Health

When one of our friends asked if it was true that Bill Gates had launched a venture with Pope John Paul II, it became clear: The Internet is messing with people's heads. And not just in terms of bogus news. A quick browse through many "health" sites will bombard you with unproven pills, "miracle" therapies for cancer, and ques-

tionable HIV cures that the Food and Drug Administration won't let us have. While you can't believe everything you download, says Tom Ferguson, M.D., a senior associate at Harvard Medical School's Center for Clinical Computing and author of Health Online, *the Internet can be a powerful resource in steering your health care decisions. In fact, Dr. Ferguson believes that the Internet will soon assume many of the roles of a doctor—and not just because it keeps us waiting.*

Why should we seek health advice through a medium like the Internet?

Because there's much more out there than advice, and because it gives people more control over their health. You can circumvent your doctor's busy schedule by using e-mail, and you can reach other experts or patients with similar problems through online conversations. Thanks to Web site–provided information and self-help guidelines, you won't have to start at ground zero when you ask your doctor about a problem.

But how can a man know he's not downloading bad advice?

Well, you can't check your brain at the door. If you have doubts about something you find on the Internet, post a question in one of the thousands of health discussion groups, such as a Usenet group called alt.health. Physicians often monitor these discussions, and off-the-wall claims don't go unchallenged. In fact, health professionals from all over the country—and many specialists—may e-mail you back. That's an empowering capability; you'll often get a more comprehensive answer online than you'll get from your doctor.

Any other tips for finding reliable health information on the Internet?

Sure. Make your first stops at sites that specialize in health topics, and try to impose standards on the information. Many fields represented on the Internet have self-appointed "gatekeepers," online experts who take it upon themselves to recommend good sites, pan bad ones, and point people toward worthwhile information.

Speaking of gatekeepers, how do your colleagues feel about the explosion of health information on the Internet? Does it cause problems?

It is a double-edged sword. Some doctors, especially those with little online experience, don't quite know what to think when a patient comes in with information they've picked up on the Internet. Others are quite 'Net-savvy and encourage their patients to become as well-educated as possible. This new technology demands a major role change for most doctors—from unquestioned guru to a partner and collaborator. Be gracious when you've learned something on the Internet or found research that you need to discuss, perhaps saying, "If you don't mind, please look over this information because I think it may be important to my situation. And maybe we could discuss these findings during my next visit."

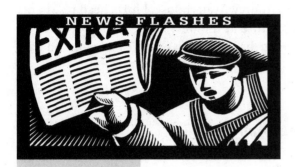

Calcium and Vitamin D
Reduce Bone Fractures As You Age

MEDFORD, Mass.—If you and your dad don't drink a few glasses of skim milk every day, you could both end up sporting more casts. Consuming more calcium and vitamin D can significantly decrease the number of bone fractures in men over 65, according to a study at Tufts University. Only 11 subjects who took 500 milligrams of calcium and 700 international units of vitamin D each day for three years suffered broken bones, compared with 26 subjects in the control group. Men over 50 need at least 1,200 milligrams of calcium a day. "Supplements aren't necessary as long as you eat at least three servings of dairy products every day," says study coauthor Susan Harris, D.Sc.

Vitamins Can Prevent Migraines

NORMAN, Okla.—Taking vitamin B_2, also known as riboflavin, helps prevent migraine headaches. Belgium Migraine Society researchers gave 54 migraine patients either 400 milligrams of vitamin B_2 or a placebo every day for three months. The subjects taking B_2 had one-third fewer migraines. "This is a safe and effective treatment for people who have two to six migraine headaches per month," says study coauthor Marc Lenaerts, M.D., of the University of Oklahoma. Ask for a prescription; 400 milligrams is a heftier dosage than you'll find over the counter.

Chocolate May Lower Risk of Heart Disease

DAVIS, Calif.—First red wine was cited as a heart protectant. Now chocolate may have the same effect. Researchers at the University of California,

Davis, discovered that milk chocolate has high levels of phenols, the antioxidants found in wine that may reduce the risk of clogged arteries and heart attack. In fact, 1½ ounces of milk chocolate, the equivalent of a candy bar, contains nearly the same amount of phenols as a 5-ounce glass of red wine. "We don't know yet if chocolate is 'good' for you, but there is hope that it may have some health benefits," says Andrew Waterhouse, Ph.D., head researcher and assistant professor of viticulture at the university. So do your heart a favor and have a low-fat chocolate bar. But do your waist a favor and have only one.

Aerobic Exercise Can Reduce Odds of Getting Diabetes

PITTSBURGH—If diabetes runs in your family, buy some running shoes. Aerobic exercise can lower insulin resistance, a condition that often leads to diabetes, in one week. In a study at the University of Pittsburgh, 11 women with insulin resistance walked and cycled for 50 minutes a day. In one week, their insulin resistance dropped by 58 percent. Exercise may improve insulin function by increasing the muscles' demand for glucose, speculates lead researcher Michael Brown, Ph.D. "These results would certainly apply to men, too."

To avoid diabetes, exercise at your target heart-rate range (subtract your age from 220, then multiply by 65 to 75 percent; it's about 120 to 140 beats per minute for a 35-year-old man) for at least 30 minutes, several times per week.

"Good" Cholesterol Level Just as Important as Total Cholesterol

MINNEAPOLIS—Just because your total cholesterol is below 200 doesn't mean you can celebrate. Men with normal total cholesterol counts but low high-density lipoprotein (HDL), or "good," cholesterol counts still had cholesterol-clogged arteries in a recent study at the Veterans Affairs Medical Center. The study found that HDL cholesterol removes buildups of the "bad" low-density lipoprotein (LDL) cholesterol. "Without enough HDL cholesterol, even normal amounts of the LDL cholesterol can build up in your arteries and cause heart disease or a stroke," says Timothy J. Wilt, M.D., associate professor of medicine at the University of Minnesota Medical School and study author. "Your total cholesterol should be less than 200, and your HDL should be more than 35," he says.

You can raise your HDL without raising your total cholesterol by eating a low-fat, high-fiber diet and exercising aerobically.

Vitamins before High-Fat Meal
May Reduce Heart Attack Risk

BALTIMORE—Did you know that eating a single fatty meal may temporarily boost your risk of having a heart attack or stroke? In a Danish study, researchers found that 18 healthy men produced about 60 percent more blood-clotting agents after they ate meals with about 55 grams of fat. However, taking 1,000 milligrams of vitamin C and 800 milligrams of vitamin E before you eat a high-fat meal like a cheese omelet, burger, or steak may reduce your chances of having a heart attack.

A study from the University of Maryland School of Medicine suggests that men who took these powerful antioxidants before they splurged on McDonald's chow (they ate an Egg McMuffin, a Sausage McMuffin and two hash browns—for a total of 790 calories and 59 grams of fat) maintained normal blood vessel function compared with the men who skipped the supplements. If you'd rather not carry pills, eat foods rich in vitamins C (strawberries and melon) and E (nuts and oils) beforehand. "The lower dosages of the vitamins that are found in food may still have a protective effect," says study author Gary D. Plotnick, M.D.

Fend Off Alzheimer's
by Keeping Blood Pressure in Check

CHICAGO—Beating high blood pressure just became a little more important. Avoiding high blood pressure may be a way to fend off Alzheimer's disease, according to research from the University of Illinois at Chicago. Researchers tracked the blood pressure of nearly 400 men and women beginning at age 70. The people who had the highest diastolic pressures (the bottom number) all developed Alzheimer's disease by age 85. Regular aerobic exercise can keep your diastolic pressure in check.

One Beer a Night Packs Health Benefits

CAMBRIDGE, Mass.—Here's some new research that may alter your beer-drinking schedule: Polishing off one six-pack per week may keep you drinking (moderately) into your eighties. Two six-packs per week, however, and last call may come way before retirement.

The white coats have long told us that drinking alcohol in moderation (no more than two drinks a night) has proven health benefits. Now Harvard researchers have offered a more sober definition: One nightly beer can help protect you from cardiovascular disease and cancer, but trouble may come if you pop a second.

Scientists chronicled the lifestyles of more than 22,000 men for 11 years and found that the risk of death, from all causes, was 28 percent lower in those who had only six or fewer drinks per week. But the risk increased 51 percent in men who had two or more drinks daily. "It's clear that small differences in alcohol consumption may make the difference between preventing and causing premature deaths," says Charles H. Hennekens, M.D., professor of medicine and lead researcher. So enjoy your microbrews. One at a time.

Garlic Is Good for Circulation

COLUMBUS, Ohio—Don't shun garlic because of its lingering odor. A diet rich in garlic makes your aorta more flexible and can increase circulation, according to researchers at Ohio State University, along with their colleagues in Mainz, Germany. They found these results after studying 49 men and 52 women who took one 300-milligram garlic supplement—or about two cloves of garlic—every day for two years. Your arteries, especially the aorta, lose elasticity as you age, says study coauthor Harisios Boudoulas, M.D. Ingesting garlic causes your body to release nitric oxide, which keeps your arteries more pliable, says Dr. Boudoulas. So keep those cloves near the stove.

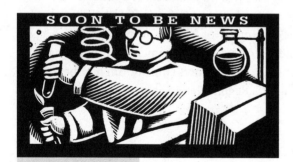

No More Talk of the Big C?

Cancer kills more than 1,500 Americans every day. It's still the Tyrannosaurus rex of diseases, with prostate, colorectal, and lung cancer being the chief man-eaters. But this will change in the next 25 years.

"The advances in fighting cancer will be phenomenal," says Edison Liu, M.D., director of the division of clinical sciences at the National Cancer Institute. Here are five promising developments that should take the bite out of cancer.

1. Early detection. Within 15 years, researchers hope to be using extremely sensitive tests of blood, urine, and saliva to detect the slightest traces of cancer proteins, says David S. Ettinger, M.D., associate director for clinical affairs and professor of oncology and medicine at Johns Hopkins Oncology Center in Baltimore. Many cancers will be diagnosed, treated, and cured years earlier than they are now.

2. Vaccines. "We'll fortify the immune system with cells that can home in on certain cancers and kill them," explains Dr. Liu. "Vaccines for liver cancer, lymphomas, melanoma, and even prostate cancer may be developed within two decades."

3. Molecular drugs. By 2015, physicians will use drugs that block only the particular molecules that allow certain cancer cells to grow. "While chemotherapy acts like an atomic bomb, the newer cancer drugs will make surgical strikes," says Dr. Liu.

4. Tumor-strangling agents. "Drugs that stop cancer from forming new blood vessels are working in the lab right now," says Mario Sznol, M.D., a physician in the cancer-therapy evaluation program at the National Cancer Institute. "These antiangiogenic agents starve tumors to death." Such drugs may significantly reduce cancer deaths—and even halt advanced cancers—as early as 2010.

5. Killer genes. Gene therapy can be used to fight cancer, too, says Dr. Liu. Snuffing out the cancer-causing genes in prostate, colon, and pancreatic cells—or introducing kamikaze genes that direct the malignant cells to die—may short-circuit the disease by 2015.

The biggest element in reining in cancer is already in our control. "Throw every other medical breakthrough out the window," says Dr. Liu. "If men stop smoking today, that'll be the most significant public health event of the twenty-first century."

Vitamin E to the Rescue?

A study at Columbia University in Morningside Heights, New York, found that high doses of vitamin E may delay the progression of Alzheimer's disease. After two years, subjects taking 2,000 international units of vitamin E daily showed 25 percent less functional deterioration than subjects taking a placebo. "Vitamin E may protect brain neurons from free radical damage," says Mary Sano, Ph.D., associate professor of clinical neurology at the university. However, such high dosages of vitamin E can be toxic.

Ongoing studies are trying to determine if lower dosages offer similar protection.

An End to Warts?

Genital warts are a result of a common group of sexually transmitted viruses. Some of these viruses can cause cervical cancer and have even been linked to cancer of the penis. But researchers are testing a vaccine that may prevent infection from the human papillomaviruses (HPV) that cause genital warts. A form of this vaccine can safely prevent infections in animals. "We're hoping that it will work in humans as well," says study leader Richard C. Reichman, M.D., director of the infectious-diseases unit at the University of Rochester School of Medicine and Dentistry in New York.

If clinical trials are successful, an HPV vaccine could be available in three to five years.

Pushing Aspirin Aside?

A four-year study showed that clopidogrel, a drug that prevents blood clotting, is more effective in preventing recurrences of heart attacks and strokes than aspirin and has fewer side effects. "This drug is better than aspirin at blocking clot formation," says Jonathan Plehn, M.D., director of the cardiac ultrasound laboratory at Dartmouth-Hitchcock Medical Center in Hanover, New Hampshire. In a study of more than 19,000 people who used heart-drug therapy, clopidogrel was significantly more protective than aspirin in preventing further attacks. And, unlike aspirin, it doesn't cause stomach bleeding.

The drug is expected to be submitted for approval by the Food and Drug Administration soon.

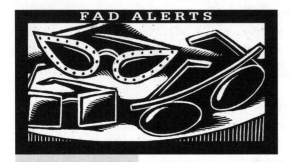

FAD ALERTS

Home Blood Pressure Monitors

An easy way to monitor your health—while minimizing your contact with doctors—is to check your blood pressure every month. With the new breed of high-tech, electronic devices on the market, you'd think that process would be easier than ever. But is it? We rolled up our sleeves to find out.

First, a registered nurse took our blood pressures using the old pressure-band-and-stethoscope method. Then she measured us using four top electronic models. One editor who scored a healthy 120/76 on the old-fashioned pump gauge clocked a much higher 135/78 just minutes later on a $100 electronic monitor. The other electronic gauges also missed the nurse's readings by 10 to 15 points.

The problem? Electronic models are too sensitive to small movements, says Ray Gifford, M.D., president of the National Hypertension Association, based in New York City. Standard manual models are more reliable. These gauges—the type used by doctors—sell in drugstores for under $30.

Pycnogenol

Health gurus say we need to stop those harmful oxygen molecules called free radicals from rusting our cells—now. And they're selling "super-antioxidants" that promise to roast more radicals than a Pat Buchanan rally.

Pycnogenol, a substance extracted from French pine bark and grape seeds, is among the most touted of these. Sold in health food stores for $25 per bottle, pycnogenol is supposed to increase brainpower and guard against heart disease and cancer.

"The earlier people start taking pycnogenol, the longer they'll delay the onset of diseases associated with free radical damage," says Richard A. Passwater, Ph.D., director of research at the Solgar Nutritional Research Center in Berlin, Maryland, and coauthor of *Pycnogenol: The Super "Protector" Nutrient.*

A diet rich in antioxidants is a solid idea, but no large-scale documented studies in humans support such far-reaching claims for supplements. Hit the produce department—not the pharmacy. "In addition to providing antioxidants, real fruits and vegetables will add fiber and carbohydrates to your diet," says Kristine Clark, R.D., Ph.D., director of sports nutrition at the Pennsylvania State University Center for Sports Medicine in University Park.

LipoGuard

Most men know that fish-oil and garlic supplements benefit the heart. LipoGuard, a supplement created by Viva America, contains 180 milligrams of eicosapentaenoic acid and 120 milligrams of docosahexaenoic acid (the active ingredients in fish oil) as well as 250 milligrams of garlic concentrate. In Viva's study, subjects taking 10 LipoGuard pills daily for one month cut their "bad" low-density lipoprotein cholesterol by 10 percent. The rub: 300 pills will set you back $147.50. The same amount of generic fish-oil and garlic supplements costs about $100 less. To see if LipoGuard works for you, have your cholesterol and triglycerides checked before and after taking it for three months, advises Bruce Holub, Ph.D., professor of nutrition at the University of Guelph in Ontario, Canada. "If the numbers don't change, you're wasting money."

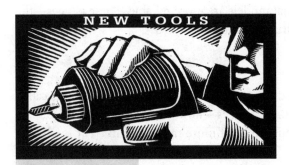

Germ-Killing Covering

Calcium-Hydroxide Paint

A fresh coat of paint could turn your house into a germ-free zone. A new antibacterial paint can kill 99 percent of bacteria and viruses within an hour of contact, for at least four years. Hospitals will likely buy tankers of this calcium-hydroxide paint to reduce the almost two million infections that are contracted in hospitals each year. "It'll be especially beneficial in air-conditioning ducts, which transmit airborne bacteria and allergens," says inventor Bill Mallow, a scientist at Southwest Research Institute in San Antonio, Texas.

More Eye Protection

UV-Absorbing Contact Lenses

Yet another way to protect your peepers: Eye-care companies are marketing new contact lenses that block harmful ultraviolet (UV) light. These extended-wear contacts, coated with UV-absorbing chemicals, block up to 90 percent of UV rays and cost about the same as normal contacts, according to Robert E. Neger, M.D., assistant clinical professor of ophthalmology at the University of California, San Francisco. "And they don't let light in from the sides, the way sunglasses can," Dr. Neger says.

Painless Plaque Fighter

Atridox

Even the words "gum scraping" are enough to make you cringe. But here's an alternative cure for gum disease: A new antibiotic gel may fight plaque and tartar—painlessly. Squirted into the pockets created by gum disease, Atridox, which contains doxycycline and a hardening agent—would seal and treat the area over the course of a week. "Then it biodegrades or is flushed away," says Charles Cox, Ph.D., vice president at Atrix Labs in Fort Collins, Colorado, developers of the gel.

Better Dental Diagnoses

Computed Dental Radiography

Besides bombarding your brain with radiation, dental x-rays have another major shortcoming: Dentists need a keen eye to find insidious problems on these tiny squares of film. But new digital x-rays yield 90 percent less radiation and use a computer to help diagnose hidden dental problems. The Computed Dental Radiography (CDR) system uses x-ray sensors instead of film, explains Howard Spielman, D.D.S., a restorative dentist in New York City. Thousands of dentists are using the CDR system.

An End to Hypothyroidism

Thyroid-Stimulating Hormone Blood Test

If you suddenly and inexplicably gain weight, lose hair, or become grouchier than a Utah militia member, it's probably not your boss's fault. You may be the unlucky owner of an underactive thyroid gland, which results in a common condition known as hypothyroidism. According to researchers at Johns Hopkins University in Baltimore, as many as 3 percent of men suffer from some degree of hypothyroidism, which can drag on for years and, if left untreated, can cause high cholesterol, heart disease, and memory loss.

Luckily, your doctor has a quick fix. "There's a safe, relatively inexpensive test that can diagnose the problem, and there's also a very effective treatment," says Paul Ladenson, M.D., director of the division of endocrinology and metabolism at Johns Hopkins. If you have any of the above symptoms, ask your doctor for a thyroid-stimulating hormone (TSH) blood test. The cost ranges from $15 to $40. If you're diagnosed with hypothyroidism, taking 150 micrograms daily of a synthetic hormone called thyroxine, or T_4, usually corrects the condition.

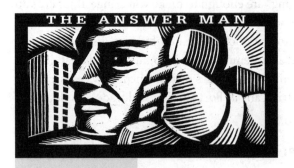

Injectable Sunscreen?

I have very pale skin, even in the summer. I read somewhere that you can get melanin injections that both darken the skin and prevent sunburns and skin cancer. True?
—R. J., McKeesport, Pa.

Melanin—a natural pigment that your body produces—does darken skin and protect against sunburn and skin cancer, says Norman Levine, M.D., chief of dermatology at the Arizona Health Sciences Center in Tucson. But it can't be injected directly.

What you may have read about is an experimental drug called Melanotan, which stimulates your body to produce more melanin. In early trials, Melanotan appears to darken skin color, says Dr. Levine, who's involved in the drug's development. However, Melanotan won't be available for at least a few years; so for now the only safe way to darken your skin is to use a self-tanning product. You'll also need a sunscreen with an SPF of at least 15 anytime you're outdoors. And make sure it's waterproof, or you'll sweat most of the protection away, says Dr. Levine.

Saw Away at a Large Prostate

My father is taking saw palmetto for his enlarged prostate. Does it make sense for me to start taking the supplement now to prevent problems down the road?
—J. P., Stillwater, Okla.

The answer depends on which doctor you talk to. "I'm taking saw palmetto as a preventive measure myself," says Steven Margolis, M.D., clinical instructor at

Wayne State University in Detroit and an alternative family physician practicing in Sterling Heights, Michigan. "I'd recommend the same to anyone with a family history of prostate enlargement."

Saw palmetto appears to block your body's ability to convert testosterone into dihydrotestosterone, the substance that causes your prostate to enlarge. So it's not much of a leap to think it could prevent your prostate from swelling in the first place.

The trouble is that no one has actually tested saw palmetto as a preventive medicine—and for every expert who thinks your plan might work, there's another who's skeptical. "There's no evidence to suggest that saw palmetto will prevent the development of prostate problems," says Glenn Gerber, M.D., associate professor of urology at the University of Chicago. "And a number of studies have suggested that taking saw palmetto may relieve symptoms but that it doesn't actually shrink the prostate."

The two doctors agree that taking saw palmetto in small doses (160 milligrams per day) probably won't hurt you and might help. Just make sure that you buy a brand that contains 85 to 95 percent saw palmetto extract; that's the minimum effective dose, according to Dr. Margolis.

The Lowdown on Chucks

Do high-top sneakers really protect your ankles any better than the conventional kind?
—A. W., West Chester, Pa.

You aren't the first to wonder about this. After studying the frequency of ankle injuries in college basketball players, researchers at the University of Oklahoma in Norman concluded that high-tops don't offer any more protection than low-tops.

"The best way to avoid ankle sprains is to find a correctly fitting shoe that feels comfortable to you, regardless of whether it's a high-top or low-top," says James R. Barrett, M.D., professor of family medicine at the university and lead author of the study.

Worn-out shoes may increase the risk of sprains, according to Dr. Barrett. They're definitely ready for the trash pile when most of the tread is worn away or when you find yourself losing traction, though the internal support may break down before then. So try to replace your shoes every three to six months, depending on how often you work out in them.

Ankle-strengthening exercises and stretching the back of the ankle before play may help as well, he says. For a simple stretch, stand facing a flight of stairs, your toes on a step, your heels hanging over the edge. Lower your heels until you can feel the stretch in your Achilles tendons. Hold for 10 to 30 seconds, relax, and repeat three or four times.

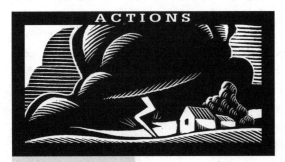

ACTIONS

Our culture puts a great deal of emphasis on curing diseases and ailments. Wouldn't it be better to prevent these problems in the first place? Of course— which is why we provide these 20 tips to keep yourself disease-free.

1. Guard the family jewels. If your mother took the antimiscarriage drug diethylstilbestrol (DES) during pregnancy—between 1938 and 1971 about 4.8 million women did—be sure to perform a monthly testicular self-exam. A study found that men whose mothers took DES while pregnant developed testicular cysts three times more often than other men. The cysts, though benign, must be checked to rule out cancer. "Ask your mother if she took DES, and report it to your doctor," says Larry I. Lipshultz, M.D., professor of urology at Baylor College of Medicine in Houston.

2. See a skin specialist. A study conducted at the University of Toronto revealed that many family physicians are uncomfortable diagnosing melanoma, a deadly skin cancer. If you think a suspicious mole may be skin cancer, see a dermatologist, not your family physician. Of 355 family physicians surveyed, 78 percent admitted they had trouble spotting early melanoma, and less than 50 percent correctly identified risk factors, such as freckles or multiple moles. A whopping 60 percent said they rarely sent patients to a specialist. So if you see something suspicious, call the dermatologist yourself.

3. Don't overdo it. Just because it's a "dietary supplement" doesn't mean it's harmless. According to a recent report, melatonin overdose is a real risk. In one case, a 66-year-old man regularly used melatonin with other sedatives. But when he quadrupled his daily dose to 24 milligrams, he felt lethargic and lost some memory, says Peter Chyka, Pharm.D., of the University of Tennessee at

Memphis. "Melatonin is an unknown," he says. "Ask your doctor or pharmacist before using it."

4. **Give them the brush off.** Next time you reach for your toothbrush, do a dry run first. According to a recent study of 129 people, "dry-brushing" your teeth before a regular brushing cuts tartar by 60 percent. The technique also cut bleeding of the gums by 50 percent, says study author Trisha O'Hehir, a registered dental hygienist in Flagstaff, Arizona. Here's how to do it: Using a dry, soft brush, start by scrubbing the insides of your bottom teeth; then hit the insides of the top ones, before working your way to the outer surfaces, says O'Hehir. Finally, rinse, spit, and brush again briefly—this time with toothpaste.

5. **Don't be shifty.** Wiped out by day's end? The reason may not be your soaring productivity. More likely you've been shifting your eyes too much. Scientists believe that darting your eyes as you work drains your brainpower and makes you tired. When your eyes refocus, concentration falters and some brain functions shut down temporarily, says Robert Abel Jr., M.D., clinical professor of ophthalmology at Thomas Jefferson University in Philadelphia. This eventually causes fatigue. You can stay more energized (and prevent sore neck muscles) by keeping all reading material at eye level and making sure that you have the correct glasses, says Dr. Abel.

6. **Let your dentist do double duty.** Next time your dentist takes an x-ray of your jaw, tell him to check your arteries, too. Researchers in California found that dental x-rays can help predict the risk of stroke and heart attack. In a study of 1,063 men, dental x-rays consistently revealed blockages in the carotid arteries, which run through the neck. That's a strong indication that the heart arteries are also blocked, says Arthur Friedlander, D.D.S., lead author of a study published in the *Journal of the American Dental Association.* "Dentists are obligated to spot these blockages and send the x-rays to the patient's physician," says Dr. Friedlander.

7. **Wash legions of germs down the drain.** Plumbing repairs could wipe out more than your wallet. A study in the *Archives of Internal Medicine* concluded that banging on the pipes can stir up otherwise idle bacteria that cause Legionnaires' disease, a serious respiratory infection. To be safe, flush out your faucets and showers for 15 minutes immediately after a plumbing repair, especially if Legionnaires' has ever broken out in your area. "And make sure that anyone with respiratory problems or a weakened immune system is out of the house," says Joseph Plouffe, M.D., study author and an infectious-disease specialist at Ohio State University Medical Center in Columbus.

8. **Don't neglect your gums.** Tartar pushes gums away from teeth, sometimes creating deep pockets in the gumline that can lead to tooth loss. According to the Academy of General Dentistry in Chicago, men are developing periodontal pockets much more frequently than women. Poor eating and brushing habits as well as smoking and drinking may explain the higher rate of this periodontal disease in men, says Charles H. Perle, D.M.D., spokesperson for the academy. Repairing the gum recession might take surgery, so spend a little more time at the sink and visit the dentist every six months.

9. **Demand a fair hearing.** By now, you've no doubt heard about the "stethoscope" study from Allegheny University in Pennsylvania. When asked to diagnose abnormal heart sounds and murmurs by listening to recordings, 453 physicians could accurately detect problems only about 20 percent of the time. Luckily, listening to the heart with a stethoscope is only one step in diagnosing health problems, says Salvatore Mangione, M.D., coauthor of the study. Still, you'd better give your doctor all the help he needs to catch cardiac ailments.

• Stay thin. Fat muffles the heartbeats your doctor needs to hear.
• Tell him about any changes in your health. They include fatigue when walking up stairs, congestion when you lie down, or fleeting chest pain. Also tell your doctor if you've ever had leg swelling, an occasional racing heartbeat, or breathlessness for no good reason.
• Finally, when shopping for a doctor, bring a harmonica and request a few bars of "Piano Man." The study found that physicians who played musical instruments discerned heart problems most accurately.

10. **Let 'er rip.** Ever wonder if your eardrums will really explode if you hold in a big sneeze? Well, that's not likely, but a smothered sneeze can still cause serious problems. "Stifling a sneeze can force infectious organisms from your nose into your ears, possibly resulting in an ear infection," says Gordon Vap, M.D., an ear, nose, and throat specialist at the ENT Medical Group of Washington, D.C. "And in rare cases, it can injure the membrane in the inner ear and damage your hearing." If you want to save your ears—but don't want to spray everyone at the salad bar—try pinching your nose when you feel the first tickle of a sneeze coming on. That might make the sensation subside. Otherwise, just let the big man blow; think of it as an orgasm for your head.

11. **Cultivate a roving eye.** Hold your hand at arm's length. Now, focusing on your thumb, move your arm in circles and figure eights as you bring your hand closer. This flexes the eye muscles and may offset time's toll on your peepers.

12. **Sniff out vitamin A.** Eat red and yellow fruits and vegetables, such as apricots, mangoes, tangerines, squash, and carrots. The vitamin A will keep your nasal lining healthy and keep your sense of smell from deteriorating prematurely.

13. **Sleep on your back.** Eight hours with your face pressed against a pillow can wrinkle your skin and, over time, cause permanent creases. If you can't sleep on your back, try face-friendly satin pillowcases.

14. **Invite antioxidants to your picnic.** Inhale more foods rich in the antioxidants C, E, and beta-carotene as well as selenium. They may help prevent lung cancer. Citrus fruits, peppers, and strawberries are rich sources of C; nuts and wheat germ are high in vitamin E; spinach, sweet potatoes, and broccoli supply beta-carotene; and seafood is full of selenium.

15. **Relax after dinner.** Your stomach needs extra blood from your muscles to properly digest a big meal. If you do something active, you interfere with digestion.

16. **Suck up abdominal strength.** To build powerful abdominal muscles, try this: Kneel with your feet crossed under your buttocks and your hands on your hips. Keeping your upper body straight, breathe out and then suck your stomach up and in as far as it will go. Hold for five seconds. Do two or three sets of 10 repetitions.

17. **Point the finger.** Place your hand palm-down on a table and spread your fingers as wide as possible. Hold the position for 10 seconds, relax, and then repeat. Do five repetitions three times a day and you'll increase your dexterity.

18. **Do the twist.** Move your hips around as if you were using a Hula Hoop. Do this for a few minutes each day and you'll increase flexibility in your pelvis. You'll have more control over the thrusting of your penis during intercourse and improved circulation in the whole region. Ukulele and grass skirt optional.

19. **Learn how to get out of bed.** Instead of jumping up to meet the day, roll onto your side and gently push with your hands to lift your torso off the mattress. Why? At night, spinal disks fill with water and expand, and the surrounding muscles tend to stiffen. One sudden movement can damage your disks.

20. **Go for a lunchtime walk.** Sunlight causes your body to produce vitamin D, which aids insulin's job of preventing elevated blood sugar levels—one of the primary causes of kidney failure.

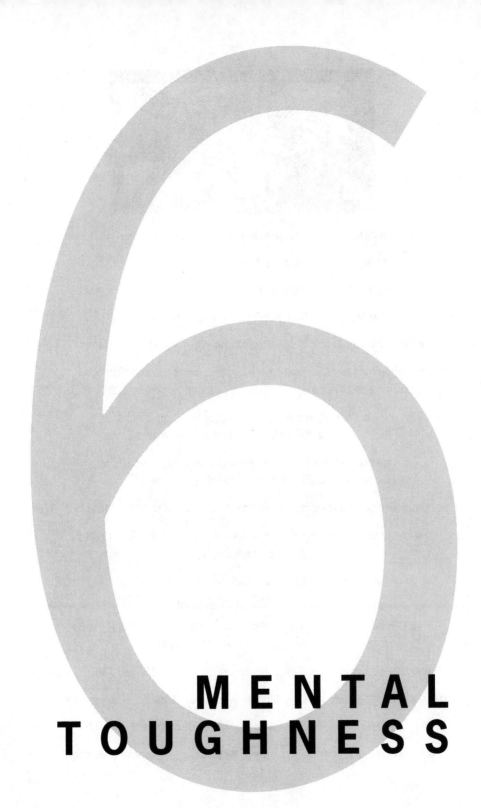

6

MENTAL
TOUGHNESS

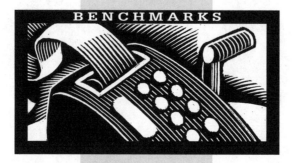

BENCHMARKS

■ Number of people who are seriously considering quitting their jobs: 2 in 5

■ Percentage of doctor visits that result from stress-related illnesses: 80

■ Percentage of baby boomers who say their lives are often out of control: 27

■ Average number of laughs a person has in a day: 17

■ Percentage of Americans who would rather be mugged than audited: 50

■ Number of Americans who have a disorder called "uncontrolled buying," which causes them to go on compulsive shopping sprees: 2,863,751

■ Cans of beer per sailor the U.S. Navy requisitions for those completing 45 straight days at sea: 2

■ Price per minute a San Francisco hotel charges guests for a phone session with its on-call psychotherapist: $2

■ Percentage of Americans who would rather vacation on short trips than long: 37

■ Percentage of people who feel that stress in moderation is not harmful, it's a fact of life: 60

■ Percentage of executives who would miss a holiday or important family event to make a business trip: 45

■ Number of Americans who credit insomnia for hampering their ability to handle stress on the job: 36 million

■ Annual cost of job stress to American industry: $200 billion to $300 billion

■ Number of people who miss work on an average day because of stress: 1 million

■ Average age at which American children develop phobias: 13.5

■ Percentage of Americans who believe they have a good sense of humor: 85

Surviving the Workday

Master stress and make it work for you.

Shortly after five o'clock on a chilly Boston morning, R. Michael Scott descends the stairs to the kitchen of his four-story South-End town house, taking pains not to wake his wife. A trim 56-year-old with a close-cropped beard, he mixes yogurt with cereal for his breakfast, chases it with coffee and a chocolate-covered doughnut as he leafs through a travel magazine, then rinses the dishes in the sink. This morning he could be any one of us, a man quietly preparing for another day at work. Except that for Scott, today's workday will be spent inside the skull of a 10-year-old girl, in a delicate and dangerous bid to save the child's life.

As R. Michael Scott, M.D., director of the section of pediatric neurosurgery at Children's Hospital in Boston, he will be in the operating room by 8:00 A.M., prepping for the operation. His patient has been flown all the way from Alabama for the surgery, which involves moving an artery from the scalp and meticulously transplanting it onto the brain's surface. If everything goes right, Dr. Scott will be operating for eight hours straight. Only when the grueling procedure is over will he begin his patient rounds, checking the progress of the many children whose futures depend on his skill and self-control.

This level of pressure would send some men hurtling toward a stress-induced meltdown. Not Dr. Scott. Despite facing life-and-death decisions on almost a daily basis, Dr. Scott has his health and his humor intact. Like other men under a lot of pressure, Dr. Scott has found ways to handle tension levels that would send most of us running to the medicine cabinet—or the liquor store. If there's a secret to coping with stress, these guys know it.

We wanted to know it, too. So we followed Dr. Scott and other highly stressed men through work time and downtime and watched their strategies for surviving the pressure cooker.

Pediatric brain surgery isn't rocket science—it's tougher. This is intricate mental and physical work, more often than not with a child's life in the balance. Every veteran surgeon has his methods of stress relief, but Dr. Scott, the president of the American Society of Pediatric Neurosurgeons, is renowned as one of the coolest and calmest, in and out of the operating room. A teaching physician at Harvard Medical School, Dr. Scott occasionally allows students to observe his procedures. During a recent surgery, with the brain of the patient exposed and Dr. Scott wielding a scalpel dangerously close to vital tissue, one such student fainted, overturning a trolley laden with surgical instruments that fell to the floor with a resounding clatter. A man in the grip of stress surely would have flinched at the racket—with potentially tragic consequences. Instead, serene and focused, Dr. Scott hardly seemed to notice.

"I'd never seen anything like it," says a doctor who was there at the time. "He's intense, yet never so stressed that he isn't perfectly polite. I'd love to know what he knows."

Creating Rituals

After an hour in his office doing paperwork, and a visit with the patient's family, Dr. Scott starts readying himself for surgery. As he steps into the cramped doctors' locker room holding a fresh pair of scrubs, he might be entering the clubhouse at nearby Fenway Park. Like an athlete, Dr. Scott has a locker; he also has his own preparation rituals that help him stay calm and focused. "It's right now, before a surgery, that my stress is the highest," Dr. Scott says. "This ritual we surgeons have of getting dressed helps me feel comfortable. It's almost like a religious rite." He pulls sanitary plastic covers over his street shoes and sticks his wallet into the front pocket of his scrub shirt. All he needs is a baseball glove.

Dr. Scott's first chore inside the operating room is picking the compact discs he'll listen to during the procedure and installing them in the CD player tucked out of the way against a wall. Though he's a trained musician who plays piano and bass for jazz bands, Dr. Scott isn't choosing the music because he likes it or because the soothing strains calm him, but because it makes him feel at home. "I want to hear music familiar to me," he says. "I know some of these CDs backward and forward." That familiarity provides a counterpoint to the potential unknowns that could arise during surgery. For this operation, he chooses Stan Getz and Joao Gilberto, Ella Fitzgerald, and Bach's Concerto in D Minor for Harpsichord, among others. On a different day, it might be different music that he knows equally well—but nothing that gets his feet tapping too much.

Concentrating on the Given

"I've planned out exactly what I want to do during the operation, down to the last detail," Dr. Scott says. "I know the instruments I'll need from the nurse and exactly the order in which I'll need them." The young girl from Alabama is suffering from a rare condition called Moyamoya disease, and her brain doesn't receive enough blood. Left untreated, the condition will likely leave her paralyzed and unable to speak.

Dr. Scott will cut through the scalp to reach the artery, open the skull and, using a microscope, attach the artery to the brain's surface with sutures thinner than a human hair. Next, he'll move to the other side of the head and graft another artery, hoping that new blood vessels will grow from the transplanted arteries into the brain. The first part of the procedure is routine—but then it happens. A few minutes into the second hour, the brain starts pulsating inside the cranium, bouncing the microscope out of focus and threatening to tear the stitches. Dr. Scott calls an audible and deftly shifts the angle of the head with a clamp, alleviating the problem. After a sigh of relief all around, he proceeds. "My day is spent getting the predictable out of the way to make room for the unpredictable," he says. "The more efficiently I can do that, the better I can handle the stress."

Dr. Scott's patients range from newborns to children in their early teens, and their parents are almost always nervous wrecks. He has to interact with the parents frequently, discussing strategies, gauging each operation's chance of success, relaying updates, and occasionally informing them of serious complications. Nothing that happens in the operating room causes him more stress than this, he says. So when Dr. Scott makes his rounds at the end of the day, he does it with a team: A half-dozen residents and fellows arrive at a patient's room simultaneously, sharing information with the family and planning treatment strategies together. Discussing these issues as a team helps to defuse the stress of dealing with sick children and their distraught families.

At home, he has his wife—a nurse at another Boston-area hospital—to listen and offer advice. "Susan can tell when I walk through the door if something is stressing me," he says. It helps that she can understand his work in detail, but the mere act of unloading the stress helps relieve it. "Don't try to be tough and keep it to yourself," he says.

Stress in the Air

It's easy to see how the twin Wasatch and Oquirrh mountain ranges dominate the Salt Lake Valley, hemming in civilization and creating a funnel for approaching airplanes. From behind the controls of a tiny private plane the size of a Volkswagen, Steve Darton points out topographical landmarks to his eight-year-old daughter, Stephany, snug in a harness in the backseat.

A few hours later, he sees these same mountain ranges. This time they're not majestic white-capped landmarks. They are altitude markers on a round, black radar screen in a dark, windowless room on the sixth floor of the airport's tower. Darton, 40, is a part of a team of air-traffic controllers that guides as many as 50 aircraft at a time through the approach procedure. A Delta Air Lines hub, Salt Lake City handles as many as 1,800 operations (takeoffs and landings) every day, and those intimidating mountains make directing traffic into Salt Lake International and seven adjacent airfields especially problematic.

In the multistage dogleg that serves as the final approach from all directions, a controller has no margin for error. "The mountains rise so steeply, so quickly, that in 10 seconds of flight time, you could go from a minimum possible height of 6,000 feet up to 11,000," Darton says. At one time, he'll have as many as a dozen planes in the air to track. He must know the type of engine and navigational equipment each aircraft carries and the way a typical crew from each airline is taught to perform; keep a mental map of the area's topography at the front of his consciousness; and remember the exact instructions he has fed to every plane he's working. He can't let his guard down for a moment. "I've seen young controllers literally shaking," says Darton. "They learn to deal with the pressure or they don't last. Stress is insidious, and it's cumulative. So you need to have a maintenance program that helps you stay ahead of it. I don't want to be playing catch-up with stress."

Pressure is always on to maintain schedules and efficiency. This means keeping the approaching planes close—but not too close. There's a minimum distance allowed by the Federal Aviation Administration (FAA), and a controller who allows planes to come any closer (called "losing separation") will lose his controller's certification. The problem is that even when one plane's operation is taking longer than planned, other planes are waiting in the sky. The controller can't simply tell them to go away. "You may be thinking about what happened a moment ago in the back of your mind, but—first and foremost—you have to make adjustments and keep on going," Darton says. "Otherwise, one incident will lead to more."

Practicing for Crunch Times

In the darkened control room, Darton guides planes into the funnel for final approach on this cloudless March evening. He needs to leave a minimum of three miles between them at the same altitude. Even a fraction of a mile too close counts as loss of separation, so many controllers make sure they give themselves plenty of room for error.

"A lot of controllers bring them in at four or five miles, but I strive for more efficient spacing—as close to three miles as I can," he says. So when traffic jams occur, ratcheting up his level of efficiency doesn't worry him—because he's already there.

During the 6:30 P.M. arrival bank of some 60 planes from all over the United States, Darton is working the "Bear" sector of Salt Lake airspace, blending streams of traffic from the north and northwest, choosing altitudes, speeds, and vector angles designed to keep the flow moving. Strips of paper, each signifying an arriving aircraft, are lined up to his right. But the unforeseen happens: Just as a small corporate plane with limited acceleration capabilities is entering the "Bear" airspace, two unscheduled F-18 Hornets request permission to leave Hill Air Force Base. In tandem, they take off, rising sharply and directly into the flight path of the slower plane.

Amidst the hum of casual conversation and the incessant beep of the radar sweep, Darton has to immediately calculate what altitude the fast-moving Hornets and the puttering Cessna will be at when their flight paths cross, laid against a background of a Frontier jet taking off eastbound and a bank of planes arriving from the northwest. But as he makes a hundred minor adjustments in his head, there's no perceptible rise in his stress level. "This is exactly what I practice for every day," he says, calmly giving radio commands and reordering his strips of paper.

Darton's breaks are FAA-mandated. But he wouldn't be able to handle an eight-hour shift, he says, without a 10- or 20-minute breather every hour and a half. "You'd see a lot more burnout than you do if we couldn't unplug and walk around," he says. "It's so important to get up and walk away for a little while and clear my head."

At least once a night, Darton descends six flights of stairs into the main passenger terminal and hikes along the concourse. But he says any scenery will do, as long as it isn't a radar screen. "Just something else to see," he says. It's a survival strategy he has taught his oldest son, Jack, a freshman at Utah State University in Logan. During dinner that night, Jack explains the wisdom of putting aside his cramming for final exams and taking in a movie. "You're more effective if you're not so worried and stressed about things," Jack declaims. Hearing that, his father nods in approval.

On the Front Line

On a balmy spring afternoon in Denver, Reuben Gomez is sweating. Not because of the double flak jacket he's wearing over his dress blues, or his balaclava and flameproof gloves. And not because the immediate-entry warrant he and 11 other officers are about to serve includes the warning that the suspected crack dealer inside is armed and dangerous. Gomez, 38, has helped execute close to a thousand of these no-knock warrants during his 12 years on the SWAT team—with as many as six in a single afternoon. He's sweating because in all that time, he has never manned the "break-and-rake" position he has been assigned on this one—removing a fortified screen door from its hinges and using a battering ram to knock the front door aside. That's his job today.

Sitting in the makeshift briefing room at SWAT headquarters, watching the surveillance video of the site that two officers have taken earlier that day, he worries about what will happen if he can't perform his task. "If I can't get the door off," he says, "the whole team has to wait, and we lose the elements of speed and surprise that are our biggest advantages. The suspect could try to escape out the back." Worse, he could stay and fight it out. It's a rare moment for Gomez, who, like most of the 33 members of Denver's elite police team, has learned to defuse his occupational stress. "We're all pretty good at it," he says. "You have to be or you wouldn't want this line of work."

The unmarked white van, intentionally battered to prevent detection, winds its way through the less-than-desirable neighborhood overlooking Mile High Stadium. Inside the van, insults are flying. The 12 team members assigned to execute this West Denver warrant deflect the building tension by picking each other apart. It gets personal, but that's the point: These men know and trust each other.

That trust is critical. As the break-and-rake man, Gomez won't be carrying a weapon when the door swings open. Like a soldier, he needs absolute belief in those to the right and left of him or he's lost. "And when you think about it, over the years we've seen many more combat situations than most people in the military have," he says. Although both the day and night SWAT teams are trained precisely the same way, their members will almost never be mixed in an operation. The reason? Unfamiliarity with each other—and a lower level of trust that can only lead to stress.

Breaking Down the Job

As the vehicle turns a corner and reduces its speed within a block of the target, the atmosphere changes and the group suddenly falls silent. The time is at hand. Gomez mentally rehearses his task once more as the van rolls to a stop, then throws open the doors and leaps out.

Knocking down the tenement door is merely the first step of the operation. He has a series of tasks to perform, from covering the door from the outside to controlling the crowd that inevitably forms at the site of a police action. But if he thinks of them all at once, he'll tense up. Instead, Gomez takes a deep breath and remembers to prioritize. Take care of the door, then move to the next duty. "Break it down like that and it's easy," he says.

That's what he's thinking between the van and the cement front steps, a distance he covers at a dead run. He grasps the door by its black iron grillwork and gets the benefit of the good luck that sometimes accompanies painstaking preparation: It's unlocked. The door swings open, and so does the second one. In an instant, the men are inside the small, sparsely furnished house, fanning out to find the suspect, the surprise complete.

It doesn't always go this well. Reuben Gomez knows what can happen when a police officer is overstressed. He saw it happen several years ago during a crisis, when an officer collapsed from the strain and had a seizure. "We had this woman hallucinating, shooting up the neighborhood from her porch because she thought she saw invaders from Mars, and all of a sudden our guy is lying out on the front lawn, convulsing," Gomez says. "It really complicated the situation."

The officer who collapsed wasn't always rigorous about physical conditioning, and the incident brought home to Gomez how essential a healthy lifestyle is to his job performance. "If it wasn't for working out and staying fit," Gomez says, "you'd have guys having heart attacks left and right." A well-built man with a linebacker's body, he does free-weight exercises several times a week for about an hour and a half. He tries to play tennis at least once a week and runs about three miles twice a week. "You prepare yourself physically for your job, knowing you're in a high-stress occupation," he says. "Sometimes, in the weight room, I push myself with that in mind."

No matter how sticky the situation during the day, Gomez rarely takes it home to his wife, a policewoman in a nearby city, and his 13-year-old son. "So much tension happens because you don't know where you stand at the end of the day," he says. "I see it with the regular units all the time. It never happens to us because we have a debriefing session after every mission. If someone has something to say about what we did or didn't do, he gets it out in the open and we talk it out. By the time we head for home, it's all behind us. There's no frustration, no bad feelings."

The West Denver mission ends in the apprehension of a suspect who had been on the loose for three years following an arrest warrant in Greeley, Colorado, and the retrieval of a large quantity of drugs and cash. At the debriefing, several questions are raised about the sequence of the entry, but mostly compliments are exchanged. Then Gomez heads to his new house in a quiet Southeast Denver area to hear about his wife's day as a police detective. "She has nobody to debrief with, so she comes home needing to talk about everything that happened," he says. "I listen because it helps relieve her stress, but I've left my work behind. That way, I have plenty of time to relax before the next mission, even if I am called at night and told to report immediately. In the meantime, I'm busy living my life."

Better Golf

Tee off with confidence with these mental tips.

Golfers are always on the brink of blowing their stacks. Here's what to do when you become teed off.

At any given moment during a round, a golfer can spiral mentally downward. Genteel banter quickly switches to explosive rage, *Caddyshack* to *Falling Down* faster than you can three-putt—maybe because you three-putt. Here's a list of the things likely to make you go ballistic on the course, and what to do about them.

Play is moving in slow motion. There is little that is more aggravating than waiting in the fairway while the foursome in front goes through its machinations: the lengthy reading of the green, the cacophony of missed putts, the dramatic head shaking. To deal with it, accept that slow play is a fact. If you're looking for fast-paced action, try shuffleboard.

The best way to deal with slow play is to strike a balance between your own playing rhythm and that of the group ahead, says Richard Coop, Ed.D., professor of educational psychology at the University of North Carolina in Chapel Hill. "Every foursome has a pattern that emerges after a few holes," says Dr. Coop. "One person puts back the flag, another stands to the side keeping score, and so on. Learn to recognize the pattern and play accordingly. Don't start your preshot routine too early and end up having to stand over the shot for a long time."

You stink. If you play only once a week with friends, you can't expect to play like a pro, says Bob Rotella, Ph.D., author of *The Golf of Your Dreams*. The best approach is to have no expectations about your score. Don't have a number in mind that you'd like to shoot—just play for the fun of it. "Golf is a game of mistakes," Dr. Rotella says. "The challenge is to not feel frustrated by them."

You're thinking too much. "You need to concentrate only for 18 to 23 seconds to execute a shot, so lose yourself in the shot, then lighten up," says Dr. Coop. "Enjoy the time with your playing companions." Or daydream about Téa Leoni, because let's face it, your playing companions aren't that enjoyable.

You're stoked. "The reason most people play competitive golf is for excitement—that rush of adrenaline on the first few holes," says Dr. Rotella. If you confuse adrenaline with stress, which is fairly common in inexperienced competitors, he believes that poor golf becomes a self-fulfilling prophecy. "You must treat adrenaline as excitement, not stress, and seek it out. Stress leads to bad play, but the reality is that the better you play, the more adrenaline you will experience."

Dr. Coop, who has worked with several tour players, says that a high level of play can occur only when accompanied by a high state of mental arousal. "However," he adds, "if you go over that line (get too pumped up), you'll start to exhibit the physical manifestations of crossing the threshold—a red face, irritability, finger tapping. You have to recognize these things and reel yourself in."

Your boss is watching. Every golfer who has lifted a driver has, at some point, felt the sting of humiliation, that sense of shame as he chunks a tee shot as the foursome behind watches. Fear of an audience—even a friendly one—contributes as much to golf stress and poor performance as slow play. "Only you can put pressure on yourself," says Joel Kirsch, Ph.D., president of the American Sports Institute in Mill Valley, California. "It's irrelevant whether your thoughts regarding the audience are positive or negative; the very fact that you have thoughts about the audience at all means you're not focused on the task at hand." Next time you get stage fright, pick one element of your swing and focus solely on it. Something like, "Take the club back slowly and low to the ground" is a good start.

Make the Sandman Your Friend

Perform great during the day by getting enough sleep at night.

We'd like you to try something, just for a month. It's simple, painless, and free, and by doing this one thing, you'll actually feel and function better. Sound good? Want to give it a shot? Here it goes: Go upstairs. Lie down. Close your eyes. Fall asleep.

It seems ridiculous at first. Of course you don't get enough sleep. Who does? Everybody you know has the same lifestyle: too many hours at work, too many social engagements to pass up, too much late-night TV. It's not a big deal.

Maybe. Maybe not. Studies suggest that a lack of sleep can interfere with our immune systems, short-circuit our growth, wilt our erections, and raise our blood pressures. Yet Americans sleep 20 percent less than their ancestors did a century ago. The National Commission on Sleep Disorders Research estimates that 60 million of us are chronically sleep-deprived; a lack of shut-eye might be the biggest health problem in America.

Why You Need Eight

We spend almost a third of our lives asleep. And yet few of us know much about sleep, and we don't get nearly enough of it. Individual needs vary, but research suggests that the average man needs at least eight hours of shut-eye each night, and like another nocturnal pleasure, he needs it regularly.

If a man misses rack time, the effects of the deficit accumulate quickly. According to one report from the Dayton Veterans Administration Hospital in Ohio, reducing sleep by just an hour and a half for a single night lowers daytime alertness by up to 33 percent. Michael Bonnet, Ph.D., director of the hospital's sleep laboratory, notes that four hours of sleep loss—two days in a row of sleeping six hours—can slow reaction times by 10 to 15 percent.

But completing your eight hours can:

Make you stronger. A study done in Great Britain showed that weight lifters who were limited to three hours of sleep a night for three days couldn't complete set numbers of curls, presses, and lifts by the second night.

In another study, researchers at the University of Kentucky in Lexington measured reduced leg strength in a group of sleep-deprived Marines.

Build and repair your body. During deep sleep, our bodies circulate 70 percent of our daily dose of human growth hormone, which is used to repair skin and build muscle and bone.

Improve your defenses. A study from the University of California, San Diego, showed that after missing five hours of sleep, healthy men produced fewer disease-fighting immune cells.

Lower your blood pressure. Though there's still debate among doctors, a small study from Japan showed that men who slept 3.6 hours a night had significantly higher blood pressure the next day.

Preserve your potency. Nocturnal erections send blood rushing into the penis, bringing with it the oxygen and nutrients needed to preserve good sexual function. Chronically depriving yourself of sleep means you're depriving your best friend of what he needs, too.

Sharpen your brain. Our ability to do useful mental work declines by 25 percent every successive 24 hours we're awake, according to scientists at the Walter Reed Army Institute of Research in Washington, D.C.

Keeping regular sleeping hours can also do the following:

Help you win. Researchers from Stanford University analyzed the outcomes of 25 years of Monday Night Football games and found that West Coast teams—who benefit from playing earlier in their day—have won two-thirds of all games with their East Coast rivals and, on average, have done so by larger margins.

Make you happier. A recent study at Brigham and Women's Hospital in Boston showed that subjects felt happier if they slept in sync with their body's internal clock. Even subjects who slept for 10 hours turned cranky when sleep times didn't match their natural cycle.

A Bad Reputation in Bed

So why don't we all relax and sleep more? Conventional wisdom says that's what lazy people do when they're busy not working. "There's almost a sense of shame around sleep," says Rubin Naiman, Ph.D., a clinical health psychologist and director of Somna Sleep Health Associates in Tucson, Arizona. It's rooted partially in our macho code: Sleep is something weaker characters do while the hero is on guard. Chronic tiredness must mean we're doing what's expected of us. "Think of how often someone wakes you with a late-night or early-morning phone call and asks, 'Were you sleeping?' The most common response is to deny it."

But there's abundant evidence that you're not receiving what you need. Just look at your nightly routine. "It ought to take you at least 5 to 10 minutes to fall asleep every night," says Dr. Naiman. "Many men say, 'My head hits the pillow and I'm out.' Well, that's like somebody saying, 'I'm a good eater. I sit down to my breakfast and it's gone in 30 seconds.' That's not the sign of a good eater. That's a sign of somebody who's starving."

Here's a checklist of other symptoms.

• You wake with an alarm clock, but only after you've repeatedly pounded the snooze button.

• You remember having more energy in your well-rested past.

- Your memory and thinking aren't as sharp as they used to be.
- You sleep late on weekends. Biologically, this makes as much sense as breathing more on the weekends.
- You rely on coffee, tea, nicotine, or other stimulants to get you through the day.

Another sign is that you fall asleep when you're bored. "Most everybody will tell you that boredom makes them sleepy," observes Thomas Roth, Ph.D., director of the sleep-disorders and research department at Henry Ford Hospital in Detroit. "That simply means they're sleep-deprived. The body is seizing that moment, and that's not productive. A well-rested person who's bored is going to find something interesting and challenging to do."

How to Repay Your Sleep Debt

"If we operated machinery like we operate the human body, we'd be accused of reckless endangerment," says James Maas, Ph.D., professor of psychology and sleep researcher at Cornell University in Ithaca, New York.

His best piece of advice about sleep: Realize that not getting enough can have serious, long-term effects on your health and productivity, so make sleep a priority. It may take some time for your body to accept your new will to snooze, so try one of these tricks, courtesy of Dr. Maas.

Keep the same hours. Set the VCR for *Homicide, Law and Order*, and all those other cop shows, and haul yourself into and out of bed the same time every day of the week. (Yes, Saturday and Sunday, too.)

Take a warm bath. After you step out of the water and cool off a bit, your body temperature will drop, a natural sleep-inducer.

Work out more. A workout makes you tired. Get it? As long as you don't pump yourself up too close to bedtime (leave at least four hours), the exertion will improve the quality of your sleep.

Skip the pills. They're addictive and won't induce needed deep sleep. Melatonin may help some people with jet lag, but there's not much evidence that it will improve the quality of sleep.

Another suggestion is to give yourself no more than 30 minutes to fall asleep once you climb into bed. If that's not enough, crawl out of bed and do something relaxing, then try again when you're feeling drowsy. It doesn't help to associate your bedroom with anything other than effortless, satisfying sleep. (Sex, of course, is the one welcome exception.)

It may take you a little while to settle into your natural sleep pattern. But then you have it made. Most experts estimate that it takes just a few days of purposeful sleeping to recover from chronic deprivation. "Sleep debt is like a loan your parents made to you in college," Dr. Naiman says. "You make a few payments, and then you are forgiven the rest."

Brain Training

Use this program and you'll be happier and sharper.

Some days—a lot of days if you're a game-show host or John F. Kennedy Jr.— your brain just seems to take a vacation. You lose your train of thought, stumble over your words, fail the bar exam again.

Launching your own national political magazine is one way to handle these brain blahs, but we have a better idea: Put your brain on a workout plan. Just like your abs, pecs, and biceps, your brain can be trained to work more efficiently. No, people on the beach won't suddenly start whispering, "Jeez, look at the brain on that guy." But if you do the right things all day long, you will be able to concentrate better, feel better, and sleep better.

Here's an all-day plan for making your brain totally buff.

When you wake up . . .

Hit the trails . . . or the racquetball court. One of the best things you can do for your brain is boost your heart rate. This brings in more oxygen, increases the brain's core temperature, and helps the chemical messengers that make the brain function. "It's like a factory powering up," says Ronald Lawrence, M.D., a neurologist and founder of the American Medical Athletic Association.

Dr. Lawrence recommends at least 30 minutes of aerobic exercise a day, six days a week. But because different kinds of exercise have different effects on your brain, your precise workout should depend on what's on your daily planner.

Hit the trails before that big presentation. "Aerobic exercise releases endorphins—literally 'the morphine within'—which have a relaxing, calming effect," says Pierce Howard, Ph.D., author of *The Owner's Manual for the Brain.*

Hit the court before that big negotiation. If you're starting your workday with something that requires a little zip—giving a pep talk to your staff, firing Janet Reno—play some early racquetball or another competitive sport. "Winning at competitive sports tends to release more testosterone, with a corresponding increase in felt aggression," says Dr. Howard.

Eat a bagel and a bowl of bran flakes for breakfast. In a 1996 study, researchers found that people who ate low-fat, high-carbohydrate breakfasts consistently were in better moods during the following three hours than those who ate high-fat, low-carbohydrate breakfasts, moderate-fat, moderate-carbohydrate breakfasts, or no breakfast at all. And it wasn't just because they found excellent prizes at the bottom of the boxes.

During the workday . . .

Put Mozart in your CD player. Several studies in the past few years have shown that listening to Mozart's piano sonatas can significantly improve abstract reasoning, at least in the short term.

Work out in your office. After burying your nose in a book or an important file for an hour, knock off for a couple of minutes of jumping jacks, pushups, or stairclimbing. Epinephrine and norepinephrine, two neurotransmitters that play a big role in converting short-term memory into long-term memory, are released whenever you subject yourself to physical or emotional stress. Scientists think this is why you can remember every detail of a car wreck.

Time your coffee break to your personality. A jolt of 200 milligrams of caffeine (the equivalent of 2 cups of coffee, 4 cups of tea, or 24 cups of cocoa) increases activity in the cerebral cortex, causing your brain's electrical activity to shift into arousal pattern. The result: a higher level of concentration. "Performance on simple tasks is faster and more accurate," says Richard Restak, M.D., a neuropsychiatrist in Washington, D.C., and author of 11 books on the brain. "Attention, problem-solving, and delayed recall are improved."

Just pay attention to the timing of that caffeine boost. Several studies have found that introverted people (quiet guys, in other words) are generally sharper when they first wake up than are extroverts, notes Dr. Howard. "As a result, an introvert performs better on morning mental tasks without coffee, while an extrovert does better with it," he says. In the evening, the pattern flips. Introverts do better in tests when they've had caffeine, while extroverts do better without.

Have paella for lunch. As the makers of Paxil (paroxetine hydrochloride), Prozac (fluoxetine hydrochloride), and Zoloft (sertraline hydrochloride) have so profitably discovered, tinkering with the level of serotonin, a neurotransmitter that plays a key role in mood, can give people a sense of well-being. Indeed, Judith J. Wurtman, Ph.D., a clinical researcher at the Massachusetts Institute of Technology in Cambridge and coauthor of *The Serotonin Solution*, says serotonin has emerged as the psychological kingmaker in the brain.

The key to keeping your serotonin in balance is your diet. Dr. Wurtman says a carbohydrate-to-protein ratio of five to one or greater will prevent your serotonin levels from dropping too low. Coincidentally, those exact proportions can be found in paella, a traditional Spanish dish of seafood and rice.

Take a walk at 3:00 P.M. Researchers have found that prolonged exposure to stress leads to the loss of neurons, particularly in the part of the brain called the hippocampus. The loss of these specialized cells can impair your memory. To fight back, look for ways throughout the day to reduce stress—take a break and go for a short walk, do some stretches at your desk, throw darts at that picture of your boss. And speaking of your boss . . .

Be like Fred. Remember how, as soon as that five o'clock whistle blew, Fred Flintstone slid down his dinosaur and got the hell out of that quarry? He must have known what researchers at Boston University School of Medicine have discovered: Overtime is bad for your brain. They studied autoworkers and found that working more than eight hours a day or more than five days a week was associated with impaired performance on several tests of attention and decision-making.

After work . . .

Tickle the ivories. You're not working late, so take up a musical instrument—it could be good for your head. In a recent study, researchers gave one group of children piano lessons, a second group computer lessons, a third group singing lessons, and a fourth group no training. The result: The piano students scored 34 percent higher than the other groups on tests of abstract reasoning.

Memorize a new poem every week. Just like your biceps, your brain becomes flabby if you don't challenge it. Unfortunately, in a world of computers and personal organizers, we're increasingly less likely to do that. "Memory is like everything else in the brain," says Dr. Restak. "It wastes away if you don't use it."

So start using yours. Go to the grocery store and shop without a list, like Dr. Restak does. Deprogram your speed dial and make yourself remember those important phone numbers. Try to get your kids' names right on the first try. You can do it. We know you can.

At night . . .

Bake a potato. And eat it with low-fat sour cream. You're watching your fat intake (thanks to the low-fat addition) and boosting your potassium level (thanks to the potato). These measures, coupled with exercise and reduced stress, help keep your blood pressure low. In the long haul, that will benefit your brain. Researchers have found that controlling systolic blood pressure (the top number) in middle age may reduce the risk for cognitive impairment as you grow old.

Take tiny doses of melatonin when you hit middle age. Until he's in his forties, a healthy man's brain makes plenty of melatonin—a hormone that helps regulate sleep and mood. But after that, production slows. As a result, doctors suggest taking synthetic melatonin when you pass into middle age. Just don't take too much. Melatonin is typically sold in pills of 0.5, 1, and 3 milligrams—way more than you need. Check with your doctor on the dosage that's right for you.

Put a 25-watt bulb in your bedroom lamp. Melatonin also plays a big role in setting your body's biological clock and determining when you fall asleep. To have an easier time dozing off, read by a weak light an hour before bedtime. Darkness stimulates the production of melatonin, and sleep generally follows in an hour or two.

Make sure you get enough sleep. Although exercise is important for the brain, so is rest. While you sleep, your brain takes the particular memories you've stored during the day and reprocesses them, extracting general knowledge from specific experiences, according to Bruce McNaughton, Ph.D., professor at the University of Arizona College of Medicine in Tucson. "We really don't know how this mechanism works, but a lot of it takes place in the hippocampus," he explains. What does that mean to the average guy? "You have another reason for getting a good night's sleep," Dr. McNaughton says.

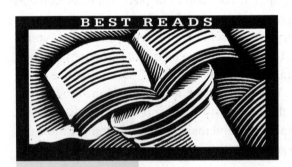

Perform under Pressure

Cool, calm, and collected. Three words that men would love to have attached to their names. Follow the tips in this excerpt from Command Respect: Cultivate the Qualities That Inspire and Impress Others *(Rodale Press, 1998) by Perry Garfinkel and Brian Paul Kaufman, and you'll soon have people commenting on how well you handle yourself.*

For the ultimate in grace under pressure, consider Bond—James Bond. No matter what the challenge—whether he's trying to rescue a bodacious babe or derail an evil genius's plan for world domination—007 always seems to emerge with the ultimate victory: hair in place and perspiration-free. (Reminder to self: Consider pitching "007 brand hair gel and after-bath splash" to merchandising.)

But when it comes down to it, a fair share of Bond's composure can be attributed to his trusty, white-haired equipment officer—the man they call "Q." It is this crotchety old chap, after all, who supplies the ingenious gizmos that consistently save Bond's urbane arse. In fact, you could argue that without Q's gadget pipeline—radio-controlled helicopters, ejector seats, assorted laser-guided, exploding, bulletproof wristwatches—Mr. Shaken, Not Stirred would have gotten his clock cleaned sequels ago.

It would be hard to find a better example of preaching to the choir than telling a red-blooded American male that gadgets are the key to coming through in the clutch. But here's something that you may not be carrying in your toolbox o' tricks: mental preparation.

"The moral is that if you have your head right, that's when you can be cool and calm. You can know that you are going to go in there and nail it—whatever you're doing," says Steven Ungerleider, Ph.D., a research psychologist and director of Integrated Research Services in Eugene, Oregon; a member of the U.S. Olympic Committee Sports Psychology Registry; and author of *Mental Training for Peak Performance.*

Going against Type

With apologies to the immortal Vince Lombardi, winning isn't the only thing—at least not when it comes to remaining cool, calm, and collected. A study of 750 men that looked at the link between personality and disease found that guys who exhibited what might be considered classic cool behavior—patience, a relaxed attitude, thoughtful speech—lived longer than the in-your-face, always-in-a-rush, highly competitive folks.

"The risk for Type A's is about the same as a moderate smoker and costs them anywhere from a couple to five or six years of their life," says Michael Babyak, Ph.D., assistant clinical professor of medical psychology at Duke University Medical Center in Durham, North Carolina. "At the root of it, Type A's seem to have a very basic insecurity about their ability and status and as a result are constantly, compulsively trying to be seen and in control. Internally, they are very fearful people."

While it once seemed that Type A's might one day rule the world, there's a trend toward cool-headedness afoot that may even land you a promotion. "People who seem highly emotional are viewed as less satisfactory employees," says Peter N. Stearns, Ph.D., author of *American Cool: Constructing a Twentieth-Century Emotional Style* and dean of the college of humanities and social sciences at Carnegie Mellon University in Pittsburgh. "Movements such as Total Quality

Management urge managerial workers and staff to identify and control vigorous emotions. They want people who are supportive of group harmony instead of those who would disrupt it."

Much of what we know about how to gradually change this kind of behavior originated in sports. But the beauty of these techniques is that they work anywhere for virtually any stressful situation. Here's how to avoid being a nervous wreck and, as a result, gain respect.

Select your skirmishes. Yes, life is a contact sport. But you don't have to smash everyone in your path, nor do you even have to compete with them. "Ask yourself: How important is it for me to win this conversation?" Dr. Babyak says. "Or better yet: Should I even walk around trying to win conversations and bowl people over? Such behavior is the opposite of staying cool—you're cranking out stress hormones all the time. And frankly, that's dangerous."

Feel the heat—and use it as fuel. You've finally found a worthy opponent, and the juices are beginning to flow. Your palms are sweaty, your heart is racing, and there's a sheepshank where your intestines used to be. Research shows that how you interpret this physiological arousal may actually determine your performance.

"If your body responds like this, you could either say to yourself, 'Man, I'm charged up and ready to go,' or 'Something is wrong,'" says Dan Gould, Ph.D., professor in the department of exercise and sport science specializing in sports psychology at the University of North Carolina at Greensboro. "You have the ability to view it as anxiety or a positive psyche, and it can make all the difference in the world in the outcome."

Enjoy oxygen. In other words, breathe! "Proper breathing not only relaxes you but also enhances performance by oxygenating your blood and energizing your brain," says Dr. Ungerleider. Since breathing right is one of the first things we stop doing properly when we're stressed, it pays to practice deep breathing at least once a day. Start by filling your lower abdomen with air as if it were a balloon. Gradually allow the air to also fill your middle abdomen and chest. Then breathe out, says Dr. Ungerleider. See? That wasn't so hard. And you probably feel calmer already.

Make a fist. Not to pound people, tough guy, but to experiment with progressive relaxation. Now it may sound like something a swami would suggest between servings of alfalfa sprouts, but progressive relaxation is just another way of describing the process of tightening and relaxing your muscles. Start right now by making a fist and squeezing it for 10 seconds. Now relax and feel the tension drain away. Applied to the rest of your muscles—either before or in the heat of battle—that same concept can help put you at ease, Dr. Ungerleider says.

Be a doom-buster. Whether it's in the boardroom or on the basketball court, we're all bombarded by negative thoughts that can make us nervous and edgy. But you can put the brakes on these notions of doom by keeping a list handy of all the reasons that you should succeed. "One power lifter I was working with had a list of the 10 reasons he should do well at nationals, even if he didn't feel right," Dr. Gould says. Some of the items on the list included: I've trained well; I'm really strong even on my weakest days; and my technique is better than ever. "It may sound gimmicky, but the list is based on reality—not just a bunch of positive affirmations, which I'm not convinced are of a whole lot of value," Dr. Gould says.

Quit complaining. Maybe you remember a *Saturday Night Live* skit featuring a family of malcontents called The Whiners. In case you missed it, their shtick was complaining about everything—in voices so annoying that you truly understood for the first time what compelled Elvis to shoot out his TV. We all know people who adopt this kind of behavior at the first sign of trouble. If this describes you, wonder no more why you don't get any respect.

"Let's say your plane is late and you're going to miss a meeting. You could sit there and complain and make everyone around you miserable, or you could take out your laptop and get some work done. And when the battery in your laptop dies, you could complain. Or you could borrow some paper and write out what you were working on. Or just catch up on some sleep. It's called making the best of the situation, and it's infinitely more healthy," Dr. Gould says.

Make adversity your ally. It's one thing to learn how to go with the flow—and frankly, that would be a big improvement for a lot of us. But another step toward being cool, calm, and collected is actually expecting the unexpected. "The really good athletes are prepared to cope with adversity," says Dr. Gould. "They realize that in sports people make bad calls. Or they get injured. Or the weather just isn't right." So how does that apply to you? You may not be able to control whether you're going to get laid off, but you can make sure that you find the best job recruiter in the area. Or talk to people who have also lost their jobs recently and find out what they've learned. And then make sure that you work as hard—or harder—getting a job as you did at your old job.

Get a cue. It doesn't get much hairier than hurtling down the side of a mountain toward a giant ramp that will propel you hundreds of feet through the air—all with the expectation that you won't be imbedded in said mountain upon return. So how do some of the top skiers and aerialists avoid stressing out before their big jump? They have what are called cue words written on the tips of their skis that remind them of what they are about to do. "They're very simple—things like 'Twist' and 'Turn and Go,'" says Dr. Gould. "They read that, and it helps them refocus on what they're about to do." You can place yours on your bathroom mirror, office bulletin board, or anywhere you need an instant reminder to stay calm.

Hang tough. We all have days—heck, maybe even a decade or two—that we wished we had just stayed in bed. Guess what: Guys who are cool to the core know this. And even when they are having a really bad day, they're banking that if they can just hang in there, you're going to falter and they're going to come out on top—again.

"Instead of really, really getting down on myself and kind of dropping into a Grand Canyon of failure where nothing goes right, I fight it and try to keep control—the best control I can under the circumstances," Dr. Gould says. "I have a bad day, but I don't have a disaster. And so when the bottom drops out on someone else, I end up winning ugly."

Go to a game. We all know that frequent exercise is a great way to blow off steam and keep the head clear. But raising Cain at a Miami Hurricane game—or any other big-time spectator sport—is a great way to release pent-up emotions that can otherwise leave you nasty, brutish, and in short, the opposite of cool, calm, and collected.

"We let athletes do all sorts of things that we don't let ourselves do," Dr. Stearns says. "They can hug each other. They can dance triumph dances over a fallen opponent. It's not the best way to experience this kind of release, but for some of us, it's the closest we'll get." Do not, under any circumstances, however, wear a block of cheese on your head.

A Stronger Memory

We're certain that most men would leap at the chance to improve their memories. Who wouldn't want to become better at remembering names, faces, appointments, and the specifics of that conversation you had with your boss last week? But there's more to building a stronger memory than recalling more details. As Fred B. Chernow puts it in this excerpt from Memory Power Plus *(Prentice Hall, 1997), there is also "learning to forget constructively."*

The world of tennis introduced us to a mind-control method originally called "yoga tennis" by Timothy Gallwey, a Harvard University–trained tennis teacher. He found that players hit their peak when they "let it happen" and directed the ball over the net first in their mind and then in actuality. This is done effortlessly. The mind is on the job, but quietly, without anxious thoughts of pressure or failure.

Today, athletes appreciate these findings, and many competitors now travel with a sports psychologist as well as a coach. But you don't have to be a professional tennis player to benefit from sports psychology when it comes to memory. Here are four basic tips adapted to strengthening your memory for the rest of your life.

1. Visualize yourself in control of your memory. See yourself remembering the dates, numbers, names, and facts necessary for your social and business success.

2. Monitor your negative thoughts. Remind yourself of the times your memory proved valuable. Don't belabor the occasional lapse of memory.

3. Shut down inner dialogues in which colleagues or authority figures tell you "you'll probably forget" or "no one can possibly remember." Dwell, instead, on those occasions when you surprised yourself and others with your memory skills.

4. Center your mind on the here and now. Stay within the concept of one thing at a time. Concentrate on each memory task as you face it, not on yesterday's or last week's memory task. Eliminate distractions; stay centered and on-task.

Avoid Leaving Memory to Chance

Too many of us leave memory to chance. We learn something and then hope that we will remember it when we need it. This is hardly good enough. It may work when your memory is at its peak in your twenties, but don't count on it later on. What you can do to prevent "losing it" in middle age and beyond is to take the advice of behavior psychologist and author B. F. Skinner and practice "good intellectual self-management."

His techniques are logical and very easy to implement. They emphasize doing something to enhance memory and not leaving memory to chance. We have paraphrased and abridged Skinner's suggestions for you.

1. Do something. If rain is expected, don't just think about it. Hook an umbrella over the knob of your front door as soon as the thought comes to mind.

2. Capture your ideas. Creative solutions and ideas frequently come to us in the middle of the night. Don't let them escape. You may not remember them in the morning. Keep a small recorder or pad and paper at your bedside.

3. Carry a memo pad. A spiral-bound, three- by five-inch memo pad in your pocket is invaluable for writing down names, numbers, and facts as they come

up throughout the day. Review them each evening and record them in a more permanent location, such as a desk calendar or a phone directory.

4. Keep it short. Speak and write in sentences that are short and to the point. Beware of going off on tangents or making digressions that make you and your listener forget your point.

5. Use an outline and stick to it. When writing a business letter, personal correspondence, or a report, draw up an outline first to guard against inconsistencies and memory lapses. Say it once and move on. You and your reader will remember it better this way.

If started early, these self-management skills will be worth their weight in gold later on in boosting memory.

Learning to Forget Constructively

Forgetting can have some major benefits in our lives. It's important to know when to forget. This is best learned early so that old age is not filled with frivolous, negative memories. We are constructive when we carefully choose which memories should be discarded.

Nature provides us with some basic forgetting skills. Without them, we would hold ourselves back. For example, a one-year-old is learning to walk. He falls and hurts his head. Fortunately, he forgets this injury the next time he has the urge to walk. If toddlers didn't forget such bumps, they'd never master the skill of walking in an upright position.

Women forget the pain of childbirth and eagerly plan another pregnancy. A 60-year-old forgets the pain of losing a mate and decides to marry again.

Yet certain pains must be remembered, and we use our judgment in deciding what should be remembered. Touching a hot pot on the stove is a memory worth recalling so that burned fingers don't become a habit.

For many, work is a haven for forgetting the pressure of a chaotic home life or a lonely, barren social life. We block out disturbing memories by immersing ourselves in a demanding schedule or task. Such escape gives us a short-term solution to our problems.

Amnesia, a disease frequently manifested on soap operas, is the blocking out of all memory by people facing unbearable tragedy. Most of us learn to handle traumatic experiences in a less dramatic way.

A technique worth learning early in life is to mix sad and vexing images with happy and satisfying memories to gain perspective. After a time, the unpleasant memories can be forgotten instead of your constantly going over them. This is an important survival tool.

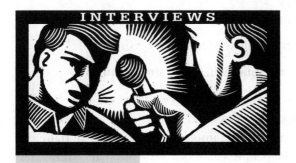

Brad Blanton on

Living a Lie-Free Life

Not many of us would consider ourselves liars. Lying *is such an ugly word, bearing a close etymologic association with other ugly words like* cheating *and* stealing. *We don't "lie." We socially lubricate, simply to make life easier for everybody. No, honey, you look good in that form-fitting dress. Yes, Mr. Moore, I can have that story on your desk by Wednesday.*

At least one person thinks we're seriously deluding ourselves. His name is Brad Blanton, Ph.D., and he advocates (and wrote a book entitled) Radical Honesty, *a lifestyle he feels can liberate us from stress, supercharge our marriages, and make the world a much brighter place. We gave this self-professed straight-shooter a chance to convince us.*

How much does the average person lie?

Well, there is a book called *The Day America Told the Truth,* written about six years ago. It's a survey of 40,000 Americans, all done in one day by electronic magic, by this big public-relations firm in New York. They found that 93 percent of the people admitted they lied regularly and habitually at work, and more than a third of the married people were having sex on the side and not telling their spouses.

And you believe that's a bad thing?

Of course. It's the source of all the stress in your life. What I've learned, based on 25 years of private practice in psychotherapy in Washington, D.C., is that lying is the primary source of depression, most anxiety disorders, most psychosomatic illnesses, most physical illnesses, and most divorces.

If you tell the truth, the experience of being on the planet is a whole lot easier, less burdensome, more nurturing; it's a more loving kind of life. And it brings you more luck, more sex, more money.

Are little white lies really detrimental?

Actually, it's the compilation of little white lies that's most harmful.

Surely, though, there are some times where you simply must lie.

If you have Anne Frank in your attic, and a Nazi knocks on the door and says, "Are there are any Jews in this house?" you should lie. If you want to tell little lies to an institution—to the government, for example—that's perfectly all right. But tell the truth to your friends, the people you work with, and your family and spouse. That's critical to your own health and well-being.

In your book, you advise couples to share graphic sexual details of past relationships and to admit when they're attracted to other people. Are you nuts?

It's unrealistic to do otherwise. The reason we have a 53 percent divorce rate is not because people are telling the truth; it's because they are lying. Complete honesty makes for a more exciting life. You actually share your life with another person. You can't have intimacy without honesty. And if you do all this phony stuff in order to protect your image in the eyes of the other person, you're playing a role in relation to them, and they are playing a role in relation to you. And playing a role all the time wears you out.

What can a guy do to make an honest man of himself?

Basically, I recommend that you find one other person and make an agreement for a definite period of time, for a month to six weeks, to just tell the truth about everything and see how it works. I recommend that you hurt people's feelings, but that you not just offend them and run off—that you stay with them. It doesn't take people more than 10 to 15 minutes to get over most hurt feelings and most anger. We can be furious at each other at 8:00, and by 8:15, we can go out and have a beer and be good friends.

Howard Gardner on
Redefining Intelligence

Remember when aptitude tests separated future Einsteins from future unemployables? Well, they still do, to an extent. Ask any guy who couldn't crack 1000 on his SATs. But educators are challenging these cut-and-dried measures of intelligence. One leader of the rebellion is Howard Gardner, Ph.D., a Harvard University psychologist who says that intelligence actually comes in eight varieties—interpersonal, intrapersonal, kinesthetic, linguistic, logical, musical, naturalistic, and spa-

tial. Those who exploit their natural strengths can go to the White House; those who ply their weaknesses are lucky if they make the white pages. Dr. Gardner's book Extraordinary Minds *presents his theories on specialized intelligence. He gave us a few tips on liberating our inner geniuses.*

Your theory says we're just as brainy as that wiseguy surgeon we met at a cocktail party. Can that possibly be true?

Well, if he works with a scalpel, I hope he has greater kinesthetic intelligence than you do. But the fact that a guy has a high I.Q. doesn't mean he's "smart." We need to ask, "Smart in what?"

You could be intelligent in school, in business, or in the arts. Intelligence is really about mobilizing your abilities to do something well, and the context determines which intelligence is most important. For example, logical intelligence is highly valued in today's society, but naturalistic intelligence—the ability to read changes and indications in the environment—was the dominant intelligence for thousands of years.

Doesn't I.Q. take all those different aptitudes into consideration?

No. For instance, Ronald Reagan probably had 50 fewer I.Q. points than Jimmy Carter or Herbert Hoover, but he was a much more effective president than either. Why? Because he had greater linguistic and interpersonal intelligence; he could motivate people. A leader's success hinges on his ability to tell moving stories and to make others believe them. I like to listen to Bill Clinton because he's a terrific storyteller.

So you're saying even the dullest among us are extremely brainy in so many ways?

Yes. All human beings are capable of high performance in something—if they utilize their dominant intelligences. Unfortunately, many people focus on their weaknesses. For instance, the lawyer who writes excellent legal briefs may be terrible in court. He may see himself as a failure. But he's really struggling against his average interpersonal intelligence and ignoring his high logical or even spatial intelligence. If he'd take advantage of his natural strengths, he'd succeed and be less frustrated.

How can a guy overcome his mental weaknesses?

Develop your strengths. If you are gifted in spatial intelligence, as Picasso was, you see abstract relationships between objects and things. This can help you view your message and audience metaphorically. The lawyer could use his spatial intelligence to look at his argument as a series of chess moves and the jurors' subtle reactions as countermoves.

What's the best way to find "hidden" intelligences?

Take a hard look at yourself and your history. Think of tasks that were easy and hard for you, and what characteristics they have in common. If you're doing extremely well in a particular facet of your career, dissect it. What skills do you use? Most important, listen to what others say about you. If someone says, "You draw well," or "You resolved that conflict easily," don't shrug it off. Take it seriously. They're giving you the most reliable clues about your natural intelligences.

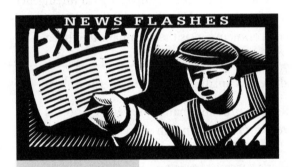

NEWS FLASHES

Brainpower Goes Down at Night

PITTSBURGH—Don't work late! Go home! Your brain downshifts into moron mode at night. Researchers at the University of Pittsburgh Medical Center gave 18 people periodic "reasoning" tests during a 36-hour study. Starting around midnight of the first day, the subjects took an average of two seconds longer to answer true-and-false questions—and that's before they were sleep-deprived. "You just can't think quickly at night," says study coauthor Tim Monk, Ph.D. This downtime invites restful sleep, he says, and nothing—not bright lights, coffee, or a nudie screen saver—will restore your daytime smarts.

Work Stress Can Slash Sperm Count

CALGARY, Alberta—Men who reported the most daily work-related stress had one-third less sperm in their ejaculate than the most relaxed subjects, according to researchers at the University of Calgary. They found this result after analyzing sperm samples from 1,469 men ages 20 to 69. Stress causes hormonal imbalances and changes in blood pressure and body temperature that may harm sperm, says study author Philip Bigelow, Ph.D. Worse, the sperm that the stressed-out men produced were sluggish swimmers. "Fortunately," says Dr. Bigelow, "if you reduce your stress level, your sperm levels should return to normal."

Type-A Behavior Could Lead to a Reduced Sex Drive

PITTSBURGH—Being highly competitive may help you get the girl, but it might also make it tough for you to keep her. Classic type-A behavior can lower your testosterone level. After examining 66 men between the ages of 41 and 61, researchers at the University of Pittsburgh found that those who showed the most competitiveness, hostility, and impatience also had the greatest decrease in testosterone with age. One possible reason: Stress produces cortisol, a hormone that suppresses testosterone, a key to a man's sex drive. More studies are needed to establish this link.

Willpower Has Its Limits

CLEVELAND—Willpower is a limited resource, according to a study from Case Western Reserve University. Researchers put students in rooms stocked with aromatic cookies, then gave them a frustrating task to complete. One group of students was told that they were allowed to eat the cookies, while another was told that they couldn't eat them. (A third, cookie-less group acted as a control.) Students who were denied the cookies quit their tasks sooner than those allowed to indulge, says project supervisor Roy Baumeister, Ph.D. The message? Dr. Baumeister says that self-control is like a muscle: When it's tired, it becomes weaker. Our opinion: Concentrate your energy on one challenge at a time. Then exercise enough so you can eat those motivational cookies when you want to.

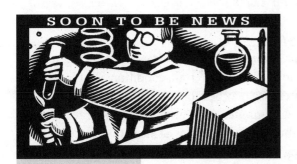

Will Memory Loss Be Just a Memory?

Drugs that boost memory are on the horizon. A study at the University of California, Irvine, reported that a drug called ampakine CX-516 more than doubled the short-term memory of 18 healthy men between the ages of 65 and 73. The drug holds brain receptors open longer, allowing more information to cross neurons. Studies on patients with Alzheimer's disease are coming. "We need to learn much more about this drug and its possible side effects," says Zaven Khachaturian, Ph.D., director of the Alzheimer Association's Ronald and Nancy Reagan Research Institute in Chicago.

Doctors believe that this fuels the hope that dementia and Alzheimer's can be reversed within 10 years.

Help to Break the Habit?

A drug may help compulsive gamblers—an estimated 7 percent of the population—control their habit. In a preliminary trial, fluvoxamine (Luvox), currently prescribed in the United States to treat obsessive-compulsive disorders, helped 7 out of 10 compulsive-gambling patients quit their wagering. "We saw patient improvement by their third week of taking the drug," says Eric Hollander, M.D., of Mount Sinai School of Medicine of the City University of New York.

A larger study is in the works.

Spit Your Way to Fewer Heart Attacks?

Stress shows up everywhere—even in your mouth. Researchers have developed a saliva test that can determine stress levels in 10 minutes. It indirectly measures the body's level of norepinephrine, a stress hormone. (Research with first-time sky divers shows the test definitely works.) "Men at risk for a heart attack could monitor their stress levels throughout the day and adjust their activities," says study leader Robert Chatterton, Ph.D., of Northwestern University Medical School in Chicago.

Researchers are hoping that this test may be in drugstores within two years.

Dial In for a Diagnosis?

Faced with patients who may be embarrassed or afraid of being stigmatized, physicians sometimes have trouble diagnosing certain conditions. But researchers say an automated telephone interview may be more successful than a clinician at identifying mental disorders. A computer-generated telephone interview was twice as likely to spot alcohol abuse and three times as likely to detect obsessive-compulsive disorder, according to a study led by Kenneth Kobak, Ph.D., a research psychologist in Middleton, Wisconsin.

Further studies are planned, though there is no word yet on when such a test might be in widespread use.

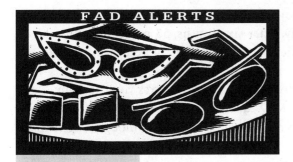

Ginkgo Biloba

Ginkgo biloba seems like the perfect male supplement. Natural-cure marketers claim that it can enlarge blood vessels, increasing blood flow. They even cite small foreign studies that suggest ginkgo improved concentration and firmed up erections. But before you pick up a $12 bottle, hold on a minute. "While many testimonials say *Ginkgo biloba* has improved mental clarity and sexual function, no large-scale clinical trial that I know has ever been done," says Arthur Jacknowitz, Pharm.D., chairman of the clinical pharmacy department at the West Virginia University School of Pharmacy in Morgantown.

In fact, when Dutch researchers investigated 40 small European studies on ginkgo, they found that only 8 followed acceptable procedures.

Because no one can patent *Ginkgo biloba*, no one stands to profit by financing a large controlled trial. So its therapeutic perks will likely remain anecdotal. Even physicians who believe that ginkgo can improve circulation warn that it's not harmless. "People should only take *Ginkgo biloba* with a physician's supervision to address a specific health problem," says Steven Margolis, M.D., clinical instructor at Wayne State University in Detroit and an alternative family physician practicing in Sterling Heights, Michigan. Side effects include easy bruising, nausea, headaches, and even reported bleeding in the whites of your eyes (if you take it with aspirin).

Kava

Kava, or kava-kava (*Piper methysticum*), is a member of the black-pepper family that Polynesians use for its calming effect. Think of it as nature's Valium, rather than another organic Prozac (such as the herb Saint-John's-wort). "Kava acts as an antianxiety agent and mild sedative, whereas Saint-John's-wort acts primarily as an antidepressant," says Raymond F. Rosenthal, M.D., an internist at the University of Hawaii in Honolulu.

In a German study, 101 subjects took either 110 milligrams of kava extract or a placebo three times a day. After six months, 53 percent of the subjects taking kava reported less anxiety, compared with 30 percent of the placebo group.

"It may release serotonin to calm you, and it relaxes your neuromuscular functions," says Ronald Podell, M.D., director of the Center for Bio-Behavioral Psychiatry in Los Angeles. It has no dangerous side effects, though long-term use can cause a skin rash.

The bottom line: "I see nothing wrong with trying kava, but you need to address the underlying source of your anxiety," says Dr. Rosenthal. If kava doesn't decrease your anxiety after three months, see your doctor. Look for kava extract at health food stores; it contains the highest level of kavalactones, the active molecule.

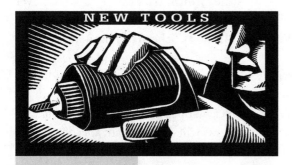

NEW TOOLS

Less Depression and Better Sleep

Serzone

Depression and sleep disturbances go hand in hand. But a new prescription drug appears to fight depression just as well as Prozac (fluoxetine hydrochloride) does—without Prozac's sleep-disrupting effects. In three studies presented at a meeting of the American Psychiatric Association, based in Washington, D.C., Serzone (nefazodone) caused fewer awakenings than Prozac and didn't affect deep sleep or dream (REM) sleep. "No antidepressant is perfect, but nefazodone is an important new one. It clearly has more favorable effects on insomnia," says Michael Thase, M.D., professor of psychiatry at the University of Pittsburgh School of Medicine. "Ask your doctor which may be best for you."

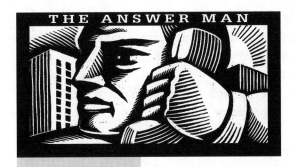

THE ANSWER MAN

A Nervous Wreck

Why do people fidget? For some reason, I can't sit still for more than a few minutes without shaking my legs or drumming my fingers on the desk. Is it physical or psychological?
—P. R., Citrus Heights, Calif.

Often, the cause of fidgeting is purely psychological. Both boredom and anxiety make some people fidget, says Steven Goldman, M.D., Ph.D., associate professor of neurology and neurological science at Cornell Medical College in New York City. Fidgeting can also have physical causes. Stimulants like caffeine and nicotine are the obvious ones, but medicines to control asthma, depression, or high blood pressure may also contribute to fidgeting, adds Dr. Goldman.

On the other hand, fidgeting can be a symptom of attention-deficit hyperactivity disorder (ADHD), says John Harvey, Ph.D., director of psychological services at the Allied Services Rehabilitation Institute in Scranton, Pennsylvania. No one knows for sure what causes ADHD, but most experts consider it a neurological condition that affects the parts of the brain that control concentration and motor activity. It's estimated that 3 to 8 percent of the adult population has ADHD. Although more boys are diagnosed with the condition than girls (at a ratio of more than five to one), adults with the condition are evenly divided. If your fidgeting is accompanied by disorganization, impulsive behavior, distractibility, mood swings, and difficulty concentrating while reading, ADHD could be the diagnosis—so check with a health professional.

Promoted out of Friends

I was just promoted, and my office buddies don't respect my new authority. How can I make them see me as their boss without looking like my title's gone to my head?
—D. P., Groton, Conn.

Sticky as your current situation is, it's also a rite of passage for all up-and-comers. To hang on to your old pals without risking a mutiny at the office, you'll need to accept that the social climate has changed. "You're making decisions that affect their lives," says James A. Autry, a management consultant and author of *Confessions of an Accidental Businessman.* "You can't share gripe sessions or lunchtime gossip anymore because you're privy to information that can violate someone's privacy." So consider it a blessing if they shut you out of the B.S. circle for awhile. But if your former cube-mates make animal noises while you're talking to the executive vice president, you need to take action.

"Immature managers always make the same mistake," says Autry. "They immediately try to demonstrate that they're the boss." Resist the temptation to assert your authority in trivial matters, he warns. If you give your buddies a hard time over an occasional long lunch, you'll end up making enemies out of the people you're managing, and then you're sunk.

Have a closed-door meeting with each of your buddies, one on one. Do this on-site—pub-talk loses its power when you return to the office. "Forget your ego and ask them for help," says Autry. "Say, 'Look, if you were in my shoes, what would you do? How would you motivate me to support you?' That'll give them a taste of what you're up against."

Your purpose is to get the job done. Period. "You don't need your pal's affection; you need him to work," says Autry. Let Joe think you're a butthead who can't handle tequila—as long as he keeps handing in crackerjack reports. He'll either come around or he won't. You want results, not mind control.

Make it a point to show up at gatherings and keep friendships alive. If you're suddenly missing in action every time your old buddies get together, you'll confirm their worst predictions about your elevation to management—and both the friendship and the work relationship will suffer.

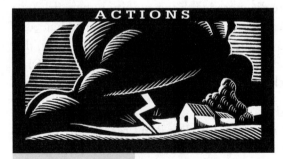

When everybody wants a piece of you, everything is out of control, and Boris Yeltsin seems to have it together better than you do, it's time to find yourself a stress-relief plan. And that doesn't mean some highly involved, stress-reducing strategy jam-packed with prolonged mantras and crystal healing. Instead, try these simple little tips.

1. Drink peppermint or lemon tea. Hell, pretend to drink it. "Research suggests that smelling the scent of lemon or peppermint can make you feel more relaxed," says Harold H. Bloomfield, M.D., coauthor with Robert K. Cooper, Ph.D., of *The Power of 5*. Dr. Bloomfield also suggests buying potpourri for its relaxing properties. But that would mean visiting a craft shop, which is entirely out of the question. Agreed?

2. Practice one-breath meditation. "When stress arrives, sit up straight in a comfortable chair and relax your shoulders," says Dr. Bloomfield. "Consciously, take a breath and inhale deeply to open your chest, imagining that the breath is filling every cell in your body. Hold for a moment, then exhale completely, releasing every bit of tension." Do this enough and it will become a reflex.

3. Try one-touch relaxation. In some meditation postures, the practitioner will place his second finger against his thumb. It's a way of capturing that relaxed moment. "Whenever you feel relaxed, remind yourself to touch those fingers together," says Dr. Bloomfield. "Once it becomes a habit, do the same thing when you're under stress or feeling anxious. You're reminding your body, using your fingers as a cue, what it's like to feel relaxed. That should ease the anxiety a bit." If not, you can still fight stress by using the same finger position to flick things at the clown in the next cubicle. Always works for us.

4. Try another breathing trick. Inhale, clench your teeth tight for five seconds, then exhale, letting your jaw muscle go loose, and say "aahhhh." "The jaw muscle is the most powerful in your body, and if you can learn to tense and then relax it, that will cause a cascading relaxation response throughout your body," says Dr. Bloomfield. Plus, squaring your jaw makes you look like Lee Majors before he grew the paunch. And you could do worse.

5. Go outside and bask in bright light. "We have a plantlike nature," says Dr. Bloomfield. (Hey, speak for yourself.) "We get a powerful surge of energy from sunlight. Spending 5 or 10 minutes in the sunshine can make a tremendous difference in your mood and stress level."

6. Crank off a super abdominal exercise. Not only is this relaxing but it also tones your gut. Best of all, it's something useful you can do while you're stuck doing something totally useless, such as idling in traffic or voting. Sit up straight and place your hands on your hips with your thumbs pointing toward your back.

Exhale slowly and completely, pushing the last air out forcefully with your lower abdominal muscles. "The more you exhale, and push out the air forcefully, the more you develop the lower abdomen," says Dr. Bloomfield.

7. Try some lyming. This is a Caribbean term that means doing nothing—guilt-free. "It gives your brain time to process information it's receiving when you're in overload," says Dr. Bloomfield. Not only does it sound multicultural but it also gives you an excuse to walk around in your underwear.

8. Offer help to save a life. Research indicates that heart attack survivors live longer if they believe they have enough help from family and friends. A study of 820 people with coronary-artery disease found that patients who felt they needed "much more help" with daily tasks were $6\frac{1}{2}$ times more likely to die within a year than those who said they didn't need help. "This is the first study that shows a powerful relationship between mortality and the sick person's perception of receiving adequate help," says Steven Woloshin, M.D., first author of the study and general internist at the Veterans Affairs Medical Center in White River Junction, Vermont. He suggests asking a sick person, "Are you getting all the help you need?"

9. Tune out stress during surgery. If you're going under the knife, consider making a musical request first. One study suggests that surgery is smoother for patients who choose the music they listen to before and during the operation. The study examined 40 patients who had had cataract surgery under local anesthesia and found that before their procedures, blood pressure soared. But within 10 minutes of listening to the music of their choice, patients' blood pressures and heart rates dropped to normal levels, says Karen Allen, Ph.D., study leader and research scientist at the State University of New York at Buffalo.

10. Find yourself, find work. Out of a job? Consider therapy. Researchers at the University of London say that psychological training can help the unemployed find work. Researchers had 199 people who were unemployed an average of two years attend either a group psychotherapy program that used the principles of cognitive-behavior therapy (CBT) or a program designed to build networking skills. After four months, 34 percent of the CBT group had found full-time work, compared with 13 percent in the networking program. Cognitive-behavior therapy helps people replace self-defeating behaviors with healthier ways of thinking through problems, researchers say.

11. **Plan a premeditated shooting.** If your jump shot or softball swing is missing its mark, try meditating before the game. In a small study, Norwegian researchers found that daily meditation can improve a shooter's accuracy. Marksmen who meditated improved their scores significantly from the previous shooting season. The relaxed mind that follows meditation may help you achieve peak performance in other sports as well, according to Erik E. Solberg, M.D., study author and sports-medicine specialist at Ullevol University Hospital in Oslo.

12. **Count to 10.** Harvard School of Public Health researchers who studied 1,305 men ages 40 to 90 found that men with the highest anger scores on a personality test were three times as likely to develop heart disease. The researchers believe that anger may trigger the release of toxic stress hormones into the blood. If you can't stop going ballistic, at least break the heart-damaging habits. "The angrier men tended to drink and smoke more, too," says study leader Ichiro Kawachi, M.D.

13. **Put on a happy face.** Lifetime happiness is an achievable goal. But for some men, the pursuit is not always easy. Investigators have found that the four common traits of happy people are self-approval, personal control of their lives, optimism, and extroverted personalities. But what if you fall short in one of these categories? "Give priority to close relationships and stay aerobically fit," says David Myers, Ph.D., professor of psychology at Hope College in Holland, Michigan. Those simple moves will head you in the right direction.

14. **Learn from your mistakes.** A study conducted by Northeastern University in Boston and the University of California, Berkeley, suggests that the way you regard your past experiences may determine your overall success. Researchers assessed 100 people at age 18 and again at 23. Self-described "ruminators" tended to "stew on past problems and generate negative feelings," says C. Randall Colvin, Ph.D., coauthor of the study. But "contemplators" used accurate recollections of past failures "to create better strategies." The lesson: Use failure to improve your performance, not to create doomsday prophecies.

15. **Cool down to avoid blowups.** We're all for working out at lunch, but not if you punch your boss's lights out afterward. If you don't take time to cool down after a workout, your anger could erupt at the wrong time, according to J. Morrow, Ph.D., professor of psychology at Iona College in New Rochelle, New York. "After an intense workout or a competitive sport, you're in a high arousal state—high emotions are transferred very easily," says Dr. Morrow. "If somebody approaches you in a marginal way, you're more likely to respond aggressively. That's called arousal transfer." To avoid assault charges, follow intense workouts with a 20- to 30-minute emotional cooldown period that begins after you reach your resting heart rate. If you don't have that much time, try some deep-breathing exercises or imagine a relaxing scene. Either way, don't make your workout mantra "I feel so pumped I could break someone in half."

16. **Torture your tormentors.** The next time a telemarketer intrudes upon your life (which will probably be any minute now), resist the temptation to just slam down the receiver. You'll walk away mad (and stressed) and Mr. Investment Wizard will call back again anyway. Instead, make a game out of getting off the phone, suggests Daniel Kegan, Ph.D., an organizational psychologist with Elan Associates in Chicago. Don't think of phone solicitations as annoyances; think of them as opportunities for amusement. Here are three different ways to start the fun.

1. Hand the phone over to a child under the age of five. Telemarketers love spending their time entertaining children!
2. Ask them if they can lend you some money. (You never know.)
3. Turn the calls into free therapy sessions! Ramble on about that fight you had with your dad, how poorly work is going, that feeling that life has no meaning. . . .

17. **Resist rushing.** One big trigger of flying anxiety is rushing. Albert Forgione, Ph.D., director of the Institute for Psychology of Air Travel in Boston, recommends arriving at least an hour ahead of your departure time for a domestic flight and two hours early for an international flight. If you're racing to get to your flight, the time anxiety can morph into other kinds of flying fear.

18. **Divide and conquer.** Humans store information in "chunks" five to nine ingredients long, according to Michael Epstein, Ph.D., chairman of the psychology department at Rider University in Lawrenceville, New Jersey. We can remember a 5-digit pin number or a 9-item grocery list. When the memory tasks get longer, Dr. Epstein suggests dividing the assignment. Instead of trying to remember 10 digits, divide the numbers into two 5-digit chunks.

19. **Summon a situation.** Our memories don't operate in a vacuum. They are often triggered by environmental cues. If you suddenly blank out on a number you usually know, it may be because you're trying to recall it in an unfamiliar situation. For example, you usually open your garage door at night. If you're without a clue as to the code at high noon, transport yourself to darkness. Imagine that you and the wife are coming home from a dinner party. Voilà, the number will appear.

20. **Diffuse your emotions.** What do you do with the rage that builds up inside you when some clown cuts you off in traffic? Try stress defusers, suggests Leon James, Ph.D., professor of psychology at the University of Hawaii at Manoa, who has studied the psychology of driving. Count to 10. Give yourself a pep talk. Make animal noises. Scream at the other guy at the top of your lungs—just keep the windows rolled up, okay? Whatever you do, avoid declarations of war. Don't use your car as a weapon. Don't speed up, slow down, or change directions to make a point of any kind.

7
CURES

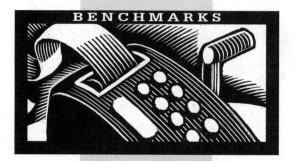

■ Number of *hourly* medication mistakes in a medium-size hospital: 60

■ Percentage of outpatients who use prescribed medicine incorrectly or not at all: 90

■ Cost of a jar of 100 aspirin tablets in Tokyo: $35.93

■ Percentage of fatal heart attack victims who don't receive cardiopulmonary resuscitation: 70

■ Number of workdays lost annually to migraine headaches: 157 million

■ Percentage of men ages 18 to 49 who have male pattern baldness, according to a recent survey: 42

■ Percentage of men ages 18 to 49 who have male pattern baldness, according to previous surveys: 33

■ Number of physicians in China: 1,832,000

■ Number of physicians in United States: 629,815

■ Percentage of U.S. hospital deaths that follow decisions to withhold treatment: 70

■ Number of annual premature deaths that could be prevented if all Americans reduced their total fat, saturated fat, and cholesterol intakes to the recommended levels: 42,000

■ Price for which a Missouri inmate offered to sell his organs to cover his legal fees: $50,000

■ Estimated number of compounds tested for every new drug that reaches the market: 10,000

■ Estimated annual percentage of deaths in the United States due to a lack of regular physical activity: 12

VITAL READING

The End of Impotence?

Viagra is promising, but it's not for everyone.

The day the Food and Drug Administration gave its blessing to a tiny blue pill capable of restoring erections to millions of men who thought they might never have sex again, they created what could well be the most exciting advance in sexual medicine since the advent of the birth control pill. Urologists are already talking about that day as if it's going to be declared a national holiday. "There's no doubt that March 27, 1998, will go down as a milestone in the history of erection treatment," says Harin Padma-Nathan, M.D., director of the Male Clinic and clinical associate professor of urology at the University of Southern California School of Medicine, both in Santa Monica.

But if you think Viagra is going to spell the end of more unpleasant treatment options, you may be assuming too much. "There will still be room for the other erection therapies, including injections, implants, and vacuum devices as well as for some exciting innovations that have yet to evolve," says Dr. Padma-Nathan. Despite its impressive performance in clinical trials and the media frenzy caused by Viagra's approval, treating impotence is not yet a one-pill-fits-all affair.

Viagra (known to many doctors by its generic name, sildenafil) works by altering levels of a chemical that controls muscle tissue in the artery walls. In fact, it was originally developed as a treatment for heart disease that didn't work out as planned. As the researchers were about to scrap the project, men who were testing the drug reported an unusual side effect: great erections.

Soon, the researchers were retooling their efforts to target impotence. They discovered that the drug's ability to relax artery muscles allowed blood to rush into the spongy tissues of the penis, causing them to expand and creating an erection.

Viagra's big advantage, besides being easy to take, is that it will only cause erections when you become aroused. "If you take the pill and walk into a business meeting, unless there are some very exciting people in that meeting, you are not going to become erect," says Laurence A. Levine, M.D., associate professor of urology and director of the Male Sexual Function and Fertility Program at Rush–Presbyterian–St. Luke's Medical Center in Chicago. That's a major departure from the injectable drugs designed to create an "automatic" erection no matter what you're thinking about.

Despite this convenience, Viagra's record is not far behind the injectables. Depending on which study you cite, the pill works for between 60 and 89 percent of men who try it. Overall, only 1 percent of men in Viagra's studies dropped out because it didn't work. Mild side effects including headache and indigestion afflicted about 10 percent of study subjects.

Because it's so easy to take, urologists will prescribe the $10-per-pill drug to most anybody who walks in their doors complaining of poor erections. "It's really going to be a good first-line treatment, especially for patients with mild to moderate impotence that are in otherwise good health," says Dr. Levine.

But for men with more severe impotence, results will not be so good. Depending on the underlying causes of their impotence, 20 to 50 percent of patients will not get sufficient erections with Viagra and will have to resort to another treatment.

Injections. It wasn't that long ago that we were heralding injectable drugs like Caverject (alprostadil) as the first reliable impotence treatments that didn't require surgery or cumbersome pre-sex vacuum treatments to create an erection. And despite the agony many men feel at the prospect of sticking their penises with needles, experts say injections will continue to have their place.

"While Viagra works quite well on men with milder forms of impotence, it works less well on men who have damage to the penile tissue because of artery disease or prostate surgery," says Irwin Goldstein, M.D., professor of urology at Boston University School of Medicine. One study showed injections were effective in 87 percent of men. And some urologists suggest injections can be used in conjunction with Viagra to deliver a double punch. In an effort to make injections easier to take, researchers developed a system called MUSE, which works by depositing a "pellet" of medicine in the tip of the penis (the urethra) via a specialized plastic plunger. Unfortunately, the approach didn't perform as well as expected, working well in only 5 to 7 percent of men. One recent study showed 98 percent of men who tried it went back to traditional injections because it either didn't work or caused pain.

Researchers at Harvard Scientific Corporation are hard at work on another urethral device that will deliver medicine in a liquid form and that they hope will cause less pain than the MUSE pellet.

Vacuum pumps. Experts believe this minimally invasive option will also continue to be useful in some men, including those on certain heart medications that cannot be mixed with Viagra. Now that high-quality vacuum pumps are available over-the-counter through drugstores and by mail order, they are also the only option that doesn't require your doctor's blessing. Dr. Padma-Nathan says pumps may make the best choice for older men who don't want to take medication.

Creams and needleless injectors. Many experts are looking forward to the day when there's an even more convenient option that can trigger an erection on contact.

Office Help

Stop these work-related pains before they strike.

With deadlines charging at us like Confederate soldiers and the boss's marching orders echoing in our ears, the absolute last thing we have time to worry about at the office is ergonomics. Like you, we're paid to pump out a quota of work in a given time. As long as the numbers are good, our boss doesn't care if we type with our chins and spend our evenings nested in a church tower. He wants results. Same with your boss, we're sure.

But sooner or later, working with poor form will cost you. The daily stiff necks, backaches, headaches, and sore wrists start out as little annoyances, but if you ignore them, they can quickly develop into painful, chronic injuries that require therapy, even surgery. Some can even result in permanent disability.

Now, we're not going to waste your time with any "sit like Joe Robot, cheerfully typing report" garbage. You're human.

You move. And aside from Johnny Carson, we've never seen a man who didn't slouch now and again at work. Instead, we offer this simple guide to the common problems that plague office workers and some expert tips on how to fix them.

Symptom: You have a stiff neck and sore shoulders by quitting time. "Your head weighs 10 to 12 pounds, and that's a bowling ball," says Adam Cobb, a physical therapist in Allentown, Pennsylvania, who treats a growing stream of corporate men who come in with chronic conditions from computer-intensive jobs. "Supporting your head for eight hours at a time is bound to strain your neck and shoulders, especially if you don't sit correctly." Massages will help, but following these four tips should eliminate the problem.

Hold your chin back. "Sitting with your head in front of your shoulders will quickly strain all of the muscles and tendons in the neck," says Cobb. It's simple gravity; without your pelvis and spine directly under it, the weight of your head pulls down on the stabilizing tissues in your shoulders and neck. Adjust the back of your chair so it supports your spine, and scoot your buttocks as far back as you can. That'll put your head and spine in line.

Keep important items nearby. Make sure you can reach your keyboard, mouse, and any other important items while keeping your elbows bent at a comfortable 90 degrees, advises Cobb. Stretching strains the shoulders.

Don't type while you're on the phone. That is, unless you're a Time-Life operator. "Flexing your head against your shoulder to hold a phone pinches the primary blood flow to the arm and brain," says Cobb. It's no joke; one woman in France sent herself to the emergency room with a torn carotid artery after cradling a phone for just a half-hour. Even if you don't keel over, you may compress nerves and numb your fingers for several minutes. We know you won't use a headset (the smartest fix), so when the phone rings, make like it's 1968 and take notes with a pen and paper. It'll give your wrists and fingers a break from the keyboard, too.

Adjust your screen low. Your neck was built to bend slightly downward throughout the day. Think of Abe in the Lincoln Memorial—that's the right angle. "Most people can't put their monitors low enough," says Chris Grant, Ph.D., an ergonomic specialist in Ann Arbor, Michigan. Place your monitor on the desktop, not on top of the computer's central unit.

Symptom: After work, your lower back feels like you've been caned. No mystery here. "You're most likely compressing your lower vertebrae by sitting with incorrect posture," says Cobb. Sitting may take a load off your feet, but it increases the pressure on your spine by 30 percent. Here are four ways to stop lower-back pain.

Move around. Staying fixed in one pose, even if it's ergonomically perfect, will eventually hurt you. "Move around even if you've found a comfortable spot," says Dr. Grant. Identify the distinct activities you perform at your desk—phoning, writing, typing, reading, eating—and make a conscious effort to do each from a different body position. "Constantly changing position helps the disks in your spine retain more fluid," says Dr. Grant. And that keeps your back more pliable.

Unwind your hamstrings. Prolonged sitting can tighten your hamstrings, which then begin to pull down on your pelvis, straining the muscles of your lower back. To alleviate the tightness, do the figure-4 stretch daily: Sit on the floor with your left leg extended in front of you, and bend the right leg so your right foot touches your left knee (your legs will form a shape like the number 4). Gently bend forward at your waist to stretch your left hamstring and hold the stretch for 10 seconds. Do this five times, then stretch your right leg.

Take short breaks, not extended lunches. Sneaking in regular hiatuses from your chair (say, every 20 minutes or so) also helps prevent backaches, says Dr. Grant. Every time you subtotal a column, take a walk. Hell, raid petty cash and go for a cappuccino.

Get rid of the bad chair. Ditch the cheap chair. Nice posture won't help if you're sitting on a folding chair from last year's sausage banquet. "An office chair should have an adjustable height and a tilting backrest," says Dr. Grant. Call the company bursar and order a work stool that would impress NASA.

Symptom: Headaches strike you every day at 3:00 P.M. Constantly looking up at your computer monitor can be a surefire cause of headaches. But if you've already lowered it, blame eyestrain. It's a common culprit; in fact, in a recent poll of 509 executives, 438 said they suffered headaches and other symptoms of eyestrain after using their computers for only two hours. You can stop afternoon headaches—and the blurry vision that accompanies them—in a few simple steps.

Stop blinding yourself. Shield your eyes with one hand. "If it feels better, your office is too bright," says Dr. Grant. Close window shades and dim the lights until you see no reflections on your monitor, and order an antiglare screen cover. That should do it.

Give your eyes a break. Position everything you need to see—computer monitor, Rolodex, calendar—three feet from your face. This will stop your eyes from refocusing thousands of times each day, says Jeffrey Anshel, O.D., an optometrist in Carlsbad, California.

Follow the 20-20-20 rule. Most computer-related eyestrain comes from staring at the monitor too intensely for too long. So give your peepers regular breaks. "Every 20 minutes, you should look at something at least 20 feet away for 20 seconds," says Dr. Anshel. This will force your eyes to refresh their focus. A tip: Whenever the phone rings or an incoming e-mail beeps, stretch your neck and look away from the monitor. Just don't ogle the new temp more than four times a day, all right?

Wear the correct glasses. Most lenses either improve vision at less than two feet or beyond five feet, to fix normal ranges of farsightedness and nearsightedness, says Dr. Anshel. This makes them useless for computer work. Ask your optometrist to prescribe lenses that are specially made for computer work.

Keep it color simple. Don't impress your co-workers with fancy screen colors. Stick with black letters on a white background, says Dr. Anshel.

Symptom: Your wrist aches so much you can barely turn a doorknob. Carpal tunnel syndrome isn't a fictional injury contrived by whining typists. "In fact, it's the most verifiable of all musculoskeletal diseases, and that includes tendinitis and golfer's elbow," says Dr. Grant. Overuse of the hands and fingers causes a painful compression of the median nerve, which runs through the carpal tunnel in the wrists. Stupidly ignore the pain, and the problem may progress until you can't pick up a coffee mug without screaming. By that time, you might need surgery to relieve the ache in your hands. If your wrists hurt during or after work, see a doctor right away. Otherwise:

Lower your keyboard—now. Position your keyboard below your belly button, directly over your upper thighs, and you won't have to worry about carpal tunnel syndrome. Resting your keyboard on your desk is a big mistake, says Cobb. It causes you to bend your wrists upward, which leaves your median nerve most vulnerable. It also forces your shoulders to stay tensed to elevate your arms, which causes back and neck pain.

Stay away from weights if you have wrist pain. "Men usually think they need to strengthen their wrists with exercise, but they really need to rest them," says Dr. Grant. "A lot of men accelerate carpal tunnel syndrome by lifting weights." If your hands ever feel numb (an important early-warning sign) or if your wrists are even a little tender, see a doctor before you start a weight training program.

Try an ergonomically correct keyboard. You've seen these; the keys are split into right-hand and left-hand angled groupings so you can type with your elbows naturally flared out. Some experts believe they can cut down on wrist and arm strain.

Protection for Your Prostate

Experts assess over-the-counter ingredients
that help the male-only gland.

Walk into any health food store and you'll see them lined up like so many tiny armies taking aim at your swollen prostate. And if it looks like the prostate-protecting herbal remedy ranks are growing, they are. A recent survey of health food stores found that sales of the prostate-friendly herb saw palmetto jumped 63 percent last year.

But more choices mean more confusion. Since the Food and Drug Administration prohibits supplement manufacturers from making specific health claims, these herb- and nutrient-packed tablets generally promise only to "nutritionally support a healthy prostate gland." Hmmm. . . . And most traditional urologists remain silent regarding herbal treatments for which there are few American studies.

So we decided to grab a handful of commonly promoted remedies and search for the few brave experts who would talk frankly. While we were encouraged by what we heard, we learned that being informed is crucial to choosing an effective over-the-counter remedy.

"I'd say more than 90 percent of my enlarged-prostate patients can be successfully treated with the right natural remedies," says Steven Margolis, M.D., clinical instructor at Wayne State University in Detroit and an alternative family physician practicing in Sterling Heights, Michigan.

And some experts believe that taking herbs can help keep the gland from sprawling in the first place. "I'm betting my own prostate on the fact that this stuff works better than any commonly prescribed drug," says James A. Duke, Ph.D., a retired economic botanist and herbal expert and author of *The Green Pharmacy*, who concocts his own herbal blend.

Such preventive measures seem prudent when you consider that 80 percent of men in their eighties have enlarged prostates (known to doctors as benign prostatic hyperplasia, or BPH). And the majority of these will suffer from at least one symptom, including urinary urgency or frequency, and an inability to completely empty the bladder. For roughly half of all men with urinary symptoms, there is an accompanying interference in sexual performance, such as limp erections, diminished ejaculation, and less-than-explosive orgasms.

That's why European doctors generally prefer herbal remedies to traditional drugs—and prescribe the natural healers routinely. In many countries, herbal products are classified as pharmaceuticals and so have been studied extensively. Urologists in France, Germany, and Italy turn to herbs before they even bring up the possibility of traditional drugs or surgery. One study estimates that 90 percent of all European prostate-enlargement prescriptions are for plant extracts.

The failure of herbal supplements to capture the support of the urologic community on this side of the Atlantic can be traced back to the almighty dollar. "Without patent rights, there's no incentive for pharmaceutical companies to spend the millions it takes to study the efficacy of these products. And without published studies, most mainstream physicians are extremely hesitant to recommend them," explains Dr. Margolis.

That's especially frustrating, given that the treatment of prostate enlargement lends itself particularly well to herbal measures since, other than how much it bothers you, an enlarged gland generally poses no medical threat. "For all but 10 percent of men—those with very large prostates that can block the outflow of urine—we treat prostate enlargement strictly for symptom relief," says Judd Moul, M.D., urologic oncologist at the Walter Reed Army Medical Center in Washington, D.C.

Inside the Capsule

In the absence of clinical studies and product regulation, personal education regarding prostate remedies is key. So, armed with our corporate credit card and a healthy dose of skepticism, we set out to sort one from another. First, we hit our local health food stores; then we started calling for information on products sent in by readers. A few days later, we had accumulated a variety of prostate remedies—enough to start dialing the experts, asking about the following ingredients.

Saw palmetto. Found in every remedy we bought, saw palmetto (*Serenoa repens*) is extracted from the berries of a palmlike shrub native to the southeastern United States. Herbal experts believe the berry acts on the prostate in much the same way as the drug Proscar (finasteride). "Both Proscar and saw palmetto work by blocking the conversion of testosterone into dihydrotestosterone (DHT), the compound that makes the prostate grow," says Richard Podell, M.D., clinical professor of nutrition and herbal medicine at the University of Medicine and Dentistry of New Jersey Robert Wood Johnson Medical School in New Brunswick. Without DHT, the prostate will slowly shrink, relieving the pressure on the urethra and making it easier to pee.

The herb has become a mainstay of prostate-enlargement treatments in France, Germany, and Italy due to 12 European clinical studies, all of which showed at least some benefit. The most recent showed that 74 percent of men taking 320 milligrams of saw palmetto a day reported improved symptoms.

Even some American researchers are jumping (tentatively) on the saw palmetto bandwagon. In a study conducted at the University of Chicago, men taking the herb reported a 30 percent improvement in symptoms after two months. "It's a small study, so it's hard to know whether every man will respond to saw palmetto. But certainly, many men felt it improved their symptoms," says lead study author Glenn Gerber, M.D., associate professor of urology at the university.

Look on the label for 320 milligrams of saw palmetto that meets the German potency standard of 85 percent fatty acids (sterols).

Pygeum. In France, 75 percent of all doctors' prescriptions for prostate enlargement are for an extract of tree bark called *Pygeum africanum*. Beta-sitosterol, the active component of pygeum, is a potent compound that has been used in the German prostate-enlargement-relieving drug Harzol and in an American cholesterol-lowering drug called Colestid (colestipol hydrochloride).

One recent study of 200 men from Ruhr University in Bochum, Germany, showed that those taking 60 milligrams a day of beta-sitosterol had a 50 percent improvement in urinary symptoms, while those on a placebo improved only 14 percent.

Our experts considered pygeum an essential component of prostate remedy, in part because it may help offset the occasional libido-lowering effects of saw palmetto.

Look on the label for at least 100 milligrams (and no more than 200 milligrams) of pygeum standardized to the German standard of at least 10 percent fatty acids (sterols).

Zinc. This common mineral is the single most important nutrient for a healthy prostate, according to Michael B. Schachter, M.D., an alternative physician practicing in Suffern, New York, and author of *The Natural Way to a Healthy Prostate.*

In one small study at the Finch University of Health Sciences/Chicago Medical School in North Chicago, 19 men with BPH were given 150-milligram zinc supplements for two months. Fourteen of their prostates shrank.

Meanwhile, researchers at the University of Edinburgh Medical School say their test-tube studies have confirmed that zinc, like saw palmetto, helps to shrink the prostate by blocking the conversion of testosterone to DHT.

Because too much zinc can deplete levels of copper and result in weakened immunity, don't take more than 50 milligrams a day unless under a doctor's supervision. Look on the label for no more than 50 milligrams of zinc. (If you take a multivitamin, check to see that your combined dose of zinc is less than 50 milligrams.)

Pumpkin seed. Originally a Ukrainian folk remedy for prostate inflammation, roasted pumpkin seeds have caught on in the United States among some men with inflamed prostates. And extracts of pumpkin seeds are showing up in prostate remedies as well. One double-blind study found that a mixture of 80 milligrams each of pumpkin seed (*Cucurbita pepo*) and saw palmetto significantly improved men's urinary symptoms in three months. Researchers believe that the active component in pumpkin seeds is the fatty acid beta-sitosterol.

Look on the label for an optimal dose of 80 milligrams of pumpkin seed or 60 milligrams of beta-sitosterol.

Flaxseed oil. This extract is packed with the healthful essential fatty acids that most men don't get enough of. Studies show that these fatty acids help to reduce inflammation in the urinary tract while boosting immune function. While that's good news for men with a prostate infection (prostatitis), it can also help to reduce the irritating effect urine can have on enlarged prostate tissue.

Look on the label for an optimum of 1,000 milligrams flaxseed oil.

Bearberry. "Bearberry is a urinary antiseptic that soothes the urinary tract and can make urine less irritating to the urethra," says Eva Urbaniak, a naturopathic physician practicing in Seattle and author of *Healing Your Prostate: Natural Cures That Work.* That's because bearberry contains arbutin, the same urinary tract–friendly compound found in cranberry juice.

Look on the label for 10 milligrams of bearberry, or *Uva ursi,* as it's sometimes referred to.

Stinging nettle. When researchers gave a few teaspoons a day of stinging nettle extract to 67 men with BPH, they found it reduced the number of times the subjects urinated nightly. And a German study put a combination formula of saw palmetto and stinging nettle head-to-head with Proscar in 516 patients suffering from BPH. After 48 weeks of treatment, the researchers concluded that their herbal formula was "therapeutically equivalent" to the drug.

Look on the label for 100 milligrams of stinging nettle or *Urtica dioica.*

Recommendations

If your symptoms are mild to moderate, consider trying a natural remedy before submitting to more powerful drugs. "These products are extremely safe, and there's no reason that a man with prostate symptoms shouldn't at least give them a try," says Dr. Margolis.

If one doesn't work, try another. "Experiment with different products. Since I see no clear evidence that more money buys you a better product, if it were my buck, I'd start with a less expensive choice," says Dr. Gerber.

Even if your prostate is healthy, you might consider starting on a reduced dose of a natural remedy now. "I'm taking a daily dose myself as a preventive measure, and I'd recommend the same to anyone with a family history of prostate enlargement," says Dr. Margolis. If this is your goal, take half the recommended daily dose, or about 160 milligrams a day of saw palmetto and 50 to 100 milligrams of pygeum, says Dr. Margolis.

Finally, even though these remedies are available over-the-counter, if it were our gland, we'd gain our doctor's blessing first. "The only way to know you're not among the 10 percent of men for whom enlargement poses a serious health threat is to see your doctor first," says Dr. Moul.

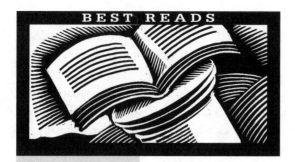

Cure the Most Common Headache

Tension headaches are literally a pain in the neck. Although they rarely cause you to stop an activity, they can certainly make life miserable. And while many men reach for the aspirin bottle when the pain comes on, this fascinating excerpt from Symptom Solver: Understanding—And Treating—The Most Common Male Health Concerns *(Rodale Press, 1997), by Alisa Bauman and Brian Paul Kaufman, reveals why that shouldn't be the first course of action, and what you can do to prevent more from coming on.*

Symptoms: Pressing, tight feeling all around the head; jaw discomfort; neck pain; and tender spots.

What it means: If you get headaches, chances are that these are the kind you get. Tension headaches cause a dull pain that makes your head feel like an overworked muscle. It's the most common kind of headache, affecting about 69 percent of men at some time during their lives.

Most tension headaches are caused by muscle tension around the temples and the back of your neck, says Frederick Freitag, D.O., associate director of the Diamond Headache Clinic in Chicago. They can also be caused by poor posture, medical problems such as arthritis, or even depression.

Some people—about 10 percent of tension-headache sufferers—get chronic headaches that may occur nearly every day. For them, over-the-counter pain remedies are often ineffective.

Though tension-type headaches and migraines are very different—migraines are more severe and generally attack only one side of the head—there's generally an overlap. People who get migraines also get tension headaches and vice versa, says Dr. Freitag.

Symptom Solver

When you feel a headache coming on, the first thing you probably do is open the medicine cabinet and reach for a painkiller like aspirin or ibuprofen. Certain brands of painkillers, however, also contain caffeine. Avoid these. While caffeine may work great for a migraine headache, it actually makes a tension headache worse, explains Marvin Hoffert, M.D., a headache specialist in private practice in Boston.

While any over-the-counter painkiller can help ease tension headaches, you might want to make ibuprofen your first choice, says Dr. Hoffert. People respond differently to different medications, so check with your doctor first. According to one study, 400 milligrams of ibuprofen is more effective than 650 milligrams of aspirin.

Here are some other things to try.

Stretch. Since tension headaches are often caused by muscle tension, stretching out those muscles can help ease the pain. For instance, if the back of your neck is tight, do slow neck stretches by holding your chin close to your chest, says Dr. Hoffert. You don't have to wait until the headache strikes. Throughout the day, periodically stretching the muscles that cause you pain can help prevent headaches from occurring.

If you can't quite tell where the tight spots are, a doctor can perform tests that pinpoint which muscles are stressed and then design an exercise and stretching program for you, says Dr. Hoffert. But we'll give you a hint. The areas usually affected are at the temples and the back of the neck.

Ice it. Putting an ice pack on the part of your head that hurts can be just as effective as taking aspirin. "If they can get to the headache when it's a dull throb, close to 80 percent of people can abort their headaches," says Fred Sheftell, M.D., director of the New England Center for Headache in Stamford, Connecticut. Cold reduces inflammation of the blood vessels that often causes the pain.

Massage it. Rub the tiny ridge between your neck and the back of your head, right behind the earlobes, for 10 to 15 minutes, says Dr. Sheftell. Then rub your temples and the back of the neck where your neck and shoulders meet. These are all prime, tight-muscle spots, and a thorough massage can help them relax and ease the pain.

Watch what you eat. Some tension headaches are triggered by ingredients in food, like the MSG (monosodium glutamate) found in many processed foods, the nitrates in lunchmeat, and the aspartame in diet sodas, says Dr. Freitag. The next time a headache strikes, think about what you ate just before. If you're able to identify a food that seems to be responsible, try avoiding it for a few weeks to see if things improve.

Sleep on schedule. Fluctuations in your normal sleep schedule—like staying up all night, for example, followed by a day in bed—can trigger tension headaches. It's best to try to keep regular hours, says Dr. Freitag.

Go easy on painkillers. If you find yourself using painkillers daily for headaches, you might be doing yourself more harm than good, cautions Dr. Hoffert. Painkillers are somewhat addictive, especially those that contain caffeine. So, eventually, they will work less effectively and actually cause more headaches to occur. If you're taking medications often to control headaches, check with your doctor.

Tune in. The best way to beat tension headaches is to listen to your body—to catch your tension and relax before the pain begins. "As you become aware of how your body talks to you, you get sophisticated enough to hear it whisper," says Joseph Primavera III, Ph.D., co-director of the Comprehensive Headache Center at Germantown Hospital and Medical Center in Philadelphia. "Then you can address the signs early on, and your body will never have to shout."

Research suggests that stopping to relax—even for as little as five minutes—at the first sign of pain may be just enough to stop a headache before it gets started.

Wash the dishes. Really. Doing mundane tasks is a great way to relax. That's because you don't have to think about what you're doing. "Nothing induces a trance quicker than a boring kind of job, like doing the dishes. You do the dishes, you drift into thinking about something else; all of a sudden the dishes are done, and you snap out of it," says Dr. Primavera.

Take small breaks. "In the real world, maybe taking a deep breath, doing a stretch, and staring out the window for a few minutes is all that you're going to get. Luckily, that's often just enough to keep you from triggering a headache," says Dr. Primavera.

Put Out the Fire

A pepperoni pizza and a pitcher of beer may sound great, but the heartburn that's sure to follow isn't any fun. But there is a way to avoid that painful burn if you're unwilling to give up the pizzafest. This excerpt from Symptom Solver: Understanding—And Treating—The Most Common Male Health Concerns *(Rodale Press, 1997), by Alisa Bauman and Brian Paul Kaufman, offers practical tips to keep the fire under control.*

Symptom: You have a painful burning sensation in your stomach and, sometimes, your chest.

What it means: You start the day with a large cup of coffee and a smoke. Then you inhale a giant Italian sub with onions and hot peppers for lunch. For dinner, you scarf down a huge plate of Buffalo chicken wings—washed down, naturally, by several pitchers of beer. And as you lie down at night, you get heartburn so bad that it brings tears to your eyes.

Of course, you know why. It was that spicy chicken wing sauce, on top of those onions and peppers that you had for lunch. Right?

Wrong.

"It's not the spice that gets you; it's the fat and the smoke and the alcohol," says Jorge Herrera, M.D., associate professor of medicine at the University of South Alabama in Mobile. "Many of these guys are overweight, too. All four things combine to give you a terrible case of heartburn."

If you're having heartburn and still smoking and eating and drinking too much, you need to—first and foremost—move out of the frat house. *National Lampoon's Animal House* was a comedy—not a lifestyle documentary. Besides, a man your age should at least have his own apartment. And you should probably see a doctor as well: There's a possibility that you're actually suffering from cardiovascular disease or having a mild heart attack.

"The pain can be similar. When in doubt, the best thing is to assume that it's the heart and have it checked," says Dr. Herrera. If you have a family history of heart problems, though, see a doctor anyway—you need to talk with him about your diet.

As for you heartburn sufferers, ever wonder why it hurts so much? In a healthy gastrointestinal tract, acid stays in the stomach, helping to break down food. The only thing separating this powerful acid and your esophagus is a small muscle that squeezes open and closed, called your lower esophageal sphincter.

Weaken that small muscle any number of ways—eating too much fat, drinking too much booze, or smoking cigarettes, for example—and stomach acid is free to lap at your tender esophagus, causing pain.

"All you need is a little bit of acid in there to cause problems, because the esophagus is not used to handling it," says Gary Green, M.D., associate team physician of intercollegiate athletics at the University of California, Los Angeles.

And athletes who overindulge in the wrong stuff and then exercise are prime candidates for big-time heartburn, Dr. Green says.

Symptom Solver

There are plenty of ways to beat the burn. Try these.

Chew gum. Saliva generated by gum chewing can help put out the fire in your esophagus, Dr. Herrera says.

Lose your love handles. Carrying just 15 percent too much weight on your frame increases your likelihood of heartburn. Some studies have shown that excessive weight can reduce the holding power of the esophageal sphincter. Those extra pounds also increase the upward pressure of stomach acids. (And until you lose the weight, lose those tight clothes, says Dr. Herrera. They can cause stomach pressure, too.)

Tilt that bed. If you have chronic heartburn, you can ease your nighttime bouts and simultaneously create a low-rent version of an adjustable bed. Simply place the two legs at the head of the bed on bricks or blocks of wood. The angle will help prevent acid from seeping from your stomach into your esophagus while you sleep, says Dr. Green.

Think before you drink. Although mugs of coffee and alcohol may top your list of favorite beverages, you can help reduce your heartburn by drinking less of both. Coffee and alcohol not only decrease the strength of the esophageal muscle but also increase stomach acid production, says William B. Ruderman, M.D., attending physician for Gastroenterology Associates of Central Florida in Clearwater.

And even switching to decaf might not help. "There are studies that show that it's not so much the caffeine as the oils in the coffee," adds Dr. Herrera. Red wine also has a reputation for causing heartburn.

Launch a pre-emptive strike. Heart set on a night of pizza and beer with the boys but worried about a major-league case of heartburn? Drop some antacid one hour before the big feast and three hours after, says Dr. Herrera. "That way, you'll blunt the acid throughout the period when it's being produced," he says. "That's the good thing about antacids. They work almost immediately. If you know that certain foods are going to cause heartburn, you can prevent it by taking an antacid before."

Trim that fat. Eating less fat can save you from heartburn. "Fatty foods delay the emptying of the stomach, so you can just imagine how that would put pressure on the esophageal muscle," says Dr. Green. Some of the worst offenders are fried foods and chocolate, he says.

Drink milk. Although not all doctors agree, some suggest that in a pinch, a glass of milk might help your heartburn. "Compared to what you can buy at the store, milk is a fairly weak antacid. But it can improve symptoms for a short time," says Dr. Herrera.

Pass on the peppermint. Ever wonder why you seem to develop heartburn after visiting a restaurant that serves peppermints with the bill? It's probably not the size of the check—although that could be a factor. Peppermint also weakens the esophageal sphincter, says Dr. Herrera.

Eat right before you exercise. Olympic records have certainly been set on some pretty weird precompetition diets, but if you have problems with heartburn, stick with carbohydrate and electrolyte solutions like Gatorade for an hour before you work out, Dr. Green says.

Mind your medication. Aspirin, anti-inflammatory pills, and certain heart, blood pressure, and asthma medications can all increase stomach acid production, Dr. Herrera says.

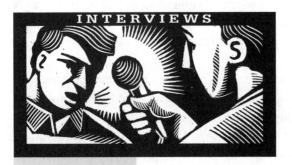

INTERVIEWS

Kevin Quirk on
Beating Sports Addiction

With the large variety of sports channels available now, most men can't wait to spend some quality time with their 25-inch TVs. But some guys lose their grips on reality, says Kevin Quirk, former Sports Illustrated *correspondent and recovering "sportsaholic." While we tend to chuckle about such a ridiculous-sounding affliction, Quirk, a support group leader and author of* Not Now Honey, I'm Watching the Game, *believes that sports addiction is a significant problem for many men. He speaks from experience. When his wife walked out on him in the middle of the 1984 Super Bowl, Quirk barely took his eyes off Joe Theismann long enough to notice.*

What's the worst example of "sports addiction" you've ever seen?

I met a sportsaholic in Michigan who took his pregnant wife to the Michigan-Michigan State game, and she went into labor in the stadium. Instead of leaving, he begged her to hold out until the game was over. "There are three doctors just in our section," he told her.

That's pathetic. But isn't the idea of an addiction to sports a bit dramatic?

I'd be the first to say it's not as serious as alcohol or drug abuse. There aren't physical consequences. But it's harmful because sports become our only emotional release. We jump for joy, scream at the ref, pray that kick through the uprights—but we shut off our emotions any other time. Some sports addicts react more strongly to their local team losing a key game than to being denied a promotion.

We watch sports and get along with women just fine. You must be talking about some real nuts.

That's the usual response I get. Guys always say, hey, I'm not nearly as bad as that guy who has eight Rotisserie-league teams and watches late-night Greco-Roman wrestling. Try this: Write down how many hours you devote to watching games and highlight shows, listening to sports on the radio, and reading the sports section. In a survey I did, most guys assumed they spent about 12 to 15 total per week. But when I asked them to keep a log, it turned out to be 35 to 40 hours. That's a full-time job.

But it's still not enough to call it an addiction.

Maybe not, but ask yourself other questions. Are you still depressed three weeks after your team loses a big game? Also, an addict treats his family differently when the game is on. Do you snap at the slightest interruption? Do you neglect things, like keeping an eye on your kid? If you answer yes to any of these, you may not be addicted, but sports may be dominating your life.

Okay, suppose our preoccupation with ESPN is cutting into our sex lives. What can we do?

Try a 2-week sports blackout. Just pretend there's a strike. If you tell yourself you'll miss only 2 weeks of sports out of 52, you'll make it. Then find out what other things you could be doing with all those hours you're wasting in front of the TV. Take up a hobby, or look into a part-time job. After 2 weeks without sports, you'll be able to make permanent changes. Cut your viewing hours to half your preblackout schedule, and watch only hometown teams.

Do you still catch a game now and then?

Absolutely. I still enjoy sports in moderation. Watching a few sporting events isn't bad; they're exciting, dramatic, and they help you connect with other guys. But they're games, and of no real consequence in the world. They shouldn't assume more importance than the real events that take place in your life.

Gregory White Smith on
Defying a Death Sentence

Ever since Brian's Song, *most men think they know the routine when the doctors tell them their time is up. You settle scores, achieve a life goal or two, then tidy your affairs with dignity until the hourglass runs out. But some people keep fighting for survival long after their physicians give up, and many—defying medical science—far outlive their expiration dates. One example: writer Gregory White Smith, author of* Making Miracles Happen. *When he was 34, physicians at the Mayo Clinic in Rochester, Minnesota, told Smith that an inoperable brain tumor would kill him within three months. That was 10 years ago.*

What was the first thing you did after hearing of your impending death?

I went back to my hotel and ate every cinnamon bun in the coffee shop, then I went for a second opinion. It was the same diagnosis. That stopped me. Going to a third doctor to hear the same thing was unthinkable. But then I had a conversation with the actor Charles Grodin, whose ex-wife had just died of cancer. He told me, "You haven't even begun to fight." And he was right. Seeing two doctors and quitting was ridiculous.

How did you fight it?

I took control. When you have a disease, you feel like the physician has all the knowledge and it's your job to sit there in your paper gown and nod. But doctors are like weathermen. They can give you a forecast about something that's likely to happen, but it's only a forecast. The more information you have, the better chance you have of changing that forecast.

Could your survival just be dumb luck?

Luck, yes. Dumb, no. I hunted down every piece of information on my condition that I could find, discovered a doctor who didn't think I was a lost cause, and eventually hit upon an experimental hormone therapy that stopped the cancer from growing.

So what exactly would be a good strategy for a man who really wants to live?

Scour the Internet to find abstracts, the library to find articles, periodicals . . . you name it. But you must realize that everything published is about three to five years behind. To find current information, you have to track down the doctors who actually conducted the studies. These people not only know the latest research but also, more important, can speculate on upcoming treatments. You probably won't get this from the local hospital, and it's the very information you need to survive.

What if even these doctors tell you there's no hope?

Regardless of what any physician might tell you, there are very few problems that don't have at least two possible treatments. The purpose of doing all this research is to come up with these options. Some treatments may be experimental, but doctors from reputable institutions are conducting trials all over the world. Find one, and beg or borrow to get in.

But won't that eventually lead you to some quack faith healer?

No. Here's my rule: Make sure every doctor you speak with is as good or better than the last one. If you start with physicians at well-known institutions, who've published research, then work your way up, you won't wind up being treated at Joe's Bait and Tackle Shop.

How do you know when you're chasing false hope?

You'll start to limit the information you're willing to listen to. You'll refuse to take a test because you're worried about the results or you won't travel to a renowned cancer center because you think, "They're not going to tell me anything new." As long as you stick with legitimate treatment, you can never look too hard. The only false hope is uninformed hope.

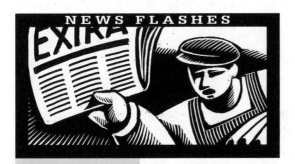

NEWS FLASHES

Important Clue Discovered in Search for Baldness Cure

NEW YORK CITY—Scientists have identified a gene missing from a Pakistani family that suffers from alopecia universalis, a rare genetic disorder that causes full-body hairlessness. While this gene does not control male pattern baldness, it is a step in the direction of finding a cure. "It's a clue, but we need a greater understanding of hair growth before we can ever apply this gene discovery to patients," says George Cotsarelis, M.D., director of the University of Pennsylvania hair and scalp clinic in Philadelphia.

The gene that the researchers, led by Angela Christiano, Ph.D., assistant professor of dermatology at Columbia University College of Physicians and Surgeons in New York City, isolated is only one of many that affect the complex hair-growth cycle, which still baffles scientists. Dr. Christiano, however, believes that patients with alopecia may one day restart hair growth by rubbing their follicles with a lotion containing the missing gene. "We're also investigating how this gene affects other hair-loss genes," she says, so a similar treatment for male pattern baldness isn't inconceivable in the future.

But don't expect one to debut in the next decade. "There are hundreds of on-going gene-therapy trials, and few have produced positive results," says David Schlessinger, Ph.D., chief of the laboratory of genetics at the National Institute on Aging in Bethesda, Maryland.

Procedure Puts an End to One Type of Dizziness

LOS ANGELES—Benign positional vertigo (BPV), a condition punctuated by bouts of dizziness, has stumped doctors for years. But this common form of vertigo can be cured in one trip to the doctor, a new study suggests. Theorizing that debris in the ear canal caused BPV, researchers rotated 15 patients in a flight simulator at an angle they predicted would clear the obstructions. All subjects reported improvement. "Your doctor can perform a similar procedure in his office," says Robert Baloh, M.D., professor of neurology at the University of California, Los Angeles, Medical Center.

Technique Wards Off Incontinence

GAINESVILLE, Fla.—Doctors say that a simple procedure can prevent urinary incontinence in men who undergo removal of the prostate. As many as one in four men who undergo radical prostatectomy loses some bladder control. When the prostate is removed, the bladder can fall into the newly created cavity, causing incontinence. Doctors using the new technique tie tissue to the bladder and lift it back into place, says Perinchery Narayan, M.D., chairman of urology at the University of Florida College of Medicine. The procedure adds about 10 minutes to the prostatectomy. "We've done it on about 35 men, and they're all doing well," says Dr. Narayan.

New Carpal Tunnel Surgery Speeds Healing

OAK PARK, Ill.—Surgeons have developed a new procedure to relieve carpal tunnel pain that requires only a tiny incision in the palm. This minimally invasive surgery can be performed in 10 minutes and costs about $1,200 (compared to $10,000 for traditional treatment), according to Manutchehr Sohaey, M.D., director of plastic and reconstructive surgery at West Suburban Hospital Medical Center. Traditional surgery to correct severe carpal tunnel pain can immobilize your hand for weeks. "With the new surgery, the patient can return to work within days and without splints," he adds.

Caffeine May Eliminate Postoperative Headaches

ROCHESTER, Minn.—Giving patients caffeine after surgery may relieve postsurgery headaches better than pain-killing drugs. Researchers say these headaches are often caused by caffeine withdrawal. Patients who were given a cup of coffee or intravenous caffeine after surgery suffered fewer postoperative headaches than those who went caffeine-free. "The equivalent of two cups of coffee or cans of cola can diminish the pain," says study leader Joseph G. Weber, M.D., an anesthesiologist with the Mayo Clinic.

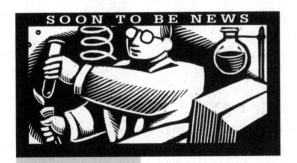

Relief for Back Pain?

If you have chronic back pain, you might have a new weapon soon. A transdermal patch may relieve back pain for up to 72 hours. The Duragesic patch delivers a continuous dose of fentanyl, a painkiller. In a study at Baylor College of Medicine in Houston, 50 patients with back pain used the patch for one month, and 43 reported significant relief. "Wearing the patch is more convenient than taking drugs every four to six hours," says study leader Richard K. Simpson, M.D.

If it passes further tests, the patch will be available by prescription for about $10 each.

Skin Bandages?

Researchers in Florida have developed a method to culture skin cells to create living "bandages." This means that soon, physicians will be able to bind wounds with biologically engineered skin and reduce healing time by as much as 66 percent. In a small trial of 11 patients, doctors treated wounds with these bandages, grafts from the patient's skin, or a polyurethane film. The bandages healed the wounds the fastest, beating the traditional grafts by half a day and the polyurethane film by three days. As the patient's skin regrows, it replaces the engineered skin, says lead researcher William H. Eaglstein, M.D., professor and chairman in the department of dermatology and cutaneous surgery at the University of Miami School of Medicine.

The new therapy is awaiting Food and Drug Administration approval.

An Acne Fighter That Slays Arthritis?

Researchers at the University of Nebraska Medical Center in Omaha have found that an acne medication can treat rheumatoid arthritis. In a study involving 46 arthritis patients, those who took 100 milligrams of minocycline twice a day found that the drug reduced joint tenderness, stiffness, and swelling by nearly half. The antibiotic may somehow protect joint cartilage, or it may even destroy the inflammatory agents that cause rheumatoid arthritis, says James O'Dell, M.D., principal study investigator.

If additional testing is successful, minocycline may be prescribed for rheumatoid arthritis within two years.

Pop a Pill after You Get the Flu?

According to a study at the University of Virginia in Charlottesville, a new oral flu treatment dramatically reduces the duration and severity of flu symptoms. "In experiments , the drug, called GS4104, inhibits the enzyme that allows the virus to replicate," says Fred Erick Hayden, M.D., a clinical investigator and professor of medicine and pathology at the university. The treatment would be given at the onset of flu symptoms and taken for about five days.

The drug is still being tested for its preventive potential and will not be available to the public for at least two years.

Help from Bloodsuckers?

A natural blood thinner created by leeches is being tested in heart attack patients. When a leech releases the blood thinner hirulog into a swimmer's body, scabs don't form, so the bloodsucker can continue to feast. Now doctors are treating heart attack patients with a synthetic form of this compound to prevent their blood from forming more clots. The new drug may replace heparin, a traditional blood thinner. "Patients treated with hirulog instead of heparin have much better results after angioplasty, a procedure that opens the blocked coronary arteries that cause heart attack," says James Chesebro, M.D., professor of medicine and director of clinical research at the Cardiovascular Institute of the Mount Sinai Medical Center in New York City.

Safe doses still need to be determined.

Nipping Strokes in the Bud?

Half a million Americans suffer strokes each year, often resulting in brain damage. But a new synthetic compound seems to limit brain damage after a stroke. When researchers at Boston University School of Medicine gave pregnanolone hemisuccinate to stroke-induced rats, the steroid stopped the destruction of neurons after a stroke. "This compound promises to treat strokes more effectively than standard drugs can," says David H. Farb, Ph.D., chairman of the department of pharmacology and study author.

Dr. Farb says the drug may be available within 5 to 10 years. Further studies are needed to assess the drug's effect on humans.

Say Good-Bye to Allergy Shots?

According to a recent study, allergy shots may soon be a thing of the past. The study, at Children's Hospital of Pittsburgh, found that a daily oral dose of encapsulated ragweed extract was more effective than a placebo in relieving sneezing, congestion, itchy throat, and runny nose after four weeks. "Past pills were ineffective because digestive enzymes destroyed them before they could be absorbed," says investigator Deborah Gentile, M.D. "But these are coated to prevent that."

Further studies are planned to determine proper dosage and long-term safety.

Acid Test for Heart Disease?

If you have high cholesterol or a heart condition, you may one day find relief from an amino acid. L-arginine may fight heart disease. A study from Stanford University School of Medicine reports that L-arginine supplements taken daily for two weeks reduced artery-clogging blood platelet clumps in 15 people with high cholesterol. "L-arginine may be converted into nitric oxide, a chemical that causes blood vessels to widen," says study leader John P. Cooke, M.D., Ph.D., director of vascular medicine at the university. Don't start taking L-arginine yet, Dr. Cooke warns.

Long-term studies are needed.

Kill the Pain before It Hurts?

If you're scheduled for an operation, ask the anesthesiologist about administering painkillers before surgery. Preliminary research at the University of Pennsylvania in Philadelphia suggests that receiving painkillers before major surgery may lessen pain and shorten recovery time. Anesthesiologists often inject an analgesic as the operation is wrapping up—well after the body has already reacted to the incision, according to study leader Allan Gottschalk, M.D., Ph.D. Starting the painkillers before surgery can reduce pain immediately after the operation and also in the weeks following, says Dr. Gottschalk.

Future studies are planned.

A Cure for Diabetes?

Sugar can be lethal to the millions of older men who develop Type II (adult-onset) diabetes. Even when treated, fluctuating blood-glucose levels can lead to heart disease, blindness, dementia, kidney failure, and loss of limbs.

But that may all change in the near future, as we approach a day when people who have diabetes won't need to inject themselves anymore. "We'll have insulin pills and inhalers within a few years," predicts Richard Marchase, Ph.D., director of the diabetes interdisciplinary research program at the University of Alabama at Birmingham.

An even more radical development: Within 25 years, physicians may routinely use gene therapy to regenerate the insulin-producing pancreatic cells or force other cells to produce insulin.

Pancreatic-cell transplants (much safer than substituting a new organ) with bio-engineered animal tissue are also coming, as is an artificial pancreas. "A small, bio-mechanical device that regulates blood sugar may be developed within two decades," says Dr. Marchase.

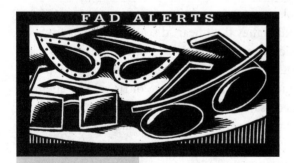

FAD ALERTS

Pain-Relieving Gel

Whether they're being hawked by Broadway Joe or Nolan Ryan, all topical pain relievers offer pretty much the same thing—temporary relief, but nothing to truly heal your muscles. Now, a new product called Perform Cool Pain Relieving Gel (endorsed by perennially sore guy Arnold Palmer) claims that its combination of a "natural herb and natural menthol" creates a chilling ice-pack effect that actually "relaxes" sore muscles.

We decided to ask some guys with physically demanding jobs and chronic aches to try using Perform. The response was unanimous: The potent-smelling, eye-tearing roll-on (think Vicks VapoRub) quickly created an "icy burn" but really did nothing to relax their stiff and aching muscles. It was a distraction, at best.

"Both of Perform's active ingredients, menthol and camphor, are found in Ben-Gay and a variety of other products," says Robert Nirschl, M.D., who operates a sports medicine clinic in Arlington, Virginia. "They irritate the skin, which diverts the attention of the pain nerves." But as far as simulating an ice pack, Dr. Nirschl says it ain't so. "Unless there's a significant change in temperature, it's highly unlikely that menthol and camphor could duplicate the therapeutic benefits of ice." So keep your cold pack. And if you'd like a distraction from your pain, stick with your trusty tube of Ben-Gay.

Sunscreen Study

 News reports on the "sunscreen-doesn't-work" study only skimmed the surface. To recap, Marianne Berwick, Ph.D., an epidemiologist at Memorial Sloan-Kettering Cancer Center in New York City, found no connection between the occurrence of cancer in 1,200 subjects and the subjects' memories of how often they used sunscreen or if they had ever been sunburned. Combining these data with other short-term studies, she concluded that sunscreen's benefit hadn't yet been scientifically proven. The media simplified this, declaring that using sunscreen is a waste of time.

That's bunk. "A number of studies show that sunscreens protect against a variety of skin cancers," says Roger Ceilley, M.D., president of the American Academy of Dermatology in Schaumburg, Illinois. Some skin cancers can take decades to develop, and strong sunscreens with sun protection factors (SPF) of 15 and higher have only been available for about 10 years. Researchers have no long-term data on sunscreen's effect against melanoma—though the disease seems to be declining in Hawaii, where sunscreen has been used regularly for a long time. One thing's certain, says Dr. Ceilley: Ultraviolet radiation triggers cancer-causing damage in cells; sunscreen can help prevent that.

"I think we'd see a lot more melanoma without sunscreen," warns Richard Essner, M.D., a cancer specialist at the John Wayne Cancer Institute in Santa Monica, California. Don't test his theory. Wear SPF 15 or higher sunblock, limit your fry time, and cover up.

Baldness Treatments

 Surf the Internet or watch late-night TV and you'll find them: quick-fix "cures" for hair loss. Infomercials bombard you with cagey before-and-after photos of men who grew hair with secret-formula $50 shampoos. Regular guys show their thatch, then earnestly touch their chests and say, "Hey, man, I was skeptical too. . . ."

Common sense tells us that most of these ads are B.S., but wishful thinking skews our judgment. Men dump an estimated $1.2 billion a year into hair-loss remedies—at least $100 million of that going toward unproven treatments, everything from vitamin pills to special shampoos. And what results did these guys get? Mainly disappointment and a growing resentment toward their Chia Pets.

Not that there isn't hope. Finasteride, which Merck is marketing as Propecia, an oral, low-dose version of the prostate drug Proscar, has joined minoxidil (Rogaine) as the second hair-loss drug approved by Food and Drug Administration (FDA). But no other product has been clinically shown to raise a single strand.

So why do thousands of men type their credit card numbers into schlocky Web sites, then anxiously await delivery of $69.95 bottles of "hair-growing" shampoo?

Blame it on *The X-Files*. Too many guys are willing to believe that the FDA is involved in a baldness plot, covering up a treatment that's growing baskets of hair somewhere else on the planet. That's why so many advertisements cite "breakthroughs" from exotic places. For example, the Web site for a product called Stop-Loss touts the product as a "Chinese herbal hair-loss treatment that has proven successful in thousands of cases in China and other countries of the world." A month's supply of capsules (taken before each meal) and a once-a-day lotion costs $180. What's in it? The ad says only that "the herbs come from a secret remedy of the Qing Dynasty Imperial doctors."

The FDA probably doesn't know what's in Stop-Loss either. The agency says it has more important concerns than deciding whether dried weeds from the Orient will grow hair. "If something that's called a baldness cure is hurting or killing people, we'll take action," explains Don McLearn, the FDA's deputy associate commissioner for public affairs. "We just don't have the resources to go after everyone." That may explain why a marketer can get away with pretty much anything, as long as the product is harmless.

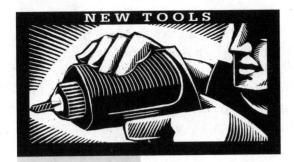

NEW TOOLS

An End to Needles

Microspheres

Hypodermic injections of drugs aren't just painful; they have to be carefully timed and administered. Ask anyone with diabetes. But soon, oral medications containing microscopic plastic beads may offer an alternative to injections. Researchers at Brown University in Providence, Rhode Island, can encapsulate drugs in tiny "microspheres" that pass right through the digestive tract into the bloodstream. The drugs can be absorbed as quickly as injections, says researcher Edith Mathiowitz, Ph.D. Microspheres, which may also deliver time-release drugs, may ultimately be used for vaccines, cancer drugs, and gene therapy.

Drink to Your Health

Echinacea Tubes

The herb echinacea can fight colds and flu when taken at first sniffle. But for the most benefit, try a liquid shot. "Liquids can be absorbed more quickly than tablets since your body doesn't have to dissolve them," says Elson Haas, M.D., director of the Preventive Medical Center of Marin in San Rafael, California. Nature's Solutions says its echinacea tubes are available in many drugstores for $10 to $12 per pack of 12. Not cheap, but each 3.5-ounce tube delivers 1,000 milligrams of echinacea, twice the amount found in many tablets.

Seeing More Clearly

Corneal-Ring Implants

For men tired of foggy lenses, the only alternatives have been contact lenses, laser surgery, or radial keratotomy. But now, physicians can correct nearsightedness by implanting a tiny plastic ring into the cornea. The 0.3-millimeter transparent polymer ring alters the curve of the eye to help it focus. "Two-thirds of patients achieve 20/20 vision, which is comparable to results from laser surgery," says George O. Waring III, M.D., professor of ophthalmology at Emory University School of Medicine in Atlanta. But unlike other procedures, corneal-ring implants are completely reversible. The surgery takes about 20 minutes and costs $2,000 per eye, compared with about $900 to $1,400 per eye for radial keratotomy.

Angina Relief

Enhanced External Counterpulsation

Angina—severe chest pain caused by poor blood flow in the heart—usually requires a surgical fix. But physicians have begun treating angina by inflating a series of cuffs on a patient's lower body, to open clogged passageways in the heart. In a study at Columbia-Presbyterian Medical Center in New York City, 71 subjects who underwent 35 one-hour sessions of "Enhanced External Counterpulsation" (EECP) for up to seven weeks cut their incidence of angina in half.

"This treatment may help expand the blood vessels around the heart," says study leader Rohit Arora, M.D. "It's also noninvasive, and the benefits last up to three years." EECP is available at 30 treatment centers in the United States.

Prostate Help without Side Effects

Flomax

Popular drugs prescribed to treat enlarged prostates were originally used to ease hypertension, so they often cause a drop in blood pressure. This can be an unwelcome side effect for men who have normal blood pressure or who are taking other hypertension medications, says Stephen N. Rous, M.D., professor of urology at the Dartmouth Medical School in Lebanon, New Hampshire. Fortunately, a newly approved drug can treat enlarged prostates without lowering blood pressure. The drug, Flomax (tamsulosin), may well be the best alternative for men who have benign prostatic hyperplasia (BPH) but who are taking other medications that lower blood pressure, says Dr. Rous.

Relief for Knee Pain

Synvisc

Sufferers of osteoarthritis, a painful joint disease, don't always find relief through therapy and traditional painkillers, such as acetaminophen. But a synthetic fluid injection seems to relieve osteoarthritic pain—without the side effects common to current treatments. Synvisc, recently approved by the Food and Drug Administration, works by replacing a natural lubricating fluid in the knee that is damaged through osteoarthritis, says Doyt Conn, M.D., senior vice president of medical affairs at the Atlanta-based Arthritis Foundation.

A study of 102 patients at the University of Calgary in Alberta showed that Synvisc relieved pain as well as standard treatments. A treatment course of three injections may protect the joint for more than eight months—just the length of a professional basketball season.

Kick the Habit for Good

Nicotine Inhalers

Still trying to quit smoking? Consider taking your medicine by inhaling it in a mist. According to one study, nicotine inhalers are just as effective as other smoking remedies, with fewer side effects. Swedish researchers followed 247 smokers as they tried to quit. After a year, those using nicotine inhalers were about 30 percent more likely to have quit than those with dummy inhalers. Side effects were minimal, researchers say, compared with such products as nicotine gums, patches, and sprays, all of which may cause irritation.

Say Farewell to Snoring

Radio Waves

If your snoring regularly lands you on the couch, listen to this: A new technique employs radio waves to treat snoring. The outpatient procedure, which takes about 20 minutes, uses radio-frequency energy to selectively destroy cells and shrink excess tissue around the palate, explains Nelson Powell, M.D., co-director of the Stanford Sleep Disorders and Research Center. "It's practically pain-free," he says. Twenty-two patients reported at least a 70 percent improvement after three to five treatments, says Dr. Powell.

Faster Recovery from Sprains

Prednisone

Doctors routinely use ibuprofen to treat ankle sprains, the most common sports-related injury. But for a speedier recovery from sprains, ask your doctor about the steroid prednisone. In a four-week study, one group of patients took prednisone—a prescription anti-inflammatory—for the first 4 days after a sprain, followed by ibuprofen for 24 days. A second group took only ibuprofen. "Difficulty walking on the injured ankle was consistently lower in the prednisone group," says Kim Edward LeBlanc, M.D., a family practice sports medicine physician in Breaux Bridge, Louisiana.

More Potent Migraine Cure

Imitrex Statdose System

Migraine victims, take note: A new self-injector gives sufferers a backup even when oral medication doesn't do the trick. The Imitrex Statdose System comes with two single-dose syringes. "With an injection, the medication gets into your system a lot quicker, and at higher concentrations," says Egilius Spierings, M.D., a neurologist and headache specialist in Wellesley Hills, Massachusetts. But relief doesn't come cheap. The prescription-only Statdose system costs about $35; oral Imitrex, about $10 per tablet.

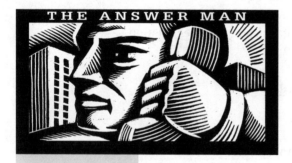

THE ANSWER MAN

Sick of the Car

Ever since I was a kid, I've suffered from motion sickness whenever I'm a passenger in a car or bus. I've taken over-the-counter medicines, but they make me drowsy. Are there any better cures?
—A. E., Laramie, Wyo.

See a doctor first. Motion sickness can be a symptom of vision problems or undiagnosed migraines, says Horst Konrad, M.D., chairman of otolaryngology at Southern Illinois University School of Medicine in Springfield. If what you have is a simple case of ride 'n' puke, be the designated driver. "Driving helps because steering and shifting gears connect you with the road," says Dr. Konrad. If that's not possible, at least sit in the front seat, and eat lightly before traveling. An acupressure wristband (also called a Sea-Band) may also help reduce nausea, although some doctors say the bands may not work on everyone.

If none of this helps, new prescription antihistamines like Allegra (fexofenadine) can minimize symptoms without drowsiness. (Antihistamines reduce oversensitivity to motion.)

A behind-the-ear patch containing the prescription medication scopalamine can also help.

Sore about Cankers

Every month, like clockwork, I get canker sores in my mouth—usually in groups of two or three, and they normally take a week to run their course. What causes them? How can I prevent them or at least get rid of them faster? —H. K., Jacksonville, Fla.

No one really knows why certain people get canker sores. It could be stress, an amino acid imbalance, or even a diet with too many acidic foods, says Cherilyn Sheets, D.D.S., clinical professor of restorative dentistry at the University of Southern California in Los Angeles. But there are ways to make sores go away faster—and relieve pain in the meantime.

- Rinse your mouth with salt water a few times a day. Mix a teaspoon of salt in an eight-ounce glass of lukewarm water, swish it around in your mouth, and spit. This may sting, but it speeds up the healing process.
- Stay away from spicy and acidic foods, such as orange juice, tomato sauce, and grapefruit. Not only do they hurt when you already have a canker sore but also they can cause a canker sore breakout, says Dr. Sheets.
- Try lysine tablets. A small study found that people who took two 500-milligram lysine tablets every six hours had their canker sores clear up 50 percent faster than those who didn't take the supplements.
- Go the prescription route. If your canker sores are particularly bad, ask your dentist to prescribe a dental paste called Kenalog (triamcinolone acetonide), says Dr. Sheets. It contains an antibiotic that helps sores heal faster.

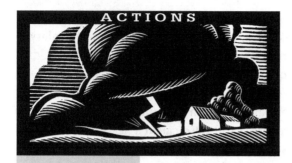

Want to get rid of some persistent hiccups? Need some hangover relief but can't take aspirin? Cures for these problems won't get front-page attention, but they would come as a relief to many men. This is why we offer these 16 tips to cure some common, and not so common, problems that afflict men.

1. Kick out her cat. If you develop asthma later in life, you may want to consider being tested for allergies. According to a recent study at Brigham and Women's Hospital in Boston, men with asthma are six times more likely to be allergic to cats, compared with non-asthmatics. Researchers say that their findings defy the long-held belief that older people aren't likely to suffer from allergy-induced asthma, and that doctors may be overlooking allergens as a cause of worsening asthma symptoms.

2. Use caution the morning after. If you can't take aspirin, choose your hangover aids carefully. Over-the-counter heartburn and indigestion remedies may make hangovers worse, says Stuart Lewis, M.D., assistant professor of clinical medicine at New York University in New York City. Such products (Alka-Seltzer Original, for example) may be hidden sources of aspirin, Dr. Lewis says, which can contribute to problems such as nausea and ulcers in certain people. "And when mixed with alcohol, aspirin can damage the stomach," says Dr. Lewis.

3. Avoid close calls. Researchers say that cell phones kept near the chest can interfere with cardiac pacemakers. "The phone's electrical signals confuse the pacemaker," says David L. Hayes, M.D., professor of medicine at the Mayo Clinic in Rochester, Minnesota. When researchers placed cell phones on maximum power over the chests of 980 pacemaker patients, they found interference 20 percent of the time (holding the phone to the ear was safe). Digital phones were nearly 10 times more likely to cause problems than analog phones.

4. Listen to lullabyes. If you suffer from insomnia, maybe you should flip on the classical station at night. In a recent study of 25 patients who reported trouble sleeping, researchers found that music by Baroque artists such as Bach and Handel helped nearly all of them fall asleep. New Age music (ask the guy with the nose ring in Sam Goody) did the trick as well. "This type of music accommodates your body rhythms and slows your heart rate," says study leader Gail C. Mornhinweg, Ph.D., associate professor of nursing at the University of Louisville. So that explains why we slept through that required music class in college.

5. **Patch a painful gut.** Even nonsmokers might benefit from nicotine patches. Researchers at the Mayo Clinic in Rochester, Minnesota, found that wearing a nicotine patch can reduce the symptoms of ulcerative colitis, a painful inflammation of the colon. In the study, 39 percent of colitis patients who wore nicotine patches improved within one month, compared to only 9 percent of a group who wore dummy patches. Nicotine seems to reduce inflammation, says William J. Sandborn, M.D., associate practice chairman in the division of gastroenterology and hepatology at the clinic.

6. **When you take ibuprofen for a headache, chase it with coffee.** According to research at the Diamond Headache Clinic in Chicago, taking caffeine and ibuprofen relieves headaches more effectively than ibuprofen alone. Among 400 headache patients, 71 percent of those who took ibuprofen and the caffeine equivalent of two cups of coffee reported complete relief, compared to 58 percent of those who took either ibuprofen or caffeine. "This combination should also relieve backaches and other muscle pain," says Seymour Diamond, M.D., director of the clinic.

7. **Don't bare your sole.** Plantar fasciitis, a rip or tear in the ligament connecting your heel to the ball of your foot—usually heals naturally in about a month. But walking even a few steps in bare feet can rupture healing tissue and prolong plantar fasciitis. Keep a pair of slip-on shoes by your bed, advises Kurt Jepson, a physical therapist from Saco, Maine. A sole limits the motion of your foot so you don't overstretch the plantar fascia ligament. "Otherwise, you may have to start the healing process again," says Jepson.

8. **Watch your eyesight.** A blow from an elbow or a basketball can give you a dull pain in your eye. Often it's not serious, but if you have blurry vision, light sensitivity, and redness, see an optometrist (or your doctor) immediately. These could signal anterior uveitis, an inflammation of the iris that can cause vision problems if not treated quickly, says John Downey, O.D., of Indiana University School of Optometry in Bloomington. An optometrist can treat the condition with anti-inflammation eyedrops, says Dr. Downey. Recovery takes about a week.

9. **Get thee to an infirmary.** If you feel a persistent, uncomfortable pressure in your chest, don't waste time blaming those burritos. Head to the emergency room. A study of 2,404 heart attack patients showed that 40 percent waited more than six hours before going to the hospital. That's too long, says Jerry H. Gurwitz, M.D., associate professor of medicine at the University of Massachusetts Medical School in Worcester. "The longer you take to seek treatment, the more heart muscle you'll lose," warns Dr. Gurwitz. "Many people simply arrive at the emergency room too late."

10. **Don't pill yourself.** If you have a persistent sore throat, see a doctor. Quick treatment could head off a nasty case of strep throat. But if your doctor doesn't think you need antibiotics, don't demand them. A study in the *British Medical Journal* found that aside from a placebo effect, antibiotics do very little to help most sore throats. More than 700 patients with sore throats were divided into groups; some received antibiotics and others didn't. The untreated healed as quickly as those who took medication. Worse, researchers warn that taking antibiotics too often can lead to "smart" bacteria that are more resilient. So lay off germ-killing drugs until they'll do some good.

11. **Ask for an ultrasound.** If you have persistent ankle pain but x-rays show nothing, request an ultrasound test. Some forms of ankle sprains can be detected only by ultrasound. "X-rays reveal only bone damage, but with ultrasound we can see what's going on in soft tissue as the patient moves his foot," says Marnix van Holsbeeck, M.D., director of musculoskeletal radiology at Henry Ford Hospital in Detroit. These hidden sprains usually hurt when a runner pushes off, says Dr. van Holsbeeck, who has used ultrasound to diagnose similar damage in Detroit Lions football players.

12. **Don't get stuck on gum.** A recent study has determined that chewing nicotine gum for a prolonged period can increase your risk of diabetes and heart disease. Twenty ex-smokers who chewed nicotine gum for a year or more had elevated levels of insulin and greater resistance to insulin, conditions that can cause Type II (adult-onset) diabetes or cardiovascular disease. Go ahead and use the gum, says Bjorn Eliasson, M.D., at the Lundberg Laboratory for Diabetes Research in Göteborg, Sweden. Just follow directions: Chew a full dose for two to three months, a lower dose for two to three more; then switch to sugarless gum.

13. **Block UV rays with zinc.** Against your better judgment, you played hoops (the skins team, naturally) at high noon without sunblock. That doesn't mean you have to suffer. Applying zinc to your skin after sun exposure may lessen sunburn. In an Australian study, hairless mice swabbed with zinc an hour after exposure to ultraviolet rays developed fewer sunburned cells. "Zinc absorbs ultraviolet energy," explains John F. Romano, M.D., a dermatologist at New York

Hospital–Cornell Medical Center in New York City and *Men's Health* magazine advisor. While a quick postburn smear will help, it's smarter to apply sunblock before venturing outside.

14. **Make a clean sweep of dandruff.** When you find flakes, don't think a dandruff shampoo will magically fix the problem. Fighting dandruff is mostly a matter of keeping the scalp moist, says Steven Greenbaum, M.D., chief of dermatology surgery at Jefferson Medical College of Thomas Jefferson University in Philadelphia. Here are his tips.

- Go easy on the dandruff shampoo. Steady use can dry your scalp and cause more flakes. Mix in a baby shampoo a few times per week.
- Buff, don't blow. Towel-drying is better for your hair.
- Relax. Stress can make you flaky. If you're a Wall Street type, relaxation exercises might keep your personal forecast free of snow.

15. **Get back in business.** Lower-back pain is a common complaint and can come from anywhere: lifting, twisting, bending, driving, slouching, stepping in a hole. Try ice and an anti-inflammatory such as Aleve. Try this exercise as well: Lie on your back and bring one knee to your chest. If it doesn't hurt too much, slowly rotate to the opposite side. Repeat with the other knee, going to the opposite side.

16. **Say, "Hic, hic, hooray."** Even doctors don't know what triggers hiccups—spasms of the diaphragm that cause sudden intakes of air. Stimulating the back of the throat may disrupt the firing of the phrenic nerves, which regulate the diaphragm's contractions, says hiccups maven Nancy Kemp, M.D., of Sonoma State University in Rohnert Park, California. Use a spoon to lift the uvula—the thing that hangs down like a punching bag, she suggests. Or, try pulling your tongue, drinking a glass of water rapidly, or swallowing dry bread. Hiccups almost always disappear within an hour or two. If they persist longer than two days, see a doctor; chronic hiccups can signify a serious medical condition.

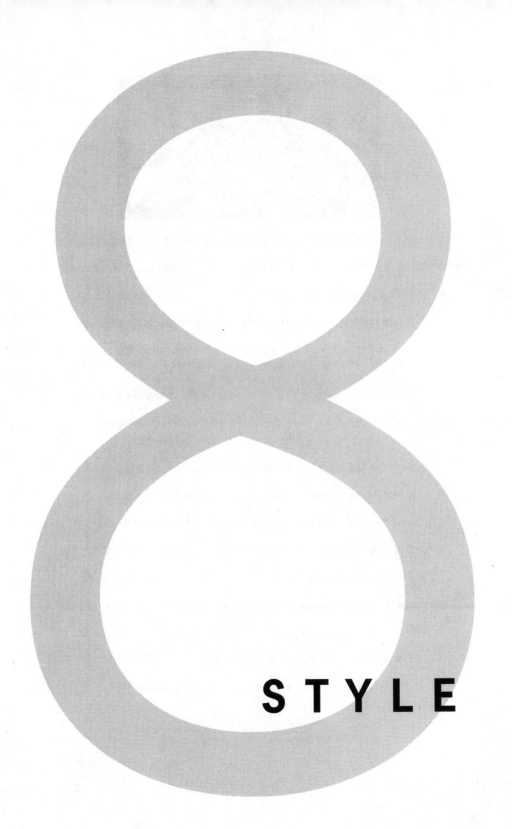

8
STYLE

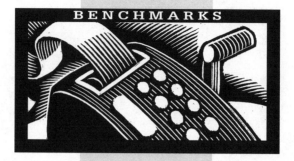

■ Percentage of men who don't use deodorant in the morning: 16

■ Percentage of Americans who believe rudeness is a critical problem in our nation: 77

■ Percentage of baby-boomer men who are concerned about facial wrinkles: 44

■ Age a man first notices that his hair is turning gray: 39

■ Percentage of men who would rather end casual day
and go back to suits full-time: 48

■ Length of time Americans 18 to 24 spend in the shower: 16.4 minutes

■ Average number of people killed each year before hair dryers
were designed to shut off when submerged in water: 17

■ Average number of articles of clothing an American male buys annually: 35

■ Percentage of men in America who "care how their feet look": 77

■ Percentage of male farmers in Iowa who own bib overalls: 41

■ Percentage of Ford Explorer owners who have never driven them off-road: 87

■ Percentage of married Americans who bathe or shower together: 63

■ Average number of injuries caused by clothing in America each year: 112,000

■ Price in dollars of a wallet crafted with platinum and diamonds: 84,000

■ Number of American men who had facelifts in 1997: 5,067

■ Average number of square inches that men shave: 48

VITAL READING

The Basics of Matchmaking

Follow these simple rules to look your best.

One day a few months back, while a few of us were playing kick-the-intern-down-the-hall, a smartly dressed managerial sort stepped in to put an end to our fun. It wasn't our recreational practices he had a beef with; it was the way we were dressed. Seems he was upset by our combination of sweatpants and cashmere sweaters. So we kicked him—but not before realizing that the guy had a point. We've seemingly bought all the right clothes, but sometimes we have a hard time matching them up. It's probably the same for you—all those stripes, all those patterns, all those shoes—why, a man could go plumb loco trying to keep them all straight. That's why we came up with 10 simple rules for making sure your clothes look like they belong together on you and not separate on three other people. These rules aren't going to put you on the cutting edge, but they can prevent you from looking like a fugitive from the circus.

Rule #1: Keep it simple. In this case, simple means solid. "People spend so much time worrying about how to put together patterns that it's amazing they overlook the simple solutions," says Alan Flusser, a New York men's fashion designer and author of *Style and the Man.* "Consider this," he says. "What is the one thing that every man looks good in, no matter what he looks like? A tuxedo. And it's only two solid colors, black and white." The point is that as long as your clothes are properly fitted and your tie is properly proportioned and knotted, you can be stylish wearing solid colors with one pattern mixed in. "If you're going with a gray suit and blue shirt, wear a tie that picks up the blue and the gray," says Flusser. "Simplistic? Yes, but you won't get in trouble."

Rule #2: Large tie patterns go with close stripes. The farther apart the stripes, the tighter the tie pattern. The mixing of stripes and other patterns is not such a daunting endeavor that you shouldn't consider it, says Warren Christopher, *Men's Health* magazine clothing and grooming editor. Just remember to keep it simple. For example, when you're matching a suit, shirt, and tie, stick to two patterns (one stripe, one nonstripe) maximum. While it's true that the more sophisticated your sense of style, the more you can get away with, you gotta walk before you run, man. So . . .

- If you want to wear a striped suit, wear a solid shirt.
- If you want to wear a striped shirt, wear a solid suit.

Okay, now you need to pick out a tie. Here's where most guys screw up.

- If the stripes on your suit or shirt are close together, go for a large pattern in the tie. A tightly patterned tie would fight for attention with the stripes.
- If the stripes on your suit or shirt have some breathing room between them, go for a tie with a small, tight pattern.

Rule #3: Solid shirts go with checked suits. "The least perilous way to stylishly wear a checked suit is to wear a solid shirt and a striped tie that matches the colors of the suit," says Flusser. "Let's use a black-and-gray checked suit, for example. Wear a crisp white shirt and a black-and-gray striped tie, and you're set."

Rule #4: Your tie should be darker than your shirt. Unless you're a hit man or a boxing promoter, your tie should almost always be darker than your shirt. "The darker the tie, the dressier it is," says Flusser. "It's the shirt's job to offer contrast from the darker suit." So let your shirt do its job.

Rule #5: Your shoes and belt should match in color and material. "You can never go wrong with this approach," says Adam Derrick, designer for To Boot New York by Adam Derrick. "It's a no-brainer." Black leather shoes, black leather belt. Brown suede shoes, brown suede belt. Fluorescent-red clown shoes, fluorescent-red water-squirting clown belt. Simple, right?

Rule #6: Your socks should match your pants more than your shoes. Fred Astaire always wore brightly colored socks when he was dancing because it drew attention to his feet. "You don't want to draw attention to your feet," says Derrick, "so the pant leg and the sock should form a line of color leading to the shoe."

Rule #7: If you're wearing a suit, bring along the right shoes. According to Derrick, if you're wearing a classic suit or serious pants and blazer combo (gray pants, blue jacket), it should be worn with a classic lace-up shoe.

Rule #8: Concentrate on the shirt if you want to go sporty. If you like the sporty, no-tie look for Friday at the office or cocktails on your yacht, start first with the shirt. "For the most simple color arrangement, go with a shirt that has two colors," says Flusser. "Let's say you start with a shirt that's a medium blue and tan combination. You could go with solid khakis to work the tan in the shirt and a navy sweater or jacket to pick up the blue."

Rule #9: Patterned sport jackets require two solids. If on that sporty, no-tie day you reach into the closet and pull out a patterned jacket, keep the rest simple. Wear a solid-color shirt that matches the lighter color in the pattern, and solid pants that relate to the darker color.

Rule #10: Beware of the seasons. Let's say you love the feel of linen pants and, while you're getting dressed to go to the office Christmas party, you think it would be really groovy if you wore your white linen pants with your favorite sweater. You have two options: Forget about it or stay home. "The lines of when you can wear certain items have become more blurred over the years," says New York–based designer Sal Cesarani. "However, there are still a few rules you should heed."

Here's a list of things that you should wear only between Memorial Day and Labor Day: linen and linen/rayon blend pants and jackets; white wool or tropical summer-weight wool; silk (or silk/rayon blend) shirts; silk jackets; seersucker pants, shirts, and jackets; madras shirts. And, if you have a fancy for white bucks, put them in the closet come Labor Day as well.

Note: If you find yourself poolside in the Caribbean, chatting up some island girl and sipping banana daiquiris, the above advice does not apply. Indeed, if that sounds like your life, maybe you should be the one giving us advice.

Select with Confidence

End the anxiety caused by ordering wine.

For the majority of guys, wine is like sex: We've been sampling it for years, and deriving tremendous pleasure from it, but we still do not come close to understanding all of its complexities. Although the fundamentals of both are simple, the accompanying stigmas are frequently the cause of great angst.

Here are a few tips that should help demystify the world of wine.

Go with what you like. Connoisseurs become so wrapped up in wine's complexities that they overlook regular wines that regular people like. When you hit something that tastes good, note the name of the winery and the variety. Wines least likely to annoy others: pinot noir (red) and chardonnay (white).

Consult others. Next time you're in a good restaurant, ask about the house wine. These wines are usually selected for their good value, broad appeal, and availability. Or ask your server what he would order. Starving artists-cum-waiters always know good value.

Make it a no-brainer. Let common sense lead you to wines that are appropriate for certain foods (for example, accompany highly flavored foods with full-bodied wines that can stand up to the pungent ingredients). The following pairings are sure to please.

Food: Spicy pasta dishes or red meats
Wine: Hearty reds: Italian Chianti, Spanish rioja, French Bordeaux, or California cabernet

Food: Subtly flavored foods such as salmon or soufflés
Wine: French Beaujolais or California pinot noir

Food: Naturally rich foods (scallops or lobster), or fish or fowl prepared with lots of butter
Wine: Crisp, dry sauvignon blanc

Food: Grilled vegetables or simply prepared fish or chicken (no butter or fat)
Wine: California chardonnay

Food: Chocolate cake
Wine: Cabernet sauvignon

No need to overspend. A typical range is $5 to $7; a splurge is $12. The company, occasion, and surroundings will do more to influence your appreciation of a wine than the money you throw at it.

Feel the cork. Sniffing won't tell you anything. Instead, feel the cork to make sure it's moist (a dry cork means air may have sneaked into the bottle and ruined the wine).

Stop letting it breathe. Older red wines improve after exposure to the air for an hour or two. But that's not necessary for your average wine, so serve it when you uncork it. The wine will naturally breathe once it's poured into a glass. If you drink it slowly, you may notice subtle changes in the characteristics of each glass as it "opens up." Being conscious of these nuances is your first step on your road to wine appreciation.

Take it easy. The French, who wrote the book on wine, accompany most of their meals with a *vin de table*, a cheap table wine blended from the winery's leftovers. That should say it all.

Wine is meant to accompany foods, but a wine and cheese party can turn into a calories and fat party. If you want to impress your date with a sophisticated first course, skip the Limburger and try something just as easy.

This foolproof tapenade (a fancy spread for bread) is perfect to serve anytime with a glass of Italian Chianti or any other hearty red wine.

Olive Tapenade
6 servings

2	cups (about 20) black Kalamata olives, pitted (available at most Middle Eastern delis)
2	teaspoons olive oil
1	clove garlic, minced
1	cup Italian parsley (no stems)
¼	cup fresh rosemary (no stems)
1	orange rind (slice off the outer portion of the orange peel with a sharp knife)
1	teaspoon freshly ground black pepper
1	skinny sourdough baguette, sliced and toasted

1. Place olives, oil, garlic, parsley, rosemary, orange rind, and pepper in a food processor. Puree.

2. Spread on toast.

Two-slice serving: 198 calories, 6 grams fat, 27 percent calories from fat

The Ins and Outs of Wool

Clothe yourself in quality pants for cold weather.

There is something particularly grown-up about a pair of wool pants—a subtle announcement that there is a section in your fashion lexicon between sweatpants and suits, that you are aware you can't go everywhere in jeans (unless you're Bruce Springsteen).

The classic wool trouser—think gray flannel—can be paired with a quality blazer and tie for dinner with your family, dinner with her family, or the odd court appearance. More rugged wool pants go to football games or away for the weekend, paired with a denim shirt and a fisherman's sweater. A quality pair can last for years—assuming that you know how to spot quality. To get that natty look, consider these fine points.

Fabric

Wool pants range from heavy to light in weight, fine to coarse in weave—the lighter, thinner fabrics being dressier.

Covert wool is a sturdy, heavier wool fabric that is casual and is seen in more casual colors such as brown or medium gray.

Flannel you've met before. It's a brushed wool, more loosely woven than a gabardine, with a napped (slightly fuzzy) surface, which may be blended with cotton or rayon.

Gabardine is one of the dressiest types of wool, a worsted fabric with a subtle twill (or rib) to the cloth.

Tropical wool is known for its light weight: "It's a plain weave fabric, ideal for warm weather" says Judith Pinder of the Wool Bureau in New York City.

Super 100s is made from Merino wool fibers, spun into an extra-fine yarn. "It's the most luxurious wool," explains Pinder, "and feels great next to the skin."

Wool crepe is a lightweight fabric often blended with polyester, rayon, or Lycra for durability and less wrinkling. "Any blended wool is great for traveling because it packs really well," says Warren Christopher, *Men's Health* magazine clothing and grooming editor.

Cut

Certain cuts can help you appear thinner and taller.

Inseam is the measurement from crotch to cuff. Your pants should be long enough for a subtle break, not a massive pooling of fabric at your shoe tops. And we know you're proud of how your socks match your tie, but if your socks show when you walk, your pants are too short.

Rise refers to the amount of fabric between the crotch and the waistband. Tall, thin bodies are well-matched to a low rise since they can carry off this lower-on-the-hip style. If you're shorter than average, avoid pants with a low rise—it will invite comparison to a penguin.

Pleats

If you're on the wide side, you might select a single or double pleat, both of which create the optical illusion of a slim waist. The *double pleat* is the most popular style and looks good on almost every body type. A *box pleat* is stitched like a square—not the best choice if you wish to deflect curious onlookers from that accident you call your midsection. The *reverse pleat*, usually seen as a double pleat, shows the tuck sewn toward the pocket rather than toward the fly. An *inverted pleat*, an upside-down pleat, is a sophisticated, V-shaped fold favored by high-end designers, such as Armani. *Flat-front*, with no pleats, is less common, partly because it can make your hips look wide and draw attention to your waist.

Cuff, Lining, Details

Manufacturers of quality wool pants observe a few niceties that you may want to keep an eye out for.

Constructed waistband. This refers to a slightly stiff waistband formed by a sturdy piece of canvas sewn between the outer wool and the cotton-lined waistband. (You'll be able to feel it—it keeps the shape of the waist intact.)

Cotton pockets. She'll appreciate it when she reaches in. For your wallet.

Crotchpiece. This vital piece of cloth (not to be confused with the lining) is sewn between the fly and the seat of the pants to prevent chafing, says Christopher. Obviously a must-have.

Cuffs. Dressy trousers should have them, preferably measuring from $1\frac{1}{2}$ inches to $1\frac{3}{4}$ inches in width. Yes, even short guys can wear them.

Helpful buttons. Look for suspender buttons and an inside button catch (the flap that buttons inside the pants) at the waist. "Suspenders and the inside button make the pant hang smoothly," says Christopher. "And to be honest, they hold the stomach in." Sign us up.

Lining. A lining is optional in trousers made of Merino wool, according to Pinder. A lining in silk or blended poly, reaching from the waist to the knees, will help other types of wool trousers hang more smoothly.

Care and Cleaning

Industry experts say that most men dry-clean clothes too often. To stave off premature aging (in your trousers), dry-clean them once or twice a season, and have them professionally steamed when they look rumpled. Frequent fliers might also consider purchasing a small portable steamer.

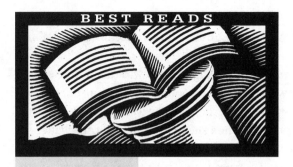

BEST READS

Buying a Suit

Just because many workplaces are moving toward a more casual dress code doesn't mean that owning a sharp, well-fitting suit is any less important. In fact, it's probably more important now since you stand out more when you do wear one. But what are the ins and outs of buying a suit? Rest easy, because in this excerpt from Paisley Goes with Nothing: A Man's Guide to Style *(Doubleday, 1995), author Hal Rubenstein lays it all out for you in the irreverent sense of humor that makes his book both educational and fun.*

You'd probably rather mow the lawn, sit through your nephew's third-grade dance recital, or have your wisdom teeth extracted with an X-Acto knife. But unless you've developed technology from an episode of *Nova* the rest of us missed, a new suit is not going to find its way into your closet unescorted. You'd love to send somebody else out to get it, wouldn't you, the same way you acquire your underwear (that only half your shorts fit correctly is merely an unfortunate coincidence). Unfortunately, you have to go out and buy it yourself. So get moving. No whining that you don't know how. Learn. There's a new world out there. Try dressing as if you're part of it.

1. Rather than embarking on your usual aimless search for the usual Harris-tweed grail, before you start wandering through the racks, decide what you are buying a suit for.

- Business travel? Then the estimable qualities are weightlessness and the ability to lose wrinkles by simply being hung for 10 minutes in a steamy bathroom. (Forget about the suit. Wouldn't you like to shake out that way?)
- Year-round usage? Remember that corduroy tends to retain beach sand.
- Determined to look more together on vacation than your kids think possible? Now, we're talking an unconstructed jacket with at least three buttons, and maybe a floppy pant leg that complements a sandal.

Knowing a suit's purpose in your wardrobe will narrow your field of vision and perhaps shorten your reenactment of the Diaspora in the men's department.

2. The more specific you can be about fabric, the better. This doesn't mean you have to know the percentage of wool to silk in a blend. Common knowledge and common sense will do for openers. Traveling while on business? Then linen is out. Find low maintenance appealing? Then linen is out. Want your money's worth with a year-round garment? Then linen is out.

What you do need to know is that many wool blends dewrinkle quickly, wool crepe being the quickest and the most comfortable. Cotton weighs nothing. Corduroy makes your butt look bigger. Polyester, born again as microfiber, but with the Sybilline capacity to adopt personalities as varied as viscose and ramie, is now pliable, resilient, occasionally luxurious, no longer the flag bearer of cheesiness. Wash and wear, however, looks and remains as cheesy as it sounds.

Note: Linen is for remaining totally cool while looking fabulously careless. However, you can sustain the effect over long periods only if you never sit down. In fact, avoid leaning, reaching, and turning too quickly. Better yet, find a convenient wall, with flattering lighting, and don't move.

3. You don't know what wool crepe or viscose is, do you? Don't worry. It's amazing how many guys reading this don't know what linen is. Nevertheless, whether you're swatch savvy or find even rudimentary classifications as cryptic as dialogue in a Frank Herbert novel, you must locate two things prior to shopping for a suit.

- At least one men's store that doesn't make you feel as if you're being judged as to whether or not you're worthy of its time.
- A salesperson in that store who likes his mission, does his homework, and most of all, listens. A savvy salesperson is the most desirable accomplice to have in tow, far more valuable than being accompanied by a male friend, which practically ensures purchasing either nothing or a duplicate of something you already own; or by a female one, which guarantees your dressing the way she sees you and permanently quashes any attempts at indulging in secret sartorial daydreams for fear of looking foolish in her eyes. As for blood relations, shop with them when you're looking for a burial plot.

Try as hard as you can to go shopping alone. Tell the others and yourself that you're going out for the paper, and just keep walking. If you're one of those fearful of being sold a bill of no-goods, how come you've no trouble tuning out an overly effusive car salesman's blasting pitch, heading off a steamrolling real estate agent, or disbelieving "Robbie," your waiter for the evening, when he perkily proclaims, "Everything is good!"? Regardless of your expertise in a particular field, a snow job always sounds like a snow job. Relax, and pay attention. You'll know when you're learning something.

4. What do you want to spend? Good-looking suits can be found at all prices, but expect to pay at least $500 retail for a suit that flatters you and offers enough quality to provide a full-day's-wearing level of comfort. The technology is such that it has become difficult to find a badly constructed suit. In fact, there are now machines used in the manufacture of "hand-tailored" suits that are actually programmed to drop stitches. But constructed well and fitting well are not synonymous. Consequently, before you put up your price ceiling, even if you have no intention of parting with this much of your paycheck, try on an expensive suit, especially if you have never done so, if only to provide you with a frame of reference as to what a suit should do for you, what it can look like on you, and what you ought to feel like in it. It's why a struggling law student test-drives a Porsche. It's the reason we have museums. You can't devise standards unless you know the range of possibilities. Is a taste of honey worse than none at all? Don't blame us.

5. Great tailors—there are only a few left (the store that employs one boasts a major asset, though you won't know that for sure until after you buy at least one suit)—can work magic.

There are two areas, though, where their powers are of no use. If a suit jacket does not fit in the shoulders—if it puckers, drops too low, or is too restricting— or if a jacket is too short or too long, *take it off.* If you can't find the same one in a different size, too bad. Shoulders are to a jacket what a foundation is to a house. You tinker with shutters, not with a foundation. Pockets, lining, and line complicate toying with jacket length. (Remember, once they start cutting, you own it. For what you're paying, it's not worth the risk.) Besides, tailoring should be about altering fit, not design. Imagine yourself a tall man who slides behind the wheel of a Toyota MR2, to discover the top of your head smashed against the moon roof as the salesman tells you, "Relax! Loosen up! Slouch!" Do not compromise. Do not be persuaded.

6. There is one less-than-obvious technical element you should be aware of— the difference between a fused and an unfused jacket. Between the fabric and the lining of the lapel, the shoulders, and the chest pieces is a layer of reinforcement. The engineering of this middle layer is an essential factor in determining price. Expensive garments utilize the insertion of one or more plies of either horsehair or regular canvas. There is not a machine yet made that can insert and secure this middle layer. An unfused jacket is always done by hand. More labor, more money. But because the horsehair or canvas remains free-floating, suspended by hand-stitching, it allows for more drape in the body, a soft roll to the lapel, more pliancy in movement.

The alternative process is called fusing, whereby a synthetic mesh canvas, treated with an adhesive, is permanently attached to the outer fabric by heat. When first developed in the 1950s, fusing approximated the it-wears-you military appeal of Michael Rennie's immobilizing spacesuit in *The Day the Earth Stood Still*. Since then, life has gotten tougher, but fusing has gotten easier. Any suit lapel that exhibits a flat, no-nonsense appearance has been fused, but the graceful roll of a featherweight wool Dolce and Gabbana suit is also made possible by advances in fusing.

The hidden drawback to fusing is lurking not within, but without, the garment: poor-quality dry cleaners. Excessive heat or harsh chemicals can cause puckering and shrinkage. Either find yourself a good dry cleaner or make up the name of an obscure Belgian designer and tell friends you're wearing him exclusively.

7. If any garment in menswear could sing out, "I'm just a suit whose intentions are good. Oh, Lord, please don't let me be misunderstood," it would be the unconstructed jacket, or "This thing has no lining," as most men refer to it. Ironically, because it's designed to be weightless as a big shirt and comfortable as an old cardigan, in many ways the unconstructed jacket is the height of tailoring. It can't rely on internal stabilizing factors, canvas backing, or any traditional ways a suit is made. All interior workings are now exposed and must be finished off, requiring more labor than if hidden by a lining. The drape and shape of the coat now rest on the inherent quality of the fabric (linen will waft appealingly, wool gabardine will hang like thinly sliced meat), the skill of the designer, and the sorcery of the tailor (though you will almost always find some reinforcement in the chest and shoulders). Want to know why an unconstructed jacket costs more than the others? This is why.

8. Looking at a suit.
- You never get more than you pay for.
- There should be no puckering or no bulk where the shoulder insets to the sleeve. If there is, it will not iron or steam out. If a salesperson promises you it will, ask to see another salesperson, permanently.
- If the desired fabric is plaid or stripes, look at the way the pattern is matched at the seams, how it is handled on the lapels, at the shoulders, and especially down the center seam in the back.
- A felt backing, not a backing of matching fabric on the underside of the lapels around the neck, is what you want.
- Look at the quality of the buttons—plastic, wood, horn—and how they're sewn on. If there is thread wound round and round between fabric and button, the buttons were probably sewn on by hand.

- Is the lining of comparable quality to that of the jacket? Is it fully sewn down? Is it sewn to the fabric at any point other than the edges, compromising movement?
- Flap pockets look best on business suits.
- All pockets and buttonholes should work.
- Look at the surgeon's cuffs. (Yes, my good man, that's what the area is called where the buttons are sewn on the sleeve, derived from times past when surgeons, usually dressed as befitting their pillar-of-the-community status, had to roll up their sleeves in emergencies and "operate.") Today, these buttons are more symbolic than functional, so it's not critical if the buttons don't work; but the evenness of their spacing (they should just touch each other) and of their finishing is an indication of craftsmanship.
- Are alterations included? Never assume.

9. Looking at yourself in a suit.
- Because good-quality menswear, especially suits in the upper price range, is about nuance and subtlety, you must try all garments on. Both parts. Stop thinking of this as such a hassle. Trying on suits is not a hassle. Chemotherapy is a hassle.
- When you go into a store, wear clothes that you can get out of easily—loose pants, slip-on shoes—and furnishings that form a blank canvas for what you're buying.
- Pick a suit shape that enhances your body type. Short and heavy? A low-slung, double-breasted jacket will make you look like Sydney Greenstreet. If you insist on double-breastedness, choose a tailored, six-button silhouette. Big hips? A low, one-button closure breaks up the girth. Short jackets make your legs look longer. Center vents do not flatter ample rear ends. The three-button jacket is the best all-around shape for all body types. Short? Wear a high-button singlebreasted in monochrome. Wide? Don't even smile at plaid, corduroy, nubbies, or cuffs. Tall and thin? Have a great time. It's not a fair world.
- Make sure the store you're in has a three-way mirror. You have to see yourself the way the world does, all 360 degrees. You wouldn't get up out of the barber's chair until he shows you the back of your head, would you? Well, you shouldn't.
- The back of the jacket collar should be flush with your neck. No dead space.
- Many men now know that you should be able to move freely in a jacket, but some go too far. There's no need to flap your arms about, unless you're too late to change for a sprint against Carl Lewis. Just bend, and reach, and see if anything pulls.

- The sleeve on a jacket should reach only to the fleshy part of the thumb. Any longer does not look hip. It looks studied and dowdy or as if you were still waiting for the director of the last version of *Lost Horizon* to yell, "Cut!"
- Suit pants should fit the same way as similarly cut dress pants sold separately. They are not supposed to be fuller because a jacket is covering them. Not everything Grandpa taught was true.
- Pants are sized by waist for a reason. It's astounding how many men wear their pants riding on their hips. If you're a Deadhead, and still into your old Landlubber jeans with the five-inch zipper, you're excused. Otherwise, hike 'em up. If you insist on being contrary, at least take your pants in at the crotch so it doesn't look as if you were smuggling contraband.
- Pants should fit in the back flat across the top of the buttocks, then follow its curve about halfway. When they follow all the way, we call them jeans, and they should cost a lot less.
- Look at your butt. Everyone else will.

10. Most men dry-clean their suits too often. The surest way to kill a good suit. The quickest way to age an inexpensive one. Do not dry-clean until a suit is visibly dirty or until you can't get the smell of cigarettes—or someone else you want to forget—out.

11. Most men iron their suits too often. Inexpensive ones often show their pedigree because overironing hastens the onset of that I-can-see-myself shininess. Buy a portable steamer and steam your suits instead. It's almost idiot-proof, certainly a lot easier to operate than an iron, while increasing a garment's longevity. And a steamer always belongs in your suitcase.

12. The two parts of a suit do not come glued together. You can and should wear them separately. Mix them, top and bottom, with other elements of your wardrobe. We used to call this stretching a buck. We now call this fashion.

What to Wear at Week's End

Ah, Casual Friday. Or, if you're really lucky, Casual Week. What was so eagerly embraced as a morale booster in the late 1980s quickly turned into confusion about the standards of casual for many men. This excerpt from Maximum Style: Look Sharp and Feel Confident in Every Situation *(Rodale Press, 1997), by Perry Garfinkel and Brian Chichester, will set you straight. From head to toe, they provide solid direction for those in need of some casual help.*

Workers may love Casual Friday, but some fashion experts fear that it may signal the decline of style in the workplace.

"Thanks to Casual Friday, corporate dress has really become a problem. We've become a nation of slobs," frets fashion expert Leon Hall of New York City, who is creative director for International Apparel Mart in Dallas, spokesperson for the Fashion Association, and a frequent fashion commentator and trend forecaster. "People say that Casual Friday is a new way of dressing, but it isn't license for sloppiness and slovenliness, and that's what has happened."

While other experts aren't so emphatic—particularly casual wear manufacturers—it's clear that Casual Friday has changed the rules about what's appropriate to wear to work. And if you want to be Joe Friday, you need to understand what the new style standards are.

A Casual Acquaintance

In many offices, Casual Friday got it's sneakered foot in the door via local charities, such as the United Way and United Cerebral Palsy. These organizations in the late 1980s and early 1990s found that employees were eager to pledge money if it meant that they could dress casually at work.

Pittsburgh-based ALCOA, the world's largest aluminum manufacturer, for example, went totally casual in September 1991 following a United Way campaign. Managers permitted employees who pledged early to the United Way to dress casually for the remainder of the fund-raising campaign. Response was so overwhelming—and productivity and morale so noticeably improved—that the company made casual dress a permanent policy.

"Casual dress can have clear advantages, at virtually no cost, for most corporations and industries," says Michael R. Losey, president and chief executive officer of the Society for Human Resource Management, a professional organization in Alexandria, Virginia.

Yet, as Losey points out, Casual Friday has caused considerable consternation, too. "Just because you're dressing casually doesn't mean that there aren't standards. In many cases, the corporate casual concept has just muddied the standards," he says.

Hall says that he knows of some companies in New York City that are so fed up with conflicting definitions of casual that they've adopted Dress-Up Friday to restore some sense of fashion order.

Losey's organization, along with Levi Strauss and Company, looked into Casual Friday by surveying 505 human resource managers nationwide in 1996. They found that:

- 90 percent of the companies allowed workers to wear casual clothing at least some of the time, which was up 27 percent from 1992
- 42 percent of the companies allow casual clothing once a week; 33 percent permit it daily
- 63 percent of all companies had a written dress policy regarding casual dress

What is the bottom line for bosses? Casual dress improves morale, is perceived as an employee benefit, saves employees money, and attracts new workers, the survey says.

According to the Society for Human Resource Management/Levi Strauss and Company survey, here's what most men wear on a designated casual day at work.

- Polo shirts, short-sleeve shirts
- Casual slacks, jeans
- Leather shoes

As a general guide, that's a pretty safe standard for a dress-down day. But does that make it the official uniform for Casual Friday? Not necessarily. Here are some tips to help you make sense of the new office anarchy.

Watch the boss. What might cut it at XYZ Advertising Agency probably won't make it past the security guard at IBM. What's appropriate varies from city to city, region to region, company to company.

"Your office might be more conservative," says Hall. "The easiest thing to do is to look around and see what the bosses are wearing. If they're not wearing sneakers, neither should you."

Tee off. T-shirts most often are a no-no on casual day, so think twice, even if your company allows them. If you opt for a T-shirt, make it plain and solid-colored, perhaps with a single breast pocket. And it doesn't matter whether your musical tastes run toward Sinatra or the Sex Pistols. Save the concert T-shirts for the weekend.

Be a trailblazer. You'll never go wrong with a blazer or sport coat. They jazz up even the most casual outfits, including jeans. And if it's too dressy, you can always take it off. "Corporate casual revolves around the sport coat. Along with a coordinating shirt and trousers, it's a definite cornerstone to a corporate casual wardrobe," says Marvin Pieland, manager and clothing consultant for Saks Fifth Avenue Club for Men in New York City.

Select a shirt. Safe shirts for casual wear include collared polo shirts, solid colors or muted prints, banded-collar shirts, denim shirts, neatly pressed oxford button-downs, and stylish rugby shirts. Stick with chambray, denim, or flannel for a softer look than standard starched cotton.

Pick the right pants. You can't go wrong with dress slacks, khakis, or chinos. Even a nice pair of jeans *might* be okay, as long as they're not the kind you'd wear horseback riding and as long as they're dressed up with an oxford shirt and blazer.

Err on the side of fashion. If you're not sure what goes in your office, dress up more than you need to. "It's safer to dress up. You can always dress down, remove your jacket, roll up your sleeves, and loosen your tie. You can't go the other way," says Ken Karpinski of Sterling, Virginia, image consultant to Fortune 500 companies, the U.S. military, and numerous corporate executives, and author of *Red Socks Don't Work.*

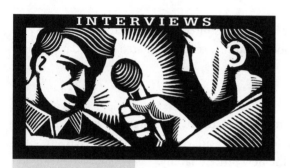

INTERVIEWS

Robert Palmer on
Dressing with Style

The son of a British naval officer, rock singer Robert Palmer learned at an early age the importance of dressing stylishly. And in a pop culture dominated by the uniform of flannel, T-shirts, and jeans, Palmer stands out as a man of impeccable style and taste. Since he launched into the pop music scene in the 1970s—and particularly since his groundbreaking music video of the early 1980s, "Addicted to Love"—Palmer has projected an image of cool sophistication. It fits him like one of his expensive Italian suits.

Dressing well and more formally than any other musician seems to come naturally to you. How did you develop your sense of style?

I grew up in Malta, a group of islands south of Sicily, and it was an international, mostly naval society. My parents used to take me out to swell evenings. They also had parties in their home, where everyone came dressed very elegantly. The people on the covers of the records they played, singers such as Billie Holiday and Nat King Cole, all dressed well, too. I never thought about not dressing well. I always recognized that some people had flair. The essence of style is to be appropriate for the situation.

How do you manage to travel around the world wearing suits?

The key is to wear trousers that don't crease. Actually, I plan ahead. I look at the week coming up and say to myself, "Well, I have shows to do in two different countries, what can I carry with me?" In general, I travel with a couple suits, a casual outfit, jacket, slacks, a few ties, and something to get there and back in.

Do you have a lot of clothes?

Yes. I usually shop in Milan, which is about an hour away from my home in Switzerland. Some of the designers there know me and what I like, so they set aside items for me. I'm very lucky, because I'm Mr. Mannequin. The samples they make for the runway are my size. I get things without a lot of markup in price.

I have a lot of white shirts. A man can't have enough white shirts. I buy them two sizes too big and then in three months they're too tight from the laundry and I throw them away.

But, you know, I also see a lot of things that are nice, but that I don't need. And if I don't need it, then I don't buy it. You should always have something in mind before you go looking.

Who are some of your favorite designers?

Most of my stuff is by Gianfranco Ferre. And you can't go wrong with Armani. The whole key is to find a designer who is thinking about your body shape and size when he's designing.

Do you wear cologne?

Yes. I wear Givenchy and Van Cleef and Arpels. Good grooming indicates self-respect. I really appreciate people who look after themselves, male or female. Of course, it has to be normal and natural, not overdone.

How important is quality?

You can really tell the difference between something that's well-made and something that isn't, especially in terms of longevity. I often have to wear something on stage that I've had on during a trans-Atlantic flight. If you've been wearing a suit for nine hours on a plane and it looks all right, then it's a well-made suit. Buying quality items is a matter of practicality.

Besides, I just really enjoy the quality of a good tailor's work, or a good cobbler's work. Sometimes I just see a good pair of shoes and go, "Whoa!"

Whose idea was it for the women in the "Addicted to Love" video to wear the same dress and makeup?

Terrance Donovan, the director's. He just told me to show up, knowing that I would arrive in a nice suit. The women in the video weren't even in the room with me when I sang. I was shot in front of a blue screen. He designed the video based on what he knows about me and my appearance. I'm not at all like that, by the way, in terms of personality. Sometimes I run the risk of being a wolf in sheep's clothing.

That's right, you really stand out in the world of rock and roll. Is that what you're aiming for?

I've just never understood the point of dressing down. I just can't think of a more comfortable alternative to trousers and a nice shirt. Music is the cult of the individual, but it's amazing how everyone wears a uniform of jeans and T-shirts. Now, everyone wears baseball caps and it's become a uniform.

So what would you do if you woke up tomorrow morning and everyone was wearing a gray suit?

I'd applaud.

David Weeks on
Eccentric People

Benjamin Franklin, Albert Einstein, Charlie Chaplin. All legendary successes. All classic eccentrics. Now, you probably won't coauthor a nation, reinvent physics, or father as many children as Chaplin, but you can still follow their examples to stay witty and virile for upward of a century. According to David Weeks, Ph.D., just a touch of eccentricity can help you cut down on stress, pump up your bank account, and even become more popular. A neuropsychologist at the Royal Edinburgh Hospital in Scotland, Dr. Weeks studied more than a thousand of the world's stranger agents during the past 12 years, and he found that eccentric people seem to have a unique formula for health and success. The coauthor of Eccentrics: A Study of Sanity and Strangeness, *he shared some of his surprising conclusions with us.*

First, what's the difference between an eccentric and a screwball?

Eccentrics are not insane, and they are not exhibitionists. They don't pay much attention to the opinions of others, good or bad, and they don't like drawing attention to themselves, though they will attempt to draw attention to their ideas. Many people whom society categorizes as weird or strange actually have a personality disorder or a psychiatric disorder. Eccentricity is neither. It's a positive, pleasant choice made by a sane person who is very aware that he is different.

What impressed you about eccentric people?

Well, they're almost entirely motivated by curiosity and intellectual stimulation. They're intelligent, creative, idealistic, and optimistic people who are happily preoccupied with a number of different hobbies and interests. And one brilliant attribute of eccentrics that I admire is that they don't see failure when it occurs—they simply race back to the drawing board with renewed conviction.

Is eccentricity a qualification for success?

It can be. Eccentricity is also very profitable in terms of brainstorming ideas. In groups, I've often witnessed one eccentric contribute more ideas than everyone else. Eccentrics specialize in creativity, and some people, especially inventors and scientists, grow very wealthy through their creativity. Eccentrics may also be more interested in the process of achievement than the achievement itself, which will let them wander off on wild tangents. This brings serendipity, a cornerstone of success.

You found that eccentric people are happier and healthier than the rest of us. They may even live longer. How so?

Eccentrics seem to be somewhat immune to depression and sickness. Pure creativity seems to offer them an invigorating intellectual stimulation, not unlike the physical gratification of sex. This constant stimulation may explain why the eccentrics we studied had slightly higher levels of growth hormone than the rest of us, which might actually make them a bit more resilient to aging. They almost always have a pronounced, even mischievous, sense of humor, which in and of itself keeps them sharp, optimistic, and engaged by friends. Last, they don't feel the stress of conformity or the fear of failing, two forces that usually preoccupy most people. Whatever their secret, it works. Most eccentrics need to visit a doctor only every decade or so.

Then how can a normal man introduce a little eccentricity into his life and realize the benefits without making people think he's nuts?

First of all, eccentricity is largely a natural predisposition, and it's extremely rare. In fact, there may be only one true eccentric for every 10,000 persons. So don't start messing your hair like Einstein or wearing a cape and top hat about town. These things are superficial. The first prescription is to question everything. Eccentrics keep a childish curiosity their whole lives. Second, don't disregard things that sound kooky. Be more inclusive in your thinking and be willing to follow tangents that interest you and others scoff at. Third, think visually. Eccentrics use vivid imagery and dreams to prime their creativity, and often explain their ideas with pictures. Last, realize that the world is wrong and you are right, and carry on merrily from that point without doubting yourself. That's the true essence of eccentricity.

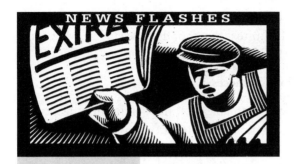

Shoe Companies Go Back to the Basics

MOUNT PROSPECT, Ill.—After experiencing some pretty flashy trends in recent years, the athletic footwear business seems to have gone back to the simple life. Walking, cross-training, tennis, and hiking shoes continue to have their devoted fans, but for the noncommitted, casual shoe buyer who goes shopping at sporting goods stores and just wants something comfortable and good-looking to work out in, it's evident that running shoes are the footwear of choice this year. Hot- or flashy-colored shoes aren't selling, but those in shades of brown are getting noticed. Sales of celebrity-endorsed shoes, other than those endorsed by Michael Jordan, have not taken off as manufacturers had hoped.

Breakthrough Technology Brings a Closer Shave

NEW YORK CITY—The Gillette Company recently launched the first and only shaving system with three progressive aligned blades, which provides men with a closer shave in fewer strokes and with less irritation. Gillette claims that its Mach3 outperforms all other razors, including the current category leader, Gillette SensorExcel, making this new system the most significant men's shaving product introduced since the first twin-blade razor, Gillette Trac II, in 1971.

The three Mach3 blades are positioned in a progressive alignment. While all three blades are in contact with the skin during a normal shaving stroke, the progressive alignment balances the pressure placed on each blade. The first blade has the lowest exposure so it can extend and cut longer hairs more comfortably. The second and third blades have progressively higher exposures, which enables each blade to extend and cut the beard hair lower along the hair shaft in a single stroke. The end result is a combination of shaving closeness, comfort, and safety.

Mach3's patented comfort edges are thinner than any other Gillette blade edges and glide through beard hairs more easily. Men should experience less drag and pull, for a more comfortable shave. The new three-blade shaving system is expected to be covered by more than 35 patents.

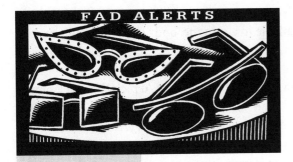

Rimless Frames

Most major designers are slimming down their eyewear lines, and rimless frames are coming back strong. They represent simplicity and come loaded with the latest in technology: corrective lenses that are barely noticeable on either side of your nose, with an antireflective coating to make the lenses practically disappear from your face. Look for simple metalwork and temples connected to the lenses with real hardware, instead of the usual plastic pins that are a dead giveaway of inferior quality. The new rimless frames are incredibly light and rest on your nose very comfortably.

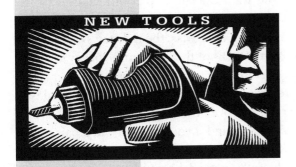

Scents to Energize You

Sports Colognes

We've long noticed that spritzing on a clean, crisp "sports" cologne after a workout and steaming shower makes us more alert. Turns out there's science behind that sensation. "Olfactory researchers have found that colognes with citrus and green notes, which smell like grass, can make you feel more energetic," says Annette Green, president of the Fragrance Foundation in New York City. Some sports colognes we like: Extreme Polo Sport by Ralph Lauren (3.4 ounces, $48). This spicy cologne has a subtle lemon scent that wakes you up—

and almost makes you feel like you can run faster. Hilfiger Athletics by Tommy Hilfiger (3.4 ounces, $45) is available in a cologne, body shampoo, and muscle-soothing soak. The sharp aroma is a combination of citrus and green woody scents.

If we had to run to a wedding after we ran a 5-K, we'd pick Nautica Competition (4.2 ounces, $45). The cologne has a rich, lasting scent. The Nautica line includes aftershave, moisturizer, shower gel, soap, and deodorant.

Stop Facial Bleeding

Nik-Aid

Styptic pencils are handy, but they leave a chalky film and don't work so well on those major arterial gashes that ruin collars. Nik-Aid, a $3 liquid styptic roll-on that leaves no residue, works better. An editor who routinely shows up wearing toilet paper on his face gave Nik-Aid a try, and it stopped his daily hemorrhaging immediately.

Comfortable, Durable Pants

Khakis

When we were young pups and wanted a sturdy pair of khakis, we knew where to go: to the nearest Army and Navy store for a pair of surplus 100 percent cotton-twill pants left over from the Big One. Alas, the military switched to a polyester blend some years back, and stocks of those beautiful, baggy originals were exhausted years ago. Luckily, before the last pair disappeared, former ad executive Bill Thomas created a replica and began manufacturing the khakis in Reading, Pennsylvania. We heartily approve of the results. These are the most comfortable khakis you'll find anywhere, and if you can wear out a pair, you're living too dangerously, pal. Bills Khakis come in several styles, including a pleated version, but our favorite is still the full-cut Model #1, a plain-front, button-fly model in $8\frac{1}{2}$-ounce prewashed cotton ($90).

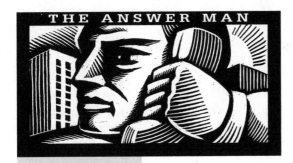

THE ANSWER MAN

Losing His Shirt

I work in retail and I'm always reaching for things, so my shirt comes untucked about a hundred times a day. What can I do about this? And should shirts be tucked straight down, or should they be untucked enough to cover your belt?
—B. N., Albuquerque, N.M.

"Most men who can't keep their shirts tucked in just need longer shirttails," says Frank Childers, corporate tailored-clothing coordinator for Nordstrom. Two brands with longer-than-average shirttails are Nordstrom's own collection of dress shirts and Faconnable, he says. As for your second question, shirts should be tucked straight down. When you move around, the shirt will pull out just slightly—enough to feel comfortable while still looking good.

Putting His Best Foot Forward

What sort of socks belong with jeans and casual footwear? Are white cotton socks acceptable?
—P. L., Buffalo

White athletic socks work with sneakers, says Elena Hart, fashion marketing director of the Fashion Association in New York City, but the key word is athletic. Wear them only when you're exercising, unless you want people to think you're an out-of-work aerobics instructor. "Bright white socks are very conspicuous with loafers and lace-ups," Hart says. "You run the risk of looking a little goofy." Subtler off-white socks, on the other hand, work just fine. (In case you're wondering, black socks work only with black jeans.)

"Even better, look for wool, cable-knit hiking socks that are somewhat rugged-looking," Hart suggests. Gold Toe and Joe Boxer make socks that are perfect for casual wear, she says. "Your best bet with jeans is to stick with socks in solid colors, like gray or dark blue," she recommends.

Smelling Fresh

I have a few bottles of cologne that are two to five years old. Does this stuff have a shelf life?
—B. F., Boise, Idaho

"Most colognes last approximately two years," says Joyce Kendall, vice president of product marketing for Ralph Lauren Fragrances. "If you notice the cologne has darkened significantly, that's a sign that it has gone bad." Other signs include a detectable vinegar or wine scent, or a date who bolts from your car at a stoplight.

If you'd rather not spring for a new bottle every two years, try keeping your cologne in any cool, dark place, such as the refrigerator. "It lasts almost forever when you do this," says Kendall, "because heat and light are the factors that cause cologne to deteriorate." If you typically grab any bottle in the refrigerator and drink without hesitation, try stowing your cologne in the dresser, rather than on it.

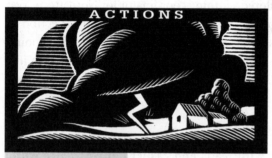

Projecting a positive image is much more than making your socks match your belt and keeping lime green out of your wardrobe. There are a whole mix of elements that go together to form that image. From the way you carry yourself to how you handle clothing emergencies, here are some tips to look sharp.

1. Stand up straight. To improve your posture, practice this exercise: When standing, push your heels into the floor. "This causes you to flex your diaphragm, lift your breastbone, and keep your chin level to the floor," says Lillian Brown, media consultant for celebrities and several U.S. presidents. "You turn your body upward, which conveys authority and confidence." And by not slouching or looking downward, you eliminate shadows and take advantage of the light—whether it's coming from the sun, a television camera, or an oncoming tractor trailer. "When you flex your diaphragm, which is the source of power for your voice, you allow greater use of your vocal instrument," says Brown, author of *The Polished Politician*. You'll look and sound like you're 10 years younger—which, unless you're 22, is pretty cool.

2. **Buy a new tie.** But not just any new tie. Pick one that matches your eyes and helps call attention to them—you'll always look better if you follow this simple rule. And if the tie that best matches your eyes is red, maybe you should be going out a little less.

3. **Inspect your closet.** Got a lot of relatively new stuff that you don't wear much? "If you are always buying something new, then you aren't spending very much for anything," says Brown. "And you won't feel good when you wear it." Her solution: investment dress. Buy an expensive, perfectly fitting suit—and wear it a lot. "A suit made of fine fabric, along with a custom-made shirt, makes you feel great. If you wear something that's ho-hum, then you'll feel ho-hum." Make it elegant and understated, a good dark gray or navy color. Sure, this costs money, but you'll keep the stuff for years.

4. **Look at your face.** Check out your complexion in the harsh light of the men's room. If your skin looks less than perfect, you could be doing something to undermine your visage. "Foods or a certain activity may aggravate your complexion," says John F. Romano, M.D., a dermatologist at New York Hospital–Cornell Medical Center in New York City and *Men's Health* magazine advisor. If your skin is acting up, take an inventory. Ask yourself the following questions.

Am I drinking too much coffee? "For some people, daily caffeine can cause breakouts," says Dr. Romano.

Am I washing my hands? If you're working on the engine of your vintage AMC Pacer, then touching your face with greasy hands, you're asking for a zit party.

Have I been eating a lot of shellfish lately? "Shellfish contain iodine, which can cause some people to break out," says Dr. Romano.

Is it cold outside? "Wearing wool scarves and turtlenecks can irritate your skin, too," says Dr. Romano.

5. **Seek out a new barber.** Let's face it, if you look lousy, it's probably not your fault. (Just keep telling yourself that over and over again until it takes.) What you need is a fresh perspective. "Look through a magazine, find a style you like, and take it to a stylist," says David Chapa, the guy who slices and dices the hair of seductive rebounder Dennis Rodman. "If you don't know a stylist, ask a friend or co-worker whose hair looks good where he has it cut. Word of mouth is still the best way to find a haircutter." That, and a lot of money.

6. **Get to the bottom of things.** You fixed the top, now go ahead and fix the bottom. Whether you know it or not, people look at your shoes. A lot. See, shoes serve as a fast-acting character barometer. If your new boss doesn't know much about you, he'll check out your shoes. If you're sporting a classic style that costs more than $100 and they're nicely shined, you pass. If they're a pair of beat-up high-tops that smell funny, you're probably a pizza-delivery guy—or you will be very, very soon.

7. **Go through your address book.** "You'll find many people you've lost touch with whom you might actually miss," says Warren Farrell, Ph.D., author of *Why Men Are the Way They Are.* "Check out the Christmas-card list, if you have one." Then write down the phone numbers of the folks you'd like to talk to or have a beer with. Call a few of them today.

8. **Act like a tourist in your own town.** Think of all the stuff nearby that people buy high-priced airline tickets to fly and see—the same stuff you'd never go near because it's oh-so-touristy. Screw your cynicism, head to the tourism office, pick up some brochures, and hit the town. Eat at restaurants you rarely visit. Buy some nifty clothes. Visit your hometown's equivalent of the Statue of Liberty. Check into a swanky hotel. Best of all, this stunt allows you to get away with a practice usually reserved for tourists and the homeless: accosting complete strangers. Curiosity and confusion, laid out sincerely before the nurturing gaze of a fetching young damsel, work like a charm.

9. **Get the spot out.** When Shakespeare wrote, "Out, damned spot!" he wasn't referring to his malcontent dog. He was trying to scour a deodorant stain out of his last clean frilly shirt. We can relate. That's why we offer remedies for typical guy-messes, courtesy of the book *The Stain and Spot Remover Handbook,* by Jean Cooper.

Antiperspirants on shirts. Try a sponge soaked in diluted ammonia, or apply rubbing alcohol to the stain and cover the area with an absorbent pad dampened with alcohol. Then rinse with very hot water and wash the shirt.

Scuff marks on shoes. Apply a little toothpaste to a damp rag and wipe away.

Gravy on the rug. Quickly mix a teaspoon of mild detergent, a teaspoon of white vinegar, and a quart of warm water. Apply to the stain, let it dry, and then vacuum.

Coffee and tea stains in coffeepots. When that nasty tannin residue cakes up in the bottom of your coffeepot, use Borax to wipe out the pot. Borax also removes stains from carpets, so try it on the gravy, too.

10. **Taper your full-cut shirts.** Unless you have the build of a Ken doll, many of your off-the-rack garments could probably stand a nip or tuck from your tailor. Tapering your baggy shirts will instantly make you appear thinner.

11. **Buy a bunch of shirts with subtle patterns.** A closetful of single-color dress shirts is a sure sign of a rut. A discreet pinstripe isn't just snazzier; it'll force new ties into the rotation.

12. **Lose that gel.** It makes your hair look stiff and slimy. Instead, pick up a pommade styling product (Paul Mitchell's Foaming Pommade, for example), which will give you a more relaxed look.

13. **Purchase a pair of black cap-toe shoes.** The kind with a slightly matte finish (not mirror-shines) will strengthen your best suit but still work with Dockers on Friday. Give those tired wing-tips to that former Congressman in the mailroom.

14. **Don't mix stiff business wear with casual clothes.** Even on Friday, silk ties and thin nylon socks don't belong with burly cotton gear. Same goes for point-collar dress shirts and chinos. And please, throw out those college sweat-shirts—nobody is going to confuse you with an undergraduate, sport.

Credits

"The Kings of Outdoor Grilling" on page 68 was adapted from *The von Hoffmann Bros.' Big Damn Book of Sheer Manliness* by Todd von Hoffmann and Brant von Hoffmann. Copyright © 1997 by Todd von Hoffmann. Reprinted by permission of General Publishing Group, Inc.

"Developing Willpower" on page 132 from *Break the Weight Loss Barrier* by Dr. James Meschino and Dr. Barry Simon. Copyright © 1997. Reprinted with permission of Prentice Hall. Permission for United Kingdom granted by Prentice Hall Canada, Inc.

"A Stronger Memory" on page 208 from *Memory Power Plus* by Fred B. Chernow. Copyright © 1997. Reprinted with permission of Prentice Hall.

"Buying a Suit" on page 274 from *Paisley Goes with Nothing* by Hal Rubenstein with Jim Mullen. Copyright © 1995 by Hal Rubenstein and Jim Mullen. Used by permission of Doubleday, a division of Bantam Doubleday Dell Publishing Group, Inc. Permission for United Kingdom granted by International Creative Management, Inc.

Index

Boldface references indicate photographs. Prescription drug names are denoted with the symbol Rx.

HIV, 109
HMB, 41
Home gym machines,
35–36
Honesty vs. lying,
211–12
Hormones. *See also specific
types*
headaches and, 165
sex, 99–105
weight loss and, 128
Human papillomavirus
(HPV), 114, 176
Hydration, 52. *See also* Water
intake
Hypertension. *See* High
blood pressure
Hypothyroidism, 179–80

I

Ibuprofen, 258, 261
Ice treatment, 164, 240,
263
avoiding, 52
Imitrex statdose system
(Rx), 258
Immune system
L-glutamine and, 39
low-fat diet and, 137
sleep and, 198
stress and, 163
weight training and, 39
Impact Bag golf aid, 44
Impotence, 229–31
assertiveness and, 153
biking and, 151
cures
current, 229–31
in development, 110,
231
Melanotan II, 111
Incontinence, 248
Indigestion. *See* Heartburn
Indole-3-carbinol, 64
Inflammation, 58–59
Inhibitions, sexual, 94–98

In-laws, managing, 107–8
Insomnia, 260–61
Insulin, 59, 128–29, 172,
252
Intelligence, 212–14
Internet, health information
on, 169–71
Intracytoplasmic sperm
injection, 114
I.Q., 212–14
Iron, 73, 140

J

Jackets, sport, 269, 281
Jet lag, 59, 200
Jet Skis, 39–40
John Daly Power Groove
golf aid, 43–44
Juices, 84

K

Kava-kava, 217–18
Kenalog (Rx), 259
Khakis, 288
Kidneys, 57, 185
Kidney stones, 85
Kingsford Charcoal
Briquets, grilling
food with, 69–70
Kissing, 92–93, 115
Knee pain, 158–59, 257
Kosher food, 80

L

Lactobacillus acidophilus, 85
Lactobacillus bulgaricus, 85
Lactose intolerance, 85
L-arginine, 251
LDL, 150–51, 172
Lean Cuisine Cafe Classics,
79–80
Legionnaires' disease, 183

L-glutamine, 39
Libido, 98–105, 215
Life cereal, 71
Lifetime of Sex, A, 98–105
LipoGuard, 177–78
Liver, immune function and,
163
Low-density lipoprotein
(LDL), 150–51, 172
Low-oxygen training, 42
Lubricant, penile, 154
Lunchtime workout, 22–26
Lung problems, 57–58
cancer, 185
Luvox (Rx), 216
Lycopene, 77
Lying vs. honesty,
211–12
Lymphocytes, 163
Lysine tablets, 259

M

Mach 3 shaver, 286
MacroChem, 110
Magnesium, 84
Marriage, 105–8
Massage, 153, 240
Master Putt golf aid, 45
Maximum Style, 279–82
Meat
in diet, 66–67
kosher, 80
mail-order, 78
marinating, 84
wound healing and, 59
Medications. *See also specific
types*
acne, 250
allergy, 84
weight loss, 140
Medicine ball, 47–48
Medi-Ject, 110
Meditation, 221
sports and, 223
Melanin, 180
Melanoma, 182, 253